Success *from the* Start

Business Principles for
Massage Therapists

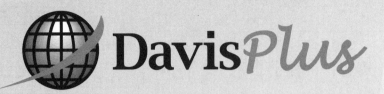
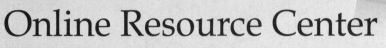
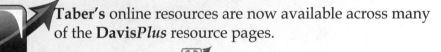

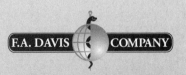

Success
from the
Start

Business Principles for
Massage Therapists

Debra Koerner
Co-founder
imassage, Inc.

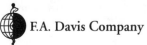

F.A. Davis Company • Philadelphia

F. A. Davis Company
1915 Arch Street
Philadelphia, PA 19103
www.fadavis.com

Printed in the United States of America

Last digit indicates print number: 10 9 8 7 6 5 4 3 2 1

Acquisitions Editor: Christa Fratantoro
Manager of Content Development: George W. Lang
Developmental Editor: Karen Carter
Design and Illustration Manager: Carolyn O'Brien

As new scientific information becomes available through basic and clinical research, recommended treatments and drug therapies undergo changes. The author(s) and publisher have done everything possible to make this book accurate, up to date, and in accord with accepted standards at the time of publication. The author(s), editors, and publisher are not responsible for errors or omissions or for consequences from application of the book, and make no warranty, expressed or implied, in regard to the contents of the book. Any practice described in this book should be applied by the reader in accordance with professional standards of care used in regard to the unique circumstances that may apply in each situation. The reader is advised always to check product information (package inserts) for changes and new information regarding dose and contraindications before administering any drug. Caution is especially urged when using new or infrequently ordered drugs.

Library of Congress Cataloging-in-Publication Data

Koerner, Debra.
  Success from the start: business principles for massage therapists / Debra Koerner.
      p. ; cm.
  Includes index.
  ISBN 978-0-8036-2575-4
  I. Title.
  [DNLM: 1. Massage—organization & administration. 2. Career Choice. 3. Marketing of Health Services—methods. 4. Marketing of Health Services—organization & administration. 5. Professional Practice—organization & administration. WB 357]

  615.822—dc23

                              2012041346

This book is first and foremost dedicated to the more than 300,000 massage therapists who are doing the work every day to help people live healthier and happier lives. My hope is that you are following your bliss at this very moment and find as much satisfaction with your career as your clients do in receiving the work. I wrote this book hoping to assist you on your personal journey, whether you are a current student at a massage school or a seasoned practitioner who is imagining a deeper understanding of your career.

I also dedicate this book to Eric Stephenson, co-founder of imassage, Inc. His passion for massage therapy and providing education that helps therapists stay mentally, emotionally, and physically healthy has kept me inspired and focused during challenging times. Without his support and encouragement, I most likely would still be working in a corporate position dreaming about the day I could leave and make a meaningful difference in an industry I love.

And finally, I offer thanks to Stefanie Ashley, who helped keep things moving along when my schedule became so hectic I found it difficult to stay focused on the writing. Her contributions helped create this book.

Preface

In 2007, I happened upon a shocking massage statistic that would change the course of my career and life. According to industry research, each year about 60,000 students enter massage school to pursue becoming a massage therapist, and at the same time, more than 50,000 practitioners leave the profession. Not understanding the reason behind this high attrition rate, I discovered through further research that the top two reasons practitioners leave are physical burn-out and business naivete. Feeling drawn to make a difference on the business front, I left my corporate job and co-founded a company—imassage, Inc.—dedicated to addressing these two issues. I attended my very first American Massage Therapy Association national convention in the fall of 2007 and coincidentally had a booth next to the publisher F. A. Davis Company. I befriended the acquisition editor and in a joking manner suggested I write a business book for the massage industry so that we could affect the quality of business education at the school level. Taking me seriously, she suggested I draft a proposal. Within 6 months, we had signed a book contract and the writing began.

As a massage therapist, your individual gifts and talents are needed, now more than ever, for the continued growth of the massage profession and for the millions of people that rely on massage and bodywork as a vital part of their well-being. As research continues to validate the efficacy of touch therapies, we continue to see public demand increase. However, unless we address root problems of attrition, the demand for massage will overcome the supply of therapists providing the therapy.

My intention for this book is to help you increase your business knowledge to extend your career. I've tried to share my knowledge of business concepts in a way that appeals to the human being inside you. If this book contributes to helping you in some way successfully practice massage for as long as your heart desires, then my intention has found a home with you and for that ... I am thankful.

ORGANIZATION

Success From the Start was written to offer assistance in any area you feel you need support to be successful in your massage career. Each chapter is a progression from the previous and offers insight into all aspects of becoming a massage therapist with a thriving and healthy practice.

This book consists of 10 chapters that embody all business aspects of starting and running a successful massage practice. Launching into a new career is not always fun, so I have attempted to soften some of the tactical business items in a way that is less overwhelming.

Chapter 1: Defining Personal Success

This chapter offers guidance on the importance of going inward before going outward in your efforts to create the career of your dreams. You will explore the benefits of mindfulness, understanding your personal desire, purposefully crafting your vision, and understanding what strengths and opportunities you naturally have.

Chapter 2: Money Matters

Often our past relationship with money plays a role in our ability to give and receive money. You will be asked to go deep and see what relationship you currently have with money. The chapter also offers ideas on how you can improve your financial health and guides you in consciously allocating your income.

Chapter 3: What Every Therapist Must Know

Because of the nature of massage therapy, you must become familiar with many rules and guidelines. This chapter, although not providing specific information for every state and circumstance, offers guidance on how to stay within the business guidelines of certification, licensure, insurance, and legal matters. Not fun, but necessary.

Chapter 4: Navigating the Ethics of Business

This chapter discusses ethical considerations important to know as you seek to become successful in your massage career. You will learn about your moral compass and how you can rely on it to help guide you through tough situations. Different types of boundaries are described, and you will be asked to put thought into how they exist for you today. You will be encouraged to purposefully craft an internal and external practice infused with your own sense of ethics.

Chapter 5: Your Path as an Employee

Becoming an employee involves much more than just showing up for work every day. This chapter discusses what it takes to be successful as an employee of a business that offers massage therapy. Finding the right place to work is key to your initial success, followed by your understanding of what it takes to be a great employee. This chapter offers guidance on writing a resume, successfully navigating an interview, and getting hired into a dream job.

Chapter 6: Your Path as an Independent Contractor

A role in which massage therapists commonly find themselves is that of an independent contractor. This chapter offers advice on the technical and interpersonal aspects of achieving success in this role. You will learn about defining expectations, scheduling, generating revenue, and preparing taxes. A list of potential companies to solicit for work will help guide you as you attempt to seek work as a contractor.

Chapter 7: Your Path as an Entrepreneur

Deciding to own and run your own business can be the most exciting but riskiest way to go. This chapter discusses all the different types of businesses options available. You will be asked to assess yourself and see if you have what it takes to be a business owner. The business plan is fully explored, and this chapter offers an example and template for easing your efforts in building your first business plan.

Chapter 8: Preparing for Marketing Success

Before you open shop and begin advertising for business, it is really important that you understand what type of business you want and who you want to attract as clients. This chapter offers insight into the importance of narrowing your focus to build the business you want. You will learn about the power of differentiation and how to stand out among a sea of therapists. This chapter also offers initial advice on how to build professional marketing materials that accurately represent who you are.

Chapter 9: Filling Your Practice With Clients You Want to Work With

Now you're ready to get to the nitty-gritty aspects of marketing and acquiring new clients. You will learn to identify your competitors and set fair pricing for your products and services. Before you start dropping money on advertising, you will be asked to assess where your future clients are so that you can reach them directly. An overview of traditional and nontraditional advertising venues will be discussed. Public relations (PR) efforts are a great way to establish credibility and generate new business. You will be offered guidelines on how to successfully use PR in your practice, and you will be asked to write a press release. Social media are also explored as an option to expand your client base.

Chapter 10: Client Loyalty: Every Therapist's Pot of Gold

Probably the most important aspect of having a long-term successful business is understanding your clients' needs, fears, and expectations. When you can exceed their expectations, you are guaranteed a level of loyalty that will keep your business sustainable for a long time. In this chapter, you will learn to create an overall experience that exceeds customer expectations, to assess client satisfaction, to help ease common anxieties in new and experienced clients, and to understand clients' verbal and nonverbal communication cues. The intention of this chapter is to help you understand the importance of the softer side of massage therapy and the customer experience so that you will have a full practice for as long as you want to practice.

FEATURES

Find It on the Web: At the time of printing, these Web addresses offer additional information and support for chapter topics. You can always search for similar terms if the link becomes inactive.

Peer Profile: Real-life stories from fellow massage therapists with their advice on how they became successful and how you, too, can be successful.

Expert Profile: Industry experts offer insights to help you take your practice to the next level of success.

Key Definitions: Those terms that are most important to remember.

Pull Quotes: Important text highlighted within each chapter.

About the Author

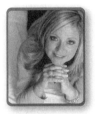

For 15 years, Debra kept the companies she worked with healthy by using her expertise in creating spectacular customer experiences. However, the 60-hour weeks this former Fortune 250 executive invested in her career had an adverse effect on her own well-being: she became an overworked insomniac on the brink of a health crisis.

After too many grab-n-go meals, scant time to exercise, and a demanding climb up the corporate ladder, Debra found herself at the doctor's office. She was handed prescriptions for everything from antacids and sleeping pills to antidepressants. Debra refused them all, walking away empty-handed, knowing she had to make career and lifestyle changes.

Motivated by her desire to create a company in the massage industry that would help therapists extend their careers, Debra risked it all and left the security of her corporate position to launch imassage, Inc., a massage education company with her partner Eric Stephenson (imassageinc.com). Her entry into the wellness industry expanded, and she began corporate-level consulting on building great employee teams and crafting exceptional guest experiences within the massage and spa industries.

In late 2010, Debra was named the Executive Director for the Destination Spa Group (DSG). This group of "whole person" spas is dedicated to the internal and external well-being of their guests. Debra is a regular presenter within the massage and spa industry and also writes articles for national print media. She has been quoted as an expert on natural health and wellness by notable media outlets, including cnn.com, *Woman's Day*, Reuters, *Massage Magazine*, About.com, and *Spa Magazine*.

Never staying still for long and fueled by a desire to make a difference in the world by bringing more awareness to natural health options, Debra created a venture titled *Journey Into Wellbeing*, a television series poised to air on PBS stations nationwide. Lacing up her hiking boots and packing her yoga mat, throughout 2013, she has trekked to health destinations across the globe in search of secrets that could turn her into something a bit more spectacular.

Journey Into Wellbeing includes some of the world's top destination spas, wellness experts, and health sanctuaries. Debra will work with on-site experts while going inward and working through the sometimes painful emotional aspects of reclaiming health. Shot on location, each episode delves into a different aspect of wellbeing—from yoga and meditation to raw foods and massage—and features expert tips to help viewers replicate the benefits at home.

In the end, Debra's journey inspires anyone who ever wondered what it would be like to finally lose those last few pounds, wake up refreshed each morning, or simply tackle stressful schedules with Zen-like calm and confident energy. To stay in touch with Debra, join the wellness journey at journeyintowellbeing.com or you can find her on Twitter Debras Journey and on Facebook at Journey Into Wellbeing with Debra K.

Contributor

Stefanie Ashley
Facilitation Services Specialist
Facilitation Center
Eastern Kentucky University
Richmond, Kentucky

Stefanie Ashley contributed writing and editing services for this book. Ashley is a facilitation services specialist at the Facilitation Center at Eastern Kentucky University, in Richmond, where she aids groups in creative problem-solving, funneling ideas into action, and conquering tough topics and challenges. Before working at the Facilitation Center, she founded Ashley Collaborative, a professional consulting firm specializing in education and training development. Ashley's background is in association management, where she worked for 11 years with the International SPA Association and National Tourism Foundation. Since 2004, Ashley has managed the development of and contributed to numerous textbooks and courses on a variety of topics, including accounting, compensation, governance, leadership, risk management, and retail management. Ashley published her first book, *Not-for-Profit Boards: A Practical Guide to Modern Governance,* in 2010. She is married to her high school sweetheart, Gillis, and has three sons—Austin, Logan, and Brennan.

Sheila Lynne Bergman
Remedial Massage Therapist, Adult and Continuing
    Education Certificate
Instructor
Department of Physiology/Pathology
Wellington College of Remedial Massage Therapies Inc.
Winnipeg, Manitoba
Canada

**Patricia Brewerton, MS, LMT, AMTA,
    NCTMB**
Adjunct Faculty and Career Development Counselor
Complementary Healthcare Department
Mount Wachusett Community College
Gardner, Massachusetts

Patricia A. Coe, MT, DC
Clinic Supervisor
Massage Therapy
National University of Health Sciences
Lombard, Illinois

Jeanne A. Dodge, MTC
Instructor and Academic Coordinator
Health Occupations/Academic Advising
Greenfield Community College
Greenfield, Massachusetts

Brian Dormer, LMT
Coordinator
Health Sciences
Georgian College
Barrie, Ontario, Canada

Sister Patricia Dowler, RN, LMT, MEd
Education Director/Clinic Director, Educator
Department of Education
Bancroft School of Massage Therapy
Worcester, Massachusetts

Pam Fitch, BA, RMT
Professor
Massage Therapy
Algonquin College
Ottawa, Ontario, Canada

**Jeane Ellen Freeman, BS, AAS, LMT,
    CFT, RMT,**
Educator and Owner
Total Body Fitness
Tucson, Arizona

Carol D. Johnson
Licensed Massage Practitioner
Former Director
Massage Therapy
Colby Community College
Colby, Kansas

**Kathleen Anne Longman, Bachelor
    of Education in Adult Education**
Registered Massage Therapist
Oshawa, Ontario, Canada

Lisa Mertz, PhD, LMT
Associate Professor
Healing Arts, Health Ed, Phys Ed, & Dance
Queensborough Community College and City
    University of New York
Bayside, New York

Paul Pozorski, MS in Higher Education
Program Director
Massage Therapy
Miller-Motte Technical College
Madison, Tennessee

Rosemary Shannon, RMT
Instructor
Massage Therapy
School of Heath Sciences
Lethbridge College
Lethbridge, Alberta, Canada

Michelle Stevenson, BS, MA
Certified Massage Therapist
Payroll Specialist
Human Resources
Northern Wyoming Community College District
Sheridan, Wyoming

Diana L. Tourney
College Instructor
Business Department
Delta-Montrose Technical College
Delta, Colorado

Denise Van Nostran, MM, BM, LMT, NCTMB
Coordinator of Massage Therapy
Division of Health Sciences
Technical College of the Lowcountry
Beaufort, South Carolina

Acknowledgments

I would like to thank Drs. Christopher and Estelle Bernabei and the Balance Health Center & Yoga Spa for allowing the use of their space for the book photo shoot.

Drs. Christopher & Estelle Bernabei
Balance Health Center & Yoga Spa
112 S 20th St.
Philadelphia, PA 19103
215.751.0344
www.balancehealthcenter.com

I would also like to thank Eric Stephenson, LHT, owner of imassage, Inc., and its chief educator, for being one of the massage therapist models.

imassage, Inc.
www.imassageinc.com

Contents in Brief

Contents

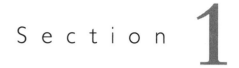

PREPARING FOR A CAREER IN MASSAGE THERAPY

Chapter

1

Defining Personal Success

"Dream lofty dreams, and as you dream, so you shall become. Your vision is the promise of what you shall one day be; your ideal is the prophecy of what you shall at last unveil."

–JAMES ALLEN

Outline

You will learn to...

- Appreciate the value of mindfulness
- Define your personal desires
- Set intentions that align with your desires
- Understand your natural tendencies
- Identify strengths and opportunities
- Finalize your vision

Key Definitions

This chapter references several key terms, which are indicated in bold. For easy reference, these terms are briefly defined here:

Action: "The bringing about of an alteration by force or through a natural agency; an act of will."*

Desire: An internal longing or hope.

Goal: A set objective you strive to achieve.

Intention: The motivation that lies beneath action.

Mindfulness: A state of being completely present and aware of your internal and external environments within the current moment.

Natural preferences: Core personality traits you prefer to function with.

PREVENT YOURSELF FROM BECOMING A STATISTIC

You are ready to embark on a successful career in massage therapy. What an exciting time! Because you are reading this book, you are also thinking about the business aspects of massage therapy—an extremely important topic that is not always embraced. Congratulations on understanding how essential a grasp of business is to your success as a massage therapist.

> As for any long trip, it is best to do some work up front to map the journey in a way that encourages success.

Each person reading this book has taken a different path to get here. People of all ages and experiences are drawn to the art of massage therapy for many reasons. If you have a strong business background, you might find setting up your business to be less challenging than will someone who has always been an employee. Although it is difficult for one book to meet everyone's needs, setting aside time to consciously plan is beneficial for people of all backgrounds. As for any long trip, it is best to do some work up front to map the journey in a way that encourages success. This book will assist you with this process.

Starting your new career with business knowledge, personal insight, and strategic **goals** will help prevent you from becoming one of the 50,000 massage therapists who leave the profession each year—a number nearly equal to those who enter the profession. Why do so many therapists leave? According to a recent report by the Associated Bodywork and Massage Professionals (ABMP), a lack of business knowledge is one of three major reasons. The following appears in the ABMP Massage Therapy Fact Sheet[1]:

> Practitioner attrition continues to be cause for concern in the massage therapy profession. ABMP estimates some 50,000 massage therapists leave the profession each year. One of the three primary factors driving this pattern:
>
> 1. As most professionals indicate they wish they had more clients, it is reasonable to conclude that at least some practitioners leave the field because of insufficient economic reward. Contributing to this may be unrealistic expectations of new graduates and a simple lack of business skill and confidence. It proves difficult for sole practitioners to reconcile their sense of higher purpose with the more mundane aspects of self-employment and the competitive realities of self-promotion.

---

*Action. Merriam-Webster Dictionary. Retrieved from http://www.merriam-webster.com/dictionary/action

ABMP cites physical demands of the profession and lifestyle changes, such as spouse relocation and maternity, as the other two reasons.

In 2010, the American Massage Therapy Association (AMTA) released similar information in their *2010 Massage Industry Research Report,* stating that an estimated 45,290 therapists left the profession in 2007, whereas more than 52,000 left in 2006. They estimate the turnover to be about 20% for a variety of reasons, the most prevalent being economic.

These statistics spurred the creation of the book you hold in your hands. This book is designed to help you address and avoid the primary, overall reason why practitioners leave— business naivety.

Now, pause for a moment to gauge your reaction to the ABMP and AMTA facts. Is it surprising to learn that there are almost as many therapists leaving the profession as entering it each year, or is this something you already knew? As the desire for natural wellness options continues to expand, a supply of trained professionals is needed to meet the demand. The International Spa Association (ISPA) reported in their *2011 U.S. Spa Industry Study*[2] that 42% of spas cited the most common problem they face is finding qualified candidates for open positions. So, again, a lack of demand does not seem to be the reason for career defection.

CONTROL YOUR DESTINY

All three reasons for attrition are preventable. Let us think about how we can avoid each one. Business naivety is within your control. If you lack business education, this is something you can strengthen through classes and by creating a support network. There are numerous educational resources available to you. Physical burnout is also within your control if you are aware that this can be an issue for massage therapists. You can learn and practice self-care such as body mechanics, exercise, and proper nutrition. Even lifestyle changes are mostly within your control. Although sudden transitions might disrupt a business, they should not be a reason for permanent departure.

The good news is that with some planning, you can have a long, successful career. Becoming aware of these risk areas is a great first step to avoiding them. Besides awareness, it is also important for you to write down the steps you will take to ensure a long career. Throughout this book, you will be asked to complete worksheets and journal your thoughts, ideas, and goals. Here's why: In an article entitled *What They Don't Teach You at Harvard Business School,*[3] Mark McCormack details a study conducted on students in the Harvard MBA program. The students were asked, "Have you set clear, written goals for your future and made plans to accomplish them?" Only 3% of the graduates had written goals and plans; 13% had goals, but they were not in writing; and the majority, 84%, had no specific goals at all. After 10 years, the members of the class were surveyed again, and the findings were astonishing. The 13% of the class who had goals were earning, on average, twice as much as the 84% who had no goals at all. Are you curious about the 3% who had clear, written goals? They were earning, on average, 10 times as much as the other 97% put together (Fig. 1–1).

> "The first and most important step toward success is the feeling that we can succeed."
> —Nelson Boswell

See Worksheet 1-1

Writing goals allows you to think through what it is you want out of life. The more specific you are, the better. A general goal might be to move to California some day, but when you set a specific goal of moving to California in 5 years, you will find yourself more likely to take the steps necessary to make this happen. Writing specific goals down and looking at them can be life changing.

MINDFULNESS: ALLOWING SPACE FOR CREATION

Before jumping into the business aspects of your future massage career, let us take a few moments to visit the concepts that permeate this book. The first is mindfulness. Have you ever started driving and gotten halfway there before you realized you could not remember anything along the way because you had been lost in thought? Maybe you have eaten dinner while watching television only to realize

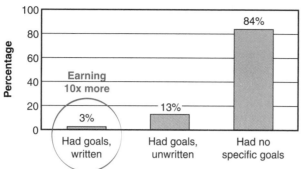

Harvard Students

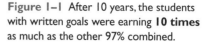

Figure 1–1 After 10 years, the students with written goals were earning **10 times** as much as the other 97% combined.

your food is gone and you do not remember tasting it. Most people have experienced times like these when your mind is off somewhere else. This is called mindlessness—not staying present in the moment or aware of what is going on around you. A habit of frequent mindlessness or a tendency to "check out" can affect your ability to make sound decisions or receive information that moves you in your desired direction.

Mindfulness, on the other hand, can be defined as being completely present and aware of your environment at this moment. Mindfulness means knowing what is going on externally while staying aware of what is going on inside. It also is the ability to pay attention without trying to change anything. Imagine that concept—accepting things as they unfold, trusting that all is happening as it should, and not using your will to change things. This is hard to do these days. With the demands of cell phones, texting, social networking, raising families, and trying to keep relationships healthy, most people find it challenging to purposefully create space to stay present.

Why would a business book start with a concept such as mindfulness? Because mindfulness has a positive impact on the many decisions you make when launching a massage career. When you learn to practice mindfulness, you begin to ask yourself, "What can I do at this moment that will bring me one step closer to where I truly want to be?" Too often, we are busy thinking about what we should have done (the past) or what we will be doing in a few years (the future). It is good to consider the past and future because they provide lessons and goals, but it is more beneficial to spend time living in the present and calculating the steps that are necessary to fulfill your aspirations. Mother Teresa put it best when she said, "Yesterday is gone. Tomorrow has not yet come. We have only today. Let us begin."

> Mother Teresa put it best when she said, "Yesterday is gone. Tomorrow has not yet come. We have only today. Let us begin."

If you are the type of person who likes clearly defined goals and projects, you might wonder, "How can staying in the present increase my chances for having a successful career?" Simply put, over time we all develop repetitive thoughts. Similar to a favorite music play list, we plug these thoughts in and hear the same predictable refrains every time. For this example, these internal thought loops are conversations we continually hold with ourselves. When these internal conversations are negative (It will never happen. I don't have the ability. I'm never going to get rich. I am not good at it.), and we never interrupt these destructive thought patterns, they become our reality. All this worrying takes energy, leaving less available neural processing power to deal with other tasks. Studies have shown that similar to physical threats, these negative thought patterns can also induce distress, dizziness, shortness of breath, sweating, and an increase in heart rate and breathing—all of which will keep you from focusing and moving confidently toward success. If you think about it, you can probably come up with some old thought conversations you have been having with yourself for years, maybe even decades.

Recent brain research shows that mental discipline and meditative practice can change the workings of the brain, allowing people to achieve more levels of awareness. A study of monks conducted by neuroscientist Richard Davidson[4] showed that meditation activated the trained minds of the monks in significantly different ways than those of untrained students. He found the movement of the waves through their brains was far better organized and coordinated than in the students. In previous studies, mental activities such as focus, memory, learning, and consciousness were associated with the kind of enhanced neural coordination found in the monks. Davidson's research is consistent with his earlier work that pinpointed the left prefrontal cortex as a brain region associated with happiness, positive thoughts, and emotions. Using functional magnetic resonance imagining (fMRI) on the meditating monks, Davidson found that their brain activity—as measured by an electroencephalogram (EEG)—was especially high in this area. Davidson concluded that meditation not only changes the workings of the brain in the short term but also quite possibly produces permanent changes. That finding, he said, is based on the fact that the monks had considerably more gamma wave activity than the control group even before they started meditating for the study.

Meditation and mindfulness go a long way in helping you pave your road to success. Once you become good at recognizing negative thoughts, you strengthen your ability to keep them from becoming your reality. Paying attention to your thoughts and purposefully interrupting negative repetitive loops will also keep you more present and better able to make decisions based on reality, not fear. One way to do this is to recognize the negative thought loop as soon as it starts and to turn it around and repetitively think the opposite. For example, if one of your consistent thoughts is "I could never do that," immediately start thinking "I could do that, I could do that, I could do that." This will strengthen your ability to stay present in all situations and recognize the mind chatter for what it is ... only thoughts.

Examples of Mindfulness

It is worth the effort to focus your thoughts on this moment. The following are examples of how you can begin to practice mindfulness during daily massage interactions.

Mindfulness Example 1: You are in conversation with one of your clients. As usual, he begins to talk about everything that is wrong in his life. You feel your energy level start to dip as his negative loop begins to lower your spirits. Normally, you might think, "I get so tired of listening to this client moan about his aches and pains." Maybe you are not even paying attention to what he is saying because you have heard it all before. Your eyes glaze over, and you begin thinking about what you will do after work, or what you will say as soon as he takes a breath. It is at this moment you can practice becoming aware of your thoughts. Bring yourself back to the moment. Focus your attention fully on what your client is saying. You do not have to feed into his angst or counter-transfer into his problems, but try to simply stay present with him and listen to what he is saying without judgment. It can be energizing for you as you develop the ability to listen without being pulled in. You will find that sometimes people just crave being listened to. Also, it is permissible to let clients go. If you find they are draining more than they are giving, then never hesitate to stop working with them. Freeing up your energy will result in other clients filling their spots.

Mindfulness Example 2: Here is another example of mindfulness that can benefit your career. Before each session, take a few moments to bring yourself to the present moment. Be aware of your breaths as you inhale and exhale. As you exhale, imagine releasing anything you are holding onto from the previous client. Approach your next client with a clean slate. After the client is on the table and you are ready to begin the session, take a moment to ground yourself and focus on her. Place your hands gently on her back, close your eyes and think to yourself, "I am here with you. I will stay in tune with you during this session. My intent is to help facilitate what you need in this moment." Take a couple of breaths and then begin the work from a place of focus and attention. The client will know

See Worksheet 1-2

you are there on more than a physical level. If your mind begins to wander during the session, simply recognize this. Do not judge yourself, but bring your awareness back to what is going on in that moment. Your thoughts will wander off, and that is fine; that is what brains do. Just try to become more aware of how much time you spend thinking about things that are not happening right now. This approach can benefit you and your client (Fig. 1–2).

THE FORMULA FOR SUCCESS

This formula will help you begin your journey toward long-term success. As reinforced by the ancient text Brihadaranyaka Upanishad IV.4.5, "You are what your deep, driving desire is. As your desire is, so is your will. As your will is, so is your deed. As your deed is, so is your destiny." To bring this to life for you, this formula contains three separate components, none of which has to do with getting your master's degree in business administration or memorizing ancient writings. It is the combination of truly understanding your innermost desires, setting an intention to fulfill those desires, and then taking action to achieve these dreams. We will fully explore each step in the formula shown in Figure 1–3.

Step 1: Clarifying Personal Desire

Desire is another term not normally associated with business textbooks. The *Merriam-Webster Dictionary* defines desire as "to long or hope for." It is something inside of us that at this moment is not fulfilled. We long to attain it and may go to great lengths to ensure this need is eventually met. Truly understanding our desire requires more reflection and less action. Taking time to think about what you really want to achieve is time well spent because it will prevent you from heading in the wrong direction early on.

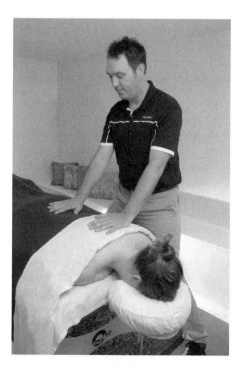

Figure 1–2 Practice a state of mindfulness before a session by bringing yourself into the present moment and approaching your client with a clean slate so that you may work from a place of focus and attention.

Desire + Intention + Action = SUCCESS

Figure 1–3 Formula for success.

From a career aspect, our desires can find fulfillment in the work we choose. We can find careers that bring us into alignment with what we seek on a personal level. Our daily tasks, though not always fulfilling in themselves, work with our desire, aligning us with what we are trying to accomplish on a deeper level. So, although we may not enjoy research, marketing, or calculating finances, all are important to maintaining a successful career in massage. These actions lead to the fulfillment of our desire. For long-term happiness, this alignment is important.

People who follow their desires are driven by deep passion to do or be something that fulfills them. Those who have managed to synchronize their desire with their actions at work are excited when they get up, and the day flies by for them. At the end of the day, they are likely to feel energized, rather than dreading the thought of doing it again. When things get tough, as they usually do at some point, it is often easier for them to navigate the rough spots. They stay focused on their desires and know things will work out. If this is you, congratulations! You are well on your way to fulfilling a deep drive for contentment.

If this is not you at this moment, you have the ability to begin the alignment process. Some of us are on a career path forged by circumstance or convenience. When this misalignment happens and our desires are not fulfilled, we can find ourselves living discontented lives and facing burnout. In fact, there can be increased health risks associated with career discontent, loss of control, and overwork. As our stress increases because of job dissatisfaction, our health can decline as a result of insomnia, anger, or other enduring issues. People who labor on in careers that do not feed their deepest drives can experience a high accumulation of stress.

You probably know someone who is similar to one of the individuals in the following examples:

- The corporate worker who has convinced herself she has to stay in an unfulfilling job because she only has 6 years until retirement.
- The autoworker whose body is continually in pain but whose financial debt generates fear that keeps him from exploring other options.
- The recently divorced mother with few marketable skills who gave up her career aspirations to raise children and now has to support a broken family.
- The massage therapist who does eight massages a day and does not have the confidence or skills to transition to a different, less taxing lifestyle.

Maybe you know someone who has lived in a similar situation for a long time. You may have noticed an unhappiness that lifts only during vacations. Most of us have lived outside our passion and allowed ourselves to stay in less-than-optimal situations because of obligation, fear, or guilt. Although being uncomfortable offers its own lessons, living this way for long periods will eventually cause something to give physically, emotionally, or financially—and force a change. Unhappiness can actually be a great chance for us to break through to a higher, more meaningful level of consciousness. When we allow ourselves to become miserable, it often forces us to take the next step toward something more fulfilling. Sometimes, it actually propels us to new states of being. That is the beauty of life. We are given countless opportunities to regroup and change direction and to make choices that will bring our hearts into alignment with our daily activities. Change and transition, though uncomfortable, are really opportunities to make new choices based on lessons learned through discomfort. Most likely, you have an experience you can reflect on that will highlight this for you. Have you ever had a horrible boss, a neglectful partner, or a lazy relative? Their influence, though uncomfortable, helped you sharpen your instincts about what works for you and what doesn't. Ideally, you learned from them not to go there again. If you didn't, they will most likely be back—perhaps in the form of another person who has similar traits to challenge your growth.

As we mature, we understand that true success is not just having a high-status title or a great paycheck. Those things are nice, but by themselves are not fulfilling. When we live our passion, those things tend to happen naturally because we believe in what we are doing. Being rewarded financially while doing something you are passionate about is a sure sign of an internal alignment of personal desires and outward action.

See Worksheet 1-3

See Worksheet 1-4

At any given moment in your life, you are in a position to consciously decide what you want to do with the rest of it. Now is the time to ensure you are planning to align your desires with your future actions. Let's start by clarifying your desires.

Step 2: Intention—Drafting a Map to Your Desires

Once you have a better understanding of what you really love and desire, you can begin to set intentions that guide you toward fulfilling these desires. When you align your intentions with your desires, you find yourself moving in the direction of your dreams, often subconsciously.

Defining Intention

What is intention? **Intention** can be defined as the motivation that lies beneath action. For example, the act of eating can be motivated by hunger or boredom. The act itself does not change, but the motivations are different and can result in different outcomes. Eating because you are bored might result in an upset stomach, overeating, or weight gain. Eating when you are hungry is simply listening to your body's cues. Some believe that intention has incredible power, especially when intentions support the desires you have defined. By thinking in positive ways and creating intentions that support your desires, you are much more likely to experience success. You are also more able to adjust and deal well when things do not seem to be going according to plan.

For leaders within organizations, the intentions behind change and initiatives are important to share. Often, company leaders make decisions that are for the good of the business, but the decisions can be seen as ill-intentioned because they affect individuals negatively. Usually, once the intentions are explained and made clear, change can move through the company more easily.

From a business perspective, intentions can set your course as you establish your career plans. A well-defined purpose provides the focus you need to stay on track when distractions crop up. When intentions are aligned with desire, there is no stopping your momentum as you move toward realizing your dreams.

Example Intentions for Entering Massage School

Why do students sign up for massage school? There are probably as many reasons as there are students. As you read through the following scenarios, notice your thoughts about each person's situation and see if any of their situations sound similar to yours. Although their actions are all the same—enrolling in massage school—their intentions look very different and will result in different outcomes.

Sara

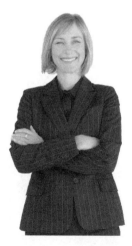

Having spent most of her career in a high-stress, corporate environment, Sara was facing burnout. She had been receiving massage for several years and out of curiosity began to discuss the career aspects of massage therapy with her therapist. After being assigned yet another work project that she did not have the personal resources to handle effectively, she resigned and entered massage school. She was nervous about leaving a secure position with benefits, but she found herself drawn to the healing aspects of massage therapy. Also, she was just tired of her corporate job and was looking for a way out. Massage school seemed to offer this.

Sara's Intentions:
Sara's intentions seem to be escaping from her current job and finding something that is more internally rewarding and less stressful.

Stan

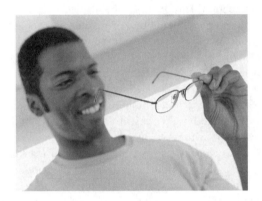

A recent high school graduate, Stan attended a career fair before his graduation. A local massage school had a table with information about the massage profession. He discovered that therapists had the potential to earn between $60 and $150 an hour and that he could graduate after only 500 hours. Not ready to jump into college full-time, which is what his parents wanted him to do, Stan thought the hourly earnings and time commitment sounded appealing, so he decided to enroll.

Stan's Intentions:
Stan seems to be focused on delaying college and making a high wage.

Margaret

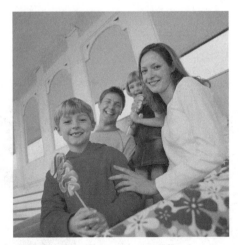

Margaret has always been drawn toward situations that put her in a nurturing role. As a young adult, she volunteered her time at nursing homes and worked with disadvantaged kids. She had enrolled in nursing school years earlier, but expanding home and child care responsibilities kept her from finishing. Still feeling a need to care for those outside of her family, she explored her options in massage therapy. She discovered a program close by at a community college. Believing she could handle the hours required while still managing her personal life, she decided to enroll.

Margaret's Intentions:

Margaret seems to really want to help people, while having the flexibility to maintain her personal life.

John

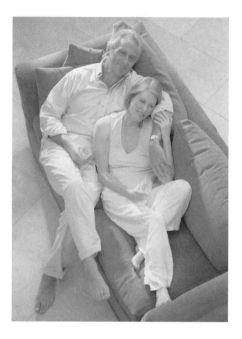

John has been married for 29 years. His wife, who was recently diagnosed with breast cancer, has been going through a hard time. Her doctor mentioned that having a weekly massage would help relax her and potentially could ease her stress level. One of John's friends had gone to massage school, and he encouraged John to look into it. John decided to enroll so that he could offer this gift to his wife.

John's Intentions:

John wants to learn skills that will help someone he loves. Although he is open to learning the art of massage therapy, he doesn't seem to want to make a career out of his newly learned skills.

As the examples demonstrate, there are many reasons why people make decisions. No one except the decision maker can know whether his or her intentions match their true internal desires. It is impossible to determine success or failure based on some formula. John, for example, might not look successful to others because he will never establish a practice or become licensed, but his personal definition of success will be met because his only true desire is to help his wife. Stan, on the other hand, might graduate and become disappointed because $100 an hour looks a lot smaller when he has to pay for all the start-up costs of opening a business, and a local spa offers him only $22 of the $90 charged for each session. If practicing massage is not his true desire, Stan will face discontentment, and life will continue to offer him opportunities to discover his real passion.

There's also the possibility that desire and intention can shift. Once she starts massage school, Margaret might find that she still wants to be a nurse. After graduation, she might decide to go back to nursing school because massage school gave her the confidence and belief that she can manage her family life and take classes at the same time. Massage school became a step on the path to her true desire, which was to become a nurse. Again, there is no right or wrong answer when clarifying intentions, but it is vital to recognize them and understand how they can impact the final outcome.

Understanding Your Own Intentions

See Worksheet 1-5

Regardless of your original intentions, it is important to clarify in your mind why you want to be a massage therapist and what your intentions are now. As you learn more about the business side of massage therapy, we will be putting these intentions in writing. All things start first as a thought or a mental creation. The second phase progresses to the physical reality, which is accomplished only by taking action. Before you begin to take the steps of creating your visions, you want to ensure you have thought everything through. You, in a sense, create the blueprint that you will refer to as you go along. It is always good to have an idea of the **goal** you are striving to achieve because it will help you take the right steps.

See Worksheet 1-6

Peer Profile 1–1

Defining Personal Success

Mary Beth Braun
CMT and Life and Health Coach, IN
One Body Therapeutic Massage, Inc.

In my 15 years of experience as a professional massage therapist, I have found a few key things that have contributed to my success. I encourage you to keep these in mind as you create your unique intention for your own success as a massage therapist. These include, but are not limited to:

- Continually work on knowing and caring for yourself
- Visualize your dream practice and write a plan
- Listen to your client and treat where the client is having pain
- Be a lifelong learner
- Become a resource for your clients

Continually Work on Knowing and Caring for Yourself
When I first began practicing, I quickly realized that in order to make a living caring for others through massage therapy, I needed to learn to care for myself. This was no easy task because I had always erred on the side of sacrificing my needs for the benefit of others. Additionally, I realized my passion and talent for massage therapy came from having a generous spirit. To be successful in caring for myself, I had to begin a journey to get to know my unique needs. Along the way, I discovered many things—a few of which I will share with you:

- I am a morning person—I thrive when I go to bed early and wake up early
- I am more productive with paperwork and thinking in the morning
- I am easily overstimulated and need to continually find ways to calm my nervous system
- I need to rest more than the average person to recharge
- I need to exercise
- I need time to be quiet and reflective
- I thrive when I connect with other massage therapy colleagues

Visualize Your Dream Practice and Write a Plan

My only vision when I first began practicing was that I wanted to help people through massage therapy. Beyond that, I didn't have a business plan or anything written down in terms of how I would get there. Essentially, I was learning as I went, which, in hindsight, made my life and practice challenging at best. I didn't receive much guidance in this area, and there weren't many people to reach out to for assistance. In the years since, I've created a written plan for my practice, and I take steps each year to accomplish my plan. Part of my plan includes enlisting the assistance of business and professional advisors—accountant, insurance agent, financial advisor, and massage mentors. Having the plan written down with specific action steps has been the key to my continued success.

Listen to Your Client and Treat Where the Client Is Having Pain

Although seemingly simple, this appears to be the missing piece in many therapists' approach to treatment. In seeking my own massage treatments, I often run across therapists who barely listen and simply do not treat my areas of concern. This is very frustrating and deters my desire to return for further sessions. Simply, learn to listen to your clients and treat them where it hurts. Be sure to manage your session time to leave enough, maybe even extra, time to treat their concern. Having said that, if the client presents with acute pain or inflammation, be sure to treat the area with lighter techniques and to address the antagonistic muscles. When in doubt, look it up or don't treat the area; however, be sure to explain to the client why you are doing so.

Be a Lifelong Learner

I never thought that my education ended once I finished massage school. I am committed to continuing my learning by attending workshops and reading professional publications and any health-related materials. With continual honing of my hands-on skills and my knowledge of health and wellness, I can serve my clients with the highest level of professionalism.

Become a Resource for Your Clients

Part of my success as a therapist is my generous nature coupled with my desire to be a resource for my clients when it comes to their health and wellness. My continued learning and commitment to make my clients the center of my practice have undoubtedly helped my success as a therapist. I have made it a point over the years to network with other health-care practitioners to refer clients for additional or adjunct treatments. By referring them out, my clients know that I have their highest quality of health in mind. In turn, they are fiercely loyal. Loyal clients have equaled a successful practice for me.

Keep these things in mind as you create your own unique vision for success. Take what works for you and leave the rest. I wish you much success as you begin your journey into the massage therapy profession.

Step 3: Action-Oriented

We have unearthed your desires and begun to set intentions toward fulfilling these desires. Now it is time to purposefully think about taking **action.** The dependable *Merriam-Webster Dictionary* defines action as "the bringing about of an alteration by force or through a natural agency; an act of will."

> "I think there is something, more important than believing: Action! The world is full of dreamers, there aren't enough who will move ahead and begin to take concrete steps to actualize their vision."
> —W. Clement Stone

This stage is too early to write exact steps; first we must spend time assessing things such as income, opportunity, and natural tendencies. Rest assured, however, that we will revisit our formula for success and outline action-oriented goals to keep you moving in the right direction. Doing this initial "nonaction" work is important because no two people have the same internal drivers, and true success rarely happens by accident.

Only frustration comes from jumping into action without first clarifying direction. You will keep moving, but maybe not toward what you really want. Then it becomes difficult to reorient yourself and start over. To ensure a smooth start, make the time to think through what you love to do and how your career can help you fulfill this.

UNDERSTANDING NATURAL TENDENCIES

We all have unique personality traits acquired through genetics and influenced by our environment. It is a good idea to thoroughly understand your natural tendencies so that you can assess and address your strengths and opportunities. In your daily life, you have probably noticed that some tasks give you energy, whereas others activities are depleting. You can observe your feelings about certain tasks and notice whether you look forward to completing them or tend to procrastinate instead of doing them. Procrastination and avoidance are sure signs of not being passionate or confident about something. Every project contains a number of activities required for it to be successful. There will be certain functions on the way to the objective you will naturally do and other portions you will resist. For example, if you decide to go back to school, you might struggle with the research necessary for finding the right school and setting up the finances to acquire a loan, but not have any problem with completing your homework and attending classes once you are a student. You may naturally fit into the role of student but struggle with the logistical arrangement part. In your massage business, your challenges might show as reluctance to pick up the phone and contact potential clients or procrastination in entering your monthly receipts into your accounting software. These areas of avoidance or resistance are called opportunity areas and usually require some sort of internal or external support. As you prepare for your career in massage therapy, knowing your strengths and opportunities will help you achieve success if you learn to relax into your strengths and support your weaker tendencies.

You are probably already aware of some of your strengths and opportunities. Others may be a little more hidden, and it does not hurt to make them clearly visible so you can purposely forge a path that includes the support required for success. When you become good at identifying your natural tendencies, you become savvy in reaching out for help in the areas needing attention. Much has been written on the risks of not understanding yourself (Box 1.1).

In terms of massage therapy, being a really good therapist does not necessarily mean you would make a good massage business owner or manager. But knowing this, in conjunction with your strengths and opportunities, gives you an edge over the 50% of new business owners who fail within the first 5 years of opening their doors.[5]

Box 1.1 The Fatal Assumption

One great resource is *The E-Myth Revisited*, written by Michael Gerber. The E-Myth explores what can happen to people who launch into entrepreneurship and then become overwhelmed by all the roles they were not prepared to play.

Carefully read what Mr. Gerber has to say about what he calls the fatal assumption.

In the throes of your Entrepreneurial Seizure, you fell victim to the most disastrous assumption anyone can make about going into business. It is an assumption made by all technicians who go into business for themselves, one that charts the course of a business—from Grand Opening to Liquidation—the moment it is made.

That Fatal Assumption is: if you understand the technical work of a business, you understand a business that does that technical work. And the reason it's fatal is that it just isn't true. In fact, it's the root cause of most small business failures." [6]

There are many tests available to help you understand all the intricate nuances that make up your personality. You can explore these tests on the Internet and decide whether you would like to complete an official test. Official testing can be a useful tool in helping you succeed by identifying your personality type (Box 1.2).

OFFICIALLY LEARNING ABOUT YOUR PERSONALITY

Many businesses have found immense value in their employees' participation in personality assessment and education. They have discovered that this knowledge helps people function more efficiently in their job roles, saving the company valuable resource dollars on management issues and addressing unhealthy teams. Having a good understanding of their employees' natural preferences helps management ensure they are placing employees in the proper roles and on the right projects. For example, a person who is naturally shy or introverted might not perform well in a position that forces him to speak to large groups, whereas someone extroverted who thrives on social interaction might excel in the role.

Personality assessment can also be beneficial for those wishing to launch their own business. Knowing your personality style can be helpful in understanding which aspect of running a business will be challenging. You can plan to support your areas needing assistance and celebrate the areas in which you are strong. As you learn more about your personality and the personalities of those closest to you, you begin to understand why people do the things they do. It may not be just to annoy you; it is often part of their natural way of being.

You will learn some basic information in this chapter about different character traits and notice which ones seem to apply to you. This is not a full assessment; if you are interested in a deeper look, do an online search for free personality tests.

UNDERSTANDING NATURAL PREFERENCES

You have probably noticed that not everyone thinks and acts like you do. Some people might appear lazy or unstable to you. Others you might resonate with and think they are diligent and good at follow-up. Often, a deeper understanding of natural preferences sheds light on the differences that exist between you and others and how your own preferences might determine how you feel about people different than you. In the 1920s, Carl Jung studied human behavior and determined that personality is not random but predictable and classifiable.

Natural preferences are the core personality traits you prefer to function with, but like your nondominant hand, you can learn to use the areas that do not come out naturally. Your environment can play a large role in determining the traits that you exhibit in the world. For example, if you were

---

Box 1.2 Personality Assessment Options

The DISC is a profile that identifies your level of Dominance, Influence, Steadiness, and Conscientiousness. Each of these types has its own ideal environment, general characteristics, individual motivations, and unique place in a team.

The Meyer's Briggs Type Indicator (MBTI) is a tool that helps identify natural traits. Through a series of questions based on natural preferences, the test defines your specific type. A fun, unofficial MBTI test can be found online at http://www.humanmetrics.com.

The Enneagram is a set of nine distinct personality types, with each number on the Enneagram denoting one type. It is common to find a little of yourself in all nine of the types, although one of them should stand out as being closest to yourself. This is your basic personality type. A couple of free Enneagram tests can be found at http://www.enneagraminstitute.com/tests_battery.asp.

a shy child but your parents encouraged you to participate in team sports or other social groups, you might overcome some of your natural introversion. However, true introverts may find the active social realm draining and require alone time to rejuvenate their resources. In this example, the base preference does not change, but you learn to adapt to your environment.

To simplify the basic personality traits and how they relate to job function, let us explore some of the notable personality functions that might impact your success or failure as a massage therapist.

Introversion and Extroversion

Taking time to assess your natural tendency toward introversion or extroversion will allow you to understand how you prefer to receive stimulation. Those who are more introverted can spend time alone and generate many new ideas and have space for creativity. Those of a more extroverted temperament might receive insight and greater awareness while in the company of others through discussion and interaction.

Starting a successful new business will sometimes require you to energetically extend yourself. These outward efforts will help you promote and expand your endeavor. For extroverts, this comes more easily because they enjoy being around people, talking with others, and sharing thoughts and ideas. For others, however, there is a preference for solitude. These quieter people find they become more creative and focused when they are alone or in small intimate groups. Outgoing people find that if they spend too much time alone, they can become lethargic and even depressed. They gain energy from being around others, preferably engaged in wonderful conversation. Although you can find introverts in highly interactive job roles, they are often labeled as shy or withdrawn. The job may require them to exhibit extrovert traits to be successful, but they can become drained inside. Occasionally, they may go missing as they remove themselves from the public arena to recharge their batteries in a private space at work or at home. If an introverted person is acutely aware of how she prefers to receive information, she can consciously build in quiet, reflective time and still be able to function in this interactive, extroverted role.

On the other side of this, you might find an extroverted, self-employed, home-based massage therapist struggling to make it. As the walls of his home close in on him, he may find his spirit wilting from lack of interaction. His motivation begins to dwindle, and he finds that he is craving interaction, even at the expense of working on his business. Extroverts crave interaction, and often the clients coming in do not provide enough social contact. It would be unprofessional to try to receive needed interaction by talking to clients during their sessions, so the extrovert suffers in silence. However, extroverts aware of these needs can purposefully build in social work time to help meet their requirement for community. Maybe they head off every morning to the local coffee shop to work on their schedule, write an article, or balance the books. Such a massage therapist might also make sure to attend community events, arrange to speak at local libraries, or attend networking meetings.

Which natural preference do you think you have? Do you like to spend time in the outer world of people and things or in your inner world of ideas and images? People with an inward preference have a tendency to reflect, take action, and then reflect again before taking more action. Outgoing people are more likely to take action, think about it, and then take more action. They draw energy from action and interaction, although this can deplete those who prefer a more introverted path.

As you view your results of the introverted or extroverted assessment, how do you think these natural traits might support or pose a challenge for your chosen career path? If you decide to open a massage practice that operates primarily from your home, then this can be supported by being more inwardly focused. The risk is that a home-based business will require solid marketing efforts, and an introverted person might find it challenging to go out and network, make contacts, and solicit business.

See Worksheet 1-7

See Worksheet I-8

Examples of jobs that might appeal to someone more introverted include private practitioner, lab analyst, and home health nurse. Examples of jobs suited for extroverts are front-desk person in a busy medical clinic, group physical therapist, and emergency medical technician.

Thinking and Feeling

These preferences determine how you make decisions. You receive information in, and through, a thinking or feeling preference. Based on your assessment of this input, you decide how to act. Logical thinkers will assess all the information and try to make an unbiased decision based on fact, often not considering whom it might impact. Those coming from a feeling preference will assess the same information and try to determine how it fits in with their value system and what impact it will have on others before making a decision. Understanding the differences in these two traits is the key to success in many relationships. Often you see a business or personal relationship develop in which one person functions from a thinking preference and the other comes from the feeling arena. The thinker often wonders why the feeler has to personalize everything and be dramatic, and the feeler wonders why the thinker is so aloof and seemingly uncaring (Fig. 1–4).

For massage therapists, there are some interesting facts related to the thinking and feeling preferences. Most practitioners in the United States are women. Almost 75% of women have a preference for making decisions based on their feeling nature. With this in mind, we can safely say that the overall workforce of massage therapists is coming from a more feeling preference than a thinking preference. This makes sense when you recognize that most massage therapists have entered the field to help others through the art of touch. Another interesting point is that when viewing people drawn to management positions, most will come from a thinking preference. They have used their skills and logic to advance in their career and often find themselves in positions such as massage franchise owner, spa director, or office manager. In this situation, we find a career-focused, logical person managing a large group of therapists who are functioning primarily from their feeling nature. If not aware of these key differences, both parties can encounter problems.

Here is a scenario on how a thinker and a feeler might handle a situation differently. A resort spa has offered a contest for its employees. The goal is to have a 25% rebooking rate for clients during

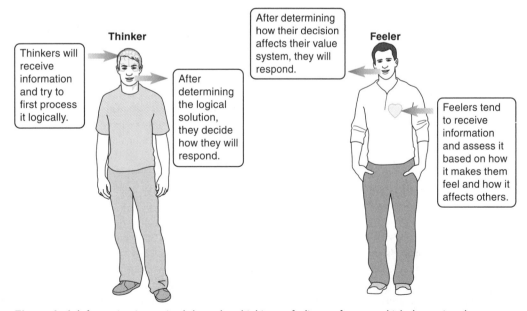

Figure I–4 Information is received through a thinking or feeling preference, which determines how decisions are made.

a 1-week time period. If the employees of the spa meet the goal, there will be an employee pizza party after hours and use of the spa amenities. At the end of the contest week, the spa has had a re-booking rate of 21%, which is 4% below the contest goal.

Thinking preference thought process: "Well, we almost made that goal. I was looking forward to the pizza party and using the salt room, but a goal is a goal. I bet if we spent some time training everyone, we could do better next time and maybe even exceed the goal. I'll have to strategize better next time."

Feeling preference thought process: "Oh no, I know Mary was really looking forward to the pizza party. I bet she will be upset when she finds out we missed the goal. I better go find her and give her a hug. I probably should have worked harder at getting my clients to rebook."

Neither way of viewing this situation is right or wrong; they are just very different ways.

As you view the results of your thinking or feeling assessment, you can better understand how these natural traits might support or pose a challenge to your chosen career path. If you are a feeler and plan on working in a very busy spa run by a thinking manager, you might feel that you are not appreciated or understood. If you are a thinker and recognize that most massage therapists are likely to be feelers, you might think twice before joining a large team of massage practitioners. You might prefer instead to be a lone therapist in the office of a chiropractor who also happens to be a thinker.

You often find thinkers in finance, science, and business careers. They prefer work environments that allow them to be analytical. They tend to avoid personal drama and on-the-job politics. Thinkers enjoy working with others who are intelligent and professional. Feelers, on the other hand, are often found in jobs related to education, health care, and the nonprofit sector. They enjoy work most when they can believe in a cause and see the positive impact they are having on others. They value warm, supportive work relationships.

Organized and Go With the Flow

The next set of preferences determines how you wish to set up your life. Do you prefer a more struc-tured and organized lifestyle, or do you love to be flexible and adapt to situations as they occur? Imagine these two preferences and how they might manifest for individuals. Let us take vacation planning as an example. People who prefer structure and dependability might be those who go online, research places to stay and things to do, and take steps to ensure the itinerary is falling nicely into place. The more spontaneous individuals might not want to plan things too far in advance, to avoid missing out on something exciting that might happen after the booking is set. They like the thought of just showing up and seeing what is going on. They might appear to those who prefer structure as procrastinators, but often they just prefer not to restrict their choices through too much organization. To them, the organizer might appear rigid and inflexible. They often trust things will fall into place at the right time and believe there is little need to structure things so far in advance. If people do not understand and respect these traits in one another, conflict can arise. If understanding exists, however, people can perform the functions that best suit their personalities. The organizer takes on the role of finding, booking, and arranging travel. The go-with-the-flow person gets to be in charge of finding activities and events once they arrive.

As you view your results of the organized or go-with-the-flow assessment, you can better understand how these natural traits might support or pose a challenge for your chosen career path. If you are an individual who craves structure, you might find that the logistical parts of massage therapy come easily to you. You can coordinate schedules, plan events, arrange your nonmassage work sessions, and keep a running list of things to do. You might be challenged when faced with unexpected situations, such as client tardiness or coworkers not completing tasks. One who prefers an easygoing lifestyle might love the "in the moment" client interaction and feel her messy work area only stimulates creativity. This person might be challenged with meeting deadlines or creating a marketing strategy before opening the doors.

See Worksheet 1-9

See Worksheet 1-10

See Worksheet 1-11

You will often find organizers in policy-making, organizational effectiveness, and scientific jobs. They prefer work environments that allow them to make and follow rules. They tend to work first and then play, and they expect others to do this as well. Easier-going people enjoy living in the moment and prefer not to be restricted by too much policy. They like to create their own work schedule and activities, trusting they will get everything done that needs to be done. You will find them in careers like firefighting, news reporting, and acting.

See Worksheet 1-12

SUPPORTING OPPORTUNITY AREAS

Let us be honest—not a single person in the world is great at everything. Success comes easier for those aware of their strengths and willing to either improve or delegate to support their opportunity areas. Your work on discovering your natural inclinations should have clarified your strengths and opportunities.

> Success comes easier for those aware of their strengths and willing to either improve or delegate to support their opportunity areas.

The first step for improvement is consciously acknowledging areas that need reinforcement. Through this recognition, you can begin looking for ways or people to assist you in improvement. Now, let us make plans to strengthen those areas you might find challenging.

See Worksheet 1-13

CHAPTER SUMMARY

There is great power in consciously deciding what you want to do. Once this decision is made, you can take steps to accomplish the goal. It is almost impossible to clearly define the steps that must be taken because life is constantly changing, but a clear focus on the destination will keep you moving in that direction. It is as if the road begins paving itself for you. Again, because of our unique differences, some will head straight for the goal and knock over anything in the way, whereas others will continue to take small steps and slowly reach the destination at their own pace, trusting they will eventually get there. You know yourself well enough to know whether you will struggle with things like bookkeeping, writing business plans, managing people, and implementing marketing strategies. If this is the case, then maybe owning your own practice is not your definition of success right now—or maybe you can move forward with that plan but find assistance with your problem areas. If reporting to another person, following policies, and wearing a uniform appall you, then maybe working in a spa might not be your best long-term choice. By understanding your desires, aligning your intentions early, and planning for action, you can prevent a lot of early missteps.

See Worksheet 1-14

BIBLIOGRAPHY

1. Associated Bodywork and Massage Professionals (2010). Massage therapy fast facts. Retrieved from http://www.massagetherapy.com
2. International SPA Association. (2011). *ISPA 2011 Spa Industry Study.* Lexington, KY: International SPA Association.
3. McCormack, M. H. (1984). *What They Don't Teach You at Harvard Business School: Notes From a Street-Smart Executive.* New York, NY: Bantam Books.
4. Kaufman, M. (2005). Meditation gives brain a charge, study finds. *Washington Post,* January 3, p. A05
5. SCORE—Counselors to America's Small Business (2009). Small biz facts & trends. Retrieved from http://www.score.org/small_biz _stats. html
6. Gerber, M. (1995). *The E-Myth Revisited: Why Most Small Businesses Don't Work and What to Do About It.* New York, NY: Harper Collins.

REVIEW QUESTIONS

1. Why do an estimated 50,000 massage therapists leave the profession each year?
   a. Business naivety
   b. Physical demands of the profession
   c. Lifestyle changes
   d. All of the above

2. Recent brain research shows that _____ and _____ can change the workings of the brain, allowing people to achieve more levels of awareness.
   a. Mental discipline; meditative practice
   b. Introversion; extroversion
   c. Thinking; feeling
   d. Natural tendencies; natural preferences

3. What does paying attention to your thoughts and purposefully interrupting negative repetitive thoughts accomplish?
   a. Keeps you more in the present moment and better able to "go with the flow"
   b. Keeps you more in the present moment and better able to make decisions based on reality
   c. Your personal definition of success
   d. A deep state of meditation

4. Desire + _____ + _____ = Long-term success and happiness
   a. Meditation; natural tendencies
   b. Strategic goals; business savvy
   c. Intention; action
   d. Feeling; thinking

5. Truly understanding our desire requires which of the following?
   a. More reflection
   b. Less reflection
   c. Less action
   d. Both a & c

6. Which of the following is an opportunity for us to break through to a higher, more meaningful level of consciousness?
   a. Adapting and changing our natural tendencies
   b. Intense desire and feeling
   c. Unhappiness and discomfort
   d. Happiness and comfort

7. What is the motivation that lies beneath action?
   a. Desire
   b. Mindfulness
   c. Success
   d. Intention

8. What provides the focus you need to stay on track when distractions crop up?
    a. Well-defined purpose
    b. Well-defined business plan
    c. Well-defined desires
    d. Well-defined personality assessments

9. Both desire and intention can shift.
    a. True
    b. False

10. Identifying that you look forward to some activities and procrastinate on others may indicate _____.
    a. Mindfulness
    b. Natural tendencies
    c. Misaligned goals
    d. Success

11. Which of the following is one reason businesses have found personality assessments valuable?
    a. So employees understand their personality type isn't suited to run a business
    b. They aid in placing employees in the proper roles
    c. They aid in placing employees on the right projects
    d. Both b & c

12. Determining personality types is often random, unpredictable, and unclassifiable.
    a. True
    b. False

13. Natural preferences are the core personality traits you prefer to function with, but you can still learn to adapt to your environment and use those traits that don't come as naturally.
    a. True
    b. False

14. Why assess your natural tendency toward introversion or extroversion?
    a. It allows understanding of how you prefer to receive stimulation
    b. It allows understanding of how you wish to set up your life
    c. It determines how you make decisions
    d. Both a & b

15. Introverts are more likely to:
    a. Take action, think about it, then take more action
    b. Reflect, take action, then reflect again
    c. Make unbiased decisions based on fact
    d. Both b & c

16. **What percentage of women are estimated to have a preference for making decisions based on their feeling nature?**

    a. 25%

    b. 50%

    c. 75%

    d. 100%

17. **Which of the following is a possible reason that managers and therapists may not always get along in a business environment?**

    a. Seventy-five percent of the employees do not have a "go-with-the-flow" tendency

    b. There is not a 50/50 split of introverts and extroverts among the managers

    c. Employees are not making decisions based on their feeling preference

    d. Often those in the management position come from a thinking preference, and the therapists come from a feeling preference

18. **Those who prefer an easygoing lifestyle may be challenged with:**

    a. Meeting deadlines

    b. A messy work area

    c. Too much corporate policy

    d. Both a & c

Worksheet 1-1   My Business Goal Sheet

Complete the following statements by writing a goal-oriented reinforcement in each blank.

Example:

To help start my business successfully, I will *read this book and complete the exercises.*

Fill in the blanks below.

To help start my career successfully, I will

To increase my business knowledge, I will

If I get stuck with a business problem, I will

To ensure I stay healthy, I will

To prevent physical burnout, I will

If my body starts to ache from practicing, I will

If I face a setback, such as a move, I will

Worksheet 1-2   Quick Mindfulness Session

Worksheet objective: To practice a brief mindfulness session and assess your response.

Read the following and then practice a brief mindfulness session. You will want to stay completely present for 1 minute without allowing your mind to wander off with random thoughts.

To begin: Allow your mind to become aware of your surroundings. Pay attention to where you are right now. Notice the noises you hear, the objects around you, and the smells. Bring awareness to your body. Are you slumping? Is your body giving you any signals you were not aware of until now? Try to stay in this state of present awareness for a full minute.

During this short exercise, I noticed

I think I could practice mindfulness for _____ minutes/hours without any difficulty.

Your mind is calmed when you rely on your senses to orient you to your surroundings. This removes the mind's constant burden of trying to figure things out. Most likely, you noticed something going on around you that you had not been aware of until you brought your mind back. Try doing this on a regular basis. Throughout the day, stop what you are doing and pay attention to what is around you. The more you do this, the more you will stay focused on your tasks at hand, and the less you will lose yourself in the memories of the past or the possibilities of the future.

Worksheet 1-3 My Happiness List

Worksheet objective: To write down what really excites you so that you can focus your energy.

Step 1: Set aside time when you will not be disturbed. Take some deep breaths, and take a few moments to clear your mind and become mindful. Envision for a moment what you are doing when you are the happiest.

Step 2: Now, write down all the things you love to do. These do not have to be massage related. Think back to past experiences, dreams, and things you do now that you truly enjoy. Write quickly and do not second guess yourself. To help your thinking, jot down answers to the following:

I love to:

Specific to massage, I love to:

I am most happy when:

Specific to massage, I am most happy when:

For others, I love to:

Specific to massage, for others, I love to:

You can come back to this page as often as you want and continue to write things down.

Worksheet I-4   Value Assessment

Another way to determine your desires is to do a quick assessment of your values. From the following list, circle the core beliefs you hold dear either "all the time" or "most of the time." After you are done, revisit the ones you have circled and list your top eight so you can reference later.

Accomplishment	Fairness	Money
Accountability	Faith	Openness
Accuracy	Faithfulness	Passion
Adventure	Family	Patriotism
Beauty	Flair	Peace, nonviolence
Being different	Freedom	Perfection
Calm, peace	Friendship	Personal growth
Challenge	Fun	Pleasure
Change	Global view	Power
Cleanliness, orderliness	Good will	Practicality
Collaboration	Goodness	Preservation
Commitment	Gratitude	Privacy
Communication	Hard work	Progress
Community	Harmony	Prosperity, wealth
Competence	Healthy living	Punctuality
Competition	Helping others	Quality of work
Concern for others	Honesty	Regularity
Connection	Honor	Reliability
Continuous improvement	Improvement	Resourcefulness
Cooperation	Independence	Respect for others
Coordination	Individuality	Responsiveness
Creativity	Inner peace, quietude	Results-oriented
Customer satisfaction	Innovation	Safety
Decisiveness	Integrity	Satisfying others
Democracy	Intensity	Security
Discipline	Justice	Self-reliance
Discovery	Knowledge	Self-thinking
Diversity	Leadership	Service to others
Ease of use	Love, romance	Simplicity
Efficiency	Loyalty	Skill
Equality	Meaning	Solving problems
Excellence	Merit	Speed

Spirit in life (using)	Teamwork	Truth
Stability	Timeliness	Unity
Standardization	Tolerance	Variety
Status	Tradition	Wisdom
Strength	Tranquility	Other: _____
Success	Trust	Other: _____

Review all the values you have circled, and narrow the list down to your top eight.

My most important values are:

1.

2.

3.

4.

5.

6.

7.

8.

Worksheet 1-5   Exploring My Intentions

Worksheet objective: To revisit your intentions when you began contemplating massage school and to fully understand what motivated you to become a massage therapist.

For the following questions, write your thoughts as they come to mind. Think back to when you were deciding to go to massage school.

Describe your first experience with massage therapy.

Think back to your first experience as a recipient of massage therapy. What were you feelings after this experience?

Describe the situation that first got you thinking about finding a massage school to attend.

Why did you pick the massage school that you did?

What excites you the most about being a massage therapist?

What makes you nervous about being a massage therapist?

How do you plan to use your massage therapy skills once you graduate?

Worksheet 1–6   Recalibrating Intentions to Match Desire

Worksheet objective: To ensure what you love to do is aligned with what you plan to do.

Now, we will check for alignment between what you love to do and the intentions you have set for yourself. Revisit your My Happiness List (Worksheet 1–3) and Value Assessment (Worksheet 1–4) and notice the values you selected and the things you love to do. In the left column, write down some of these important things. In the right column, write how these desires can be fulfilled by a career in massage therapy.

Example:

My Desire/Value (I love to . . .)	My Intention (This can be fulfilled by . . .)
Teach	I can teach at a massage school or develop continuing education programs. I can offer to give public sessions on the benefits of massage therapy at yoga studios or book stores.
Write	I can start a massage-focused blog, write educational articles for a client newsletter, or submit articles to industry periodicals.
Help others heal	I can focus my practice on working with elderly people or in a hospital. I will become an expert in working with cancer patients.
Be in nature	I can work at a destination spa, retreat center, or another location that keeps me close to nature. I will also work for them as a hiking guide.
Be around animals	I can take continuing education courses focused on animal massage and work with animals therapeutically. I will complete a program on animal massage and join a professional organization.
Be around other people	I can work at a massage franchise with 30 other therapists or a busy spa. I can work on a cruise ship or at an airport.

Now fill in the blanks for yourself. Be creative. These are not to be set in stone but will help you align your career goals to things you love to do. Also, do not let negative thoughts keep you from writing down something you think could never happen. As Henry Ford said, "Whether you think you can or think you can't … you're right."

My Desire/Value (I love to ...)	My Intention (This can be fulfilled by ...)

Now, revisit your answers in the intention column and circle any idea that really excites you or sounds appealing as a potential aspect of your career. Spend a few moments thinking about what it would be like to actually be doing what your wrote down.

Worksheet I-7   Introverted or Extroverted?

Below are some brief descriptions of interaction. Circle the descriptions that most apply to you. Remember that there are no right or wrong answers, and it is fine to have circles in both columns.

Introversion	Extroversion
Prefers to think through things before answering; sometimes thinks others speak too quickly	Often speaks before thinking; sometimes regrets not waiting to speak
Prefers a tight group of a few friends	Has a lot of friends and acquaintances
Prefers small events, quiet time, and spending time with people who are in their circle	Prefers groups, parties, and social events—the more the merrier
Viewed as reserved or shy	Viewed as approachable or outgoing
Wants others to respect their alone time and privacy	Does not mind social interruptions such as phone calls, instant messages, or e-mails
Would rather think about things and make decisions than solicit others' opinions	Enjoys asking others their opinions on decisions
Sometimes wishes for more assertiveness when asked for an opinion	Usually are early to answer questions and become impatient if other outspoken people do not allow time for speaking
Needs alone time after being in social situations—often views social interactions as draining	Tends to become bored when alone. Might need to keep the television or radio on during quiet moments to lessen the silence
More likely to work through processes quietly	Has a tendency to vocalize through processes such as speaking to the computer, talking while looking for things, or trying to involve others with the need at hand

Based on these traits, I believe I am more: (circle one)

Introverted   Extroverted

Worksheet 1-8   Strengths and Opportunities

This worksheet will help you think through the strengths you can rely on or opportunities that will require support for some basic job functions.

As a(n) _____ (Introvert or Extrovert), I will have strength or opportunity for certain job functions. Place a check under either Strength or Opportunity for each job task. Strengths tend to come naturally whereas opportunities might require support.

Job Task	Strength	Opportunity
Calling on new clients		
Offering to speak at events		
Setting up my office space		
Meeting my new business neighbors		
Hanging out with a large group of therapists		
Dedicating time to business organization at home		
Quietly writing articles for a blog		
Offering education classes to the public		
Speaking up for yourself in difficult situations		
Personal interaction with loyal clients		
Working in a solitary office with little interaction		

What other job functions might challenge you, based on your preference to be introverted or extroverted?

For areas you have identified as opportunities, spend some time assessing what you can plan now so that you will not falter once you are ready to begin your career.

Worksheet 1-9   Thinker or Feeler?

Below are some brief descriptions of how you might make decisions. Circle the ones that most apply to you. Remember that there are no right or wrong answers, and it is fine to have circles in both columns.

Thinker	Feeler
Assesses what is fair and true when deciding outcomes, even if it makes someone unhappy	Assesses the impact on others while making decisions and takes others into consideration
Can remain detached and calm during times of conflict	Can become emotional and personalize conflict
Can make tough decisions and often does not understand why others personalize it	Will back off of a logical decision if it is perceived to affect someone negatively
Prefers being right to being liked	Prefers being liked to having decisions accepted
Can be viewed as distant or unfeeling	Can be viewed as emotional or sensitive
Prefers conversations based on logic and science	Prefers conversations aimed at involving or helping others
Tends to stick with decisions because they were grounded in facts	Willing to change decisions if the result has affected someone negatively

Based on these traits, I am more: (circle one)

Thinking   Feeling

Worksheet 1-10   Strengths and Opportunities

This worksheet will help you assess the strengths you have to rely on or opportunities that will require support for some basic job functions.

As a _____ (Thinker or Feeler), I will have strength or opportunity for certain job functions. Place a check underneath either Strength or Opportunity for each job task. Strengths tend to come naturally whereas opportunities might require support.

Job Task	Strength	Opportunity
Handling client complaints		
Working for a thinking boss		
Working for a feeling boss		
Setting boundaries with coworkers		
Coaching a fellow therapist who is not following rules		
Leading team meetings		
Firing employees		
Promoting massage in your community		
Setting your massage fees		
Telling loved ones you cannot give them a massage		
Deciding on your marketing strategy		

What other job functions might challenge you, based on your preference to be a thinker or feeler?

For areas you have identified as opportunities, spend some time assessing what you can plan now so that you will not falter once you are ready to begin your career.

Worksheet 1-11   Organized or Go With the Flow?

Below are some brief descriptions of how you like to structure your life. Circle the traits that most apply to you. Remember, there are no right or wrong answers, and it is fine to have circles in both columns.

Organized	Go With the Flow
Has a schedule, prefers to stick to it, and can become upset if things do not go as planned	Is fine with spontaneity, usually works on impulse or as needed
Likes organized work spaces and has a specific place for most things	Can be viewed as messy or unorganized
Prefers not to be surprised but to have everything mapped out	Enjoys creativity, spontaneity, and the excitement of rushing to get things done
Prefers to keep things as planned	Open to new ways of doing things
Keeps lists and actually plans work based on the list—enjoys checking off things as being done	Does not enjoy being pinned down by a list of things to do, would rather deal with things as they come up
Can be annoyed when others are late or not prepared and believes most people seem to be on their own schedule	Easily distracted and can move from one thing to the next without finishing what was started
Likes it when everyone just does what they are supposed to do	Likes to make work more fun and creative

Based on these traits, I am more: (circle one)

Organized   Go With the Flow

Worksheet 1-12   Strengths and Opportunities

This worksheet will help you assess your strengths or opportunities that will require support for some basic job functions.

I am more _____ (Organized or Go With the Flow). I will have strength or opportunity for certain job functions. Place a check underneath either Strength or Opportunity for each job task. Strengths tend to come naturally whereas opportunities might require support.

Job Task	Strength	Opportunity
Meeting deadlines		
Handling emergency situations		
Writing policies for your practice		
Punctuality		
Creating business systems		
Preparing and paying taxes		
Dealing with interruptions		
Maintaining regular session notes		
Holding people accountable to policies		
Planning for and taking continuing education before your license renewal		

What other job functions might challenge you based on your preference to be an organizer or a go-with-the-flow person?

For areas you have identified as opportunities, spend some time assessing what you can plan now so that you will not falter once you are ready to begin your career.

Worksheet 1–13   Opportunity Reinforcement

Contemplating the business aspects of your massage career, write down three main opportunities you have identified and what you plan to do to reinforce them.

Example:

My Opportunity	Ideas for Reinforcement
I am shy. I don't really like to speak about myself or feel confident in what I am doing.	I will create good marketing and online materials that will help explain what I do. I will join a local Toastmaster's group to help me get comfortable with speaking in front of others.
I am not really comfortable in stating boundaries with clients when I feel they are out of line.	I will work with other therapists and role-play situations that exist in my practice so that I can be more confident when addressing issues with clients.
I absolutely do not want to deal with keeping track of all my expenses and entering them on the computer.	I will put all receipts and business papers in a box and pay or trade with a bookkeeper to enter and organize them.

Now, you try it:

My Opportunity	Ideas for Reinforcement

Worksheet I-I4   Description of My Business

Worksheet objective: To see a quick glance of how you envision your career in massage.

Now that you have worked on some self-analysis and writing, take a moment to write down your thoughts on your career plan. This most likely will change as you gain experience and figure out what you like and do not like. For now, let us see what you have in store for yourself.

I plan to offer massage therapy services within the community of _____.

I prefer to:

a. Work alone

b. Work around others

c. Have employees

d. Work from home

e. Other: _____

My immediate plan upon graduation is to:

a. Own my own business

b. Work as an employee

c. Work as an independent contractor within an established setting such as a hospital, chiropractor, or salon

d. Other:_____

I plan to specialize in the following modalities:

I would like to work with these types of clients:

Based on these decisions, my success will depend on:

Chapter 2

Money Matters

"All I ask is the chance to prove that money can't make me happy."

–SPIKE MILLIGAN

Outline

You will learn to...

- Assess how your past might affect your current relationship with money
- Improve your financial health
- Consciously allocate your money
- Determine what your income will look like as a massage therapist

Key Definitions

This chapter references several key terms, which are indicated in bold. For easy reference, these terms are briefly defined here:

Base pay: Regular income that is a fixed amount, such as a fee per service or hourly rate, which does not include additional incentives or variable pay.

Cash flow: Amount of actual cash-on-hand that is coming in and out of your bank account over a specified amount of time.

Commission: Typically a percentage of income earned by performing extra tasks such as selling products or extending service times.

Conscious allocation of money: Often referred to as a "budget," it is a financial plan for receiving and spending money over a specified amount of time. This allocation (or budget) helps an individual or company understand its financial situation and manage the inflow and outflow of resources.

Credit report: A description of a person's financial history, which includes identification and employment information, credit inquiries, payment history, and public record information, such as bankruptcies.

Credit score: A numerical score used to determine the likelihood of an individual repaying his or her debt. This score is calculated from information contained in a credit report. Credit scores range from 350 (high risk for a lender) to 850 (low risk for a lender).

Debt: Money borrowed from another person, company, or lending or financial institution with an agreement that the money will be paid back at a later time, usually with interest.

Fair Credit Reporting Act (FCRA): A federal law that requires each of the nationwide consumer reporting companies to provide consumers with a free copy of their credit report, at their request, once every 12 months.

Financial health: The condition of a person or company's finances. Similar to physical health, individuals with good financial health generally take care of their money and handle their finances with care. Those considered to have poor financial health generally do not take as much care with their finances and may be overly in debt, are slow to pay off debts, or don't make timely payments.

Gratuity: Often referred to as a "tip," it is a voluntary payment over and above the agreed-on financial obligation and usually provided for a service.

Gross income: Total revenue, before deductions and expenses.

Line of credit: A formal agreement between a person or company and a lending institution (e.g., bank), which allows the customer to easily borrow money, up to a specified maximal amount, when needed. For example, a person may establish a line of credit of $10,000 but may initially only borrow $6,000. That person still has access to the remaining $4,000, if and when needed, but generally does not pay interest on this unused portion until it is used.

Merit pay: Compensation based on internal measures such as service length, client return rate and financial performance.

Nonmassage pay: Pay earned while on duty, but not performing primary job function, such as massage.

Nonpay incentives: Items or benefits that have value, but are not money. Examples include access to free services, discounts, paid time-off, continuing education, and benefits.

Profit margin: A percentage that reflects the amount of money actually earned after all expenses have been deducted from revenue. For example, if a company has a 6% profit margin, they keep 6 cents of every dollar they receive.

Promotion pay: Extra money earned as a result of taking on more responsibility or additional roles.

Salary: An established amount of pay received in regular intervals for work or services performed. Salary payments are typically the same amounts each pay period.

EXPLORING PERSONAL FINANCES

Taking the time to realistically assess your personal finances can help you on your journey to becoming a successful massage therapist. Having an understanding of your financial status will guide decisions as you plan your career. For example, if you are interested in becoming an entrepreneur, you may need to get business loans, which require a good credit score.

It is also important to be aware of your personal financial behaviors. If you tend to treat credit cards as "free money," then you are likely to do the same professionally and might dig yourself into a deep hole. If you know that you tend to forget due dates and pay bills late, then you can take preventive steps to ensure you meet the obligations and demands of starting your own business. Strive to understand any negative tendencies and learn ways to change your habits now. When you efficiently and effectively handle your personal finances, whether you become an entrepreneur or work for someone else, you greatly reduce the stress and time spent on dealing with financial headaches (Fig. 2–1).

The Role Money Plays in Your Life

Money, cash, bills—for such small words, they have tremendous power behind them. If you have enough green pieces of paper, you can buy whatever you want: a car, a house, or even a business. Without enough of them, you may struggle to fulfill basic needs.

Have you ever thought that your life would be better if you had more money? In reality, money does not fix what needs fixing. A glimpse into the lives of lottery winners proves that. Thirty percent of them wind up filing bankruptcy after winning enormous sums of money. The truth is that money has power only because everyone agrees that these pieces of paper have a certain value.

You learn at a very early age how money can affect your life. You save coins in your piggy bank so that you can buy something special. Your parents may reward you with money for good grades or doing chores. Conversely, they might withhold money as punishment for misbehavior.

You also learn that money has incredible emotional power. As you grew up, perhaps your family gave money to help others in need. Perhaps your parents used it against each other. Maybe one parent seemed to have financial control over the other. Or, perhaps money was not visibly important in your family. You believed that everything would be provided, and somehow it always was.

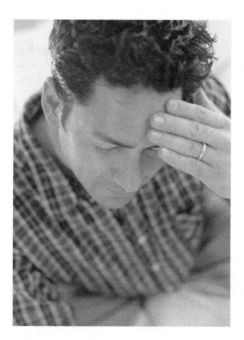

Figure 2–1 Assessing your personal financial behavior and changing any negative habits now can reduce future financial headaches.

If you were raised in an atmosphere of financial peace and security, you probably didn't feel constricted by lack of money or fear there was not going to be enough to care for your needs. Compare this to someone whose parents lived paycheck to paycheck, lost his or her home, or never had extra money to travel or invest in self-care. These grown children might view money very differently.

Your early experiences can greatly color your current views. It is worthwhile, therefore, to take some time to recall your early experiences concerning money. However, remember that as an adult, you have the ability to make your own decisions and pave your own path. Most parents did the best they could. Even if you have experienced negative feelings about money, you can learn positive things from those difficulties. So, be grateful you can now make your own choices and recognize old patterns for what they are—the past.

This book will help you begin the process of revealing how the past might affect your present situation. At the end of the chapter, you will find resources to deepen your exploration into your monetary beliefs.

The Impact of Money During Your Formative Years

See Worksheet 2-1

Your deep-rooted beliefs about money can create abundance or constrict financial growth. Plan at least 20 minutes to complete the next worksheet. Choose a time when you know you will be alone, and clear your mind of distractions before beginning. Use whatever meditative technique works for you, such as focused breathing or just sitting in silence. When you are ready, complete Worksheet 2-1.

Importance of Financial Health

The most important step you can take to ensure a healthy financial future is to understand where you are right now.

The most important step you can take to ensure a healthy financial future is to understand where you are right now. Simply knowing that **financial health** is important to long-term success is not enough. You have to understand your financial status and prepare to make changes if needed. The financial decisions you have already made—both good and bad—laid the path to your present situation. Fortunately, becoming aware of your financial health is a great way to begin the improvement process. Let us begin the process of financial self-analysis.

Credit Score

One quick and easy way to see how you are doing financially is to look at your **credit score**, which is reflected on your **credit report**. Credit reports contain details of an individual's financial history (Fig. 2–2). That information is used to calculate a numerical credit score that is used to determine whether you are likely to repay the money you borrow. Credit scores range from 350 (high risk for a lender) to 850 (low risk for a lender). The higher your score, the easier it is to borrow money when you need it and to acquire better loan rates. It is best to be at 700 or above.

You should always be aware of your credit score. This can be accomplished easily and at no cost. The **Fair Credit Reporting Act (FCRA)** allows you to obtain a free report once every year from each of the four major credit bureaus: Equifax. Experian, TransUnion, or Fair, Isaac and Company (FICO). To obtain a copy of your credit report online, visit the website of one of these companies (2-1: Find It on the Web).

Information Contained Within Your Credit Report

- **Identification and employment information:** your name, birth date, Social Security number, employer, and spouse's name are usually included. The credit reporting agency may also provide information about your previous addresses, employers, property ownership, and income.
- **Inquiries:** all inquiries into your credit by outside parties within the past year will be recorded on your report. For example, if you apply for credit, start cell phone service, or

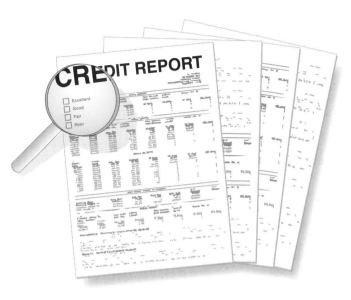

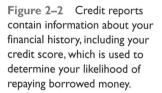

Figure 2–2 Credit reports contain information about your financial history, including your credit score, which is used to determine your likelihood of repaying borrowed money.

submit a rental application, it will likely appear on this list. Potential employers within the past 2 years who have requested your credit report are also identified.

- **Payment history**: all your various creditor accounts are included, listing the credit extended and whether you have made timely payments. Referrals to collection agencies may be noted.
- **Public record information:** events that are a matter of public record, such as bankruptcies, foreclosures, or tax liens, may appear in your report.

When you request your credit report, do not request from all agencies at the same time. Instead, stagger your requests throughout the year so as not to raise red flags. On your request, be sure to include the name of the credit bureau from which you are requesting your credit report. These agencies have additional services you might find helpful, such as e-mail alerts when your report is updated, or assistance with any disputes you might have with the content.

Improving Your Credit Score

Once you know your credit score, you can either celebrate a history of good financial decisions or begin the improvement process. Your credit score will not change overnight, but you can take

---

2-1: Find It on the Web

FREE OR INEXPENSIVE CREDIT SCORE WEBSITES

- TransUnion is a global leader in credit and information management: http://www.transunion.com
- Experian is a global leader in providing information, analytical tools, and marketing services to organizations and consumers to help manage the risk for and reward of commercial and financial decisions: http://www.experian.com
- Equifax empowers businesses and consumers with information they can trust: http://www.equifax.com
- Credit bureau scores are often called "FICO scores" because most credit bureau scores used in the United States are produced from software developed by Fair Isaac and Company. FICO scores are provided to lenders by the major credit reporting agencies: http://www.myfico.com

steps to improve it. The following are a few ideas you can implement immediately to improve your score.

- **Pay your bills early or on time.** Late payments have a major negative impact on your score. Collections are even more difficult to recover from. The more consistently you pay your bills on time, the better your credit score (Fig. 2–3).
- **If you have missed payments, get current and stay current.** Contact the company to make arrangements to catch up. Often, these companies are willing to work with you.
- **Review your credit report to determine the number of accounts that are considered active and their total value.** Even if you have a zero balance or have cut up your credit card, you still have access to a **line of credit**. Unless you have closed the account, it is considered active and is counted by firms when they decide whether to loan you money.
- **If you are having trouble making ends meet, contact your creditors or see a credit counselor.** This won't improve your credit score immediately, but if you can begin to manage your credit and pay on time, your score will gradually improve.
- **If you disagree with any of the information included in your report, file a dispute with the reporting agency.** Submit in writing the information you believe is inaccurate. Include copies (not originals) of documents that support your claim. In addition to providing your complete name and address, your letter should clearly identify each item you dispute in your report, explain why you dispute the information, provide the correct information, and request deletion or correction.
- **Be aware that paying off a delinquent account will not remove it from your credit report.** Once a **debt** goes to collection, it stays on your report for seven years.

Allure of the Credit Card

The Federal Reserve indicates that as of July 2012 Americans carry $850.7 billion in credit card debt. This works out to about $7,149 in credit card debt per household. It sounds daunting, and it is. The lure of plastic has plunged many households into financial jeopardy. Even more worrisome, credit card companies are targeting young people of high school and college age.

Buying on a whim is a momentary, exciting gratification with long-term, less-than-exciting results. The best advice is to avoid putting anything on a credit card that you cannot pay off with short notice. It is extremely difficult to dig out from under high debt and interest rates. If you currently have credit cards in use, it is a good idea to be familiar with the interest rate being assessed. Often, credit cards will raise their rates and send notifications that often go unread. Call the number on the back of your card to ensure you know the current rate and whether there are any increases coming.

Sometimes credit cards can be useful. If you are able to put all your monthly expenses on a credit card and pay the balance every month, you might earn rewards and cash back. This is a smart strategy only if you can avoid high finance charges by paying your balance in full every month. If

Figure 2–3 To improve your credit score, pay your bills early or on time.

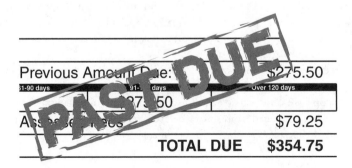

Previous Amount Due:	$275.50
	$79.25
TOTAL DUE	**$354.75**

you thoughtfully weigh the pros and cons of credit cards, you can consciously use them to assist you in your financial planning.

Conscious Allocation of Money

This section could be entitled, "Establishing a Budget," but **Conscious Allocation of Money** places the same principles in a more positive light. Much like the term "diet," which implies food intake restriction, "budget" brings to mind greater control and financial tightening.

In reality, a budget is merely a way to understand your financial situation—money coming in, money going out, and how you manage this inflow and outflow of resources. A budget helps you become conscious of your financial processes and gives you the insight to make sound decisions. Worksheets 2-2 and 2-3 will help guide you through the process of understanding your income and current obligations. On completion, you can consciously decide whether you are making good decisions.

Everyone has natural tendencies. Some are born with a sense of organization that lends itself to strong money management skills, whereas others tend to not spend a lot of energy organizing or planning. However, everyone benefits from a good understanding of current financial status.

Also, each person has a unique life situation, making it more difficult for some to assess monthly spending and earning potential. If you have a dual income or do not handle your own finances, this is still a good exercise. Just do your best when estimating monthly finances. To help with this process, save or print out your bank statements, credit card invoices, bills, and income statements for 6 weeks. These can help fill in any blanks you might encounter when completing the worksheet. Also, many credit cards will total and categorize expenses for you. Visit your credit card's website to set up an online account and access the various reporting tools they provide.

The worksheet provided here is relatively simple. Many people have never actually taken the time to write down the facts about their income, purchases, and obligations. The first time you go through this process, you might be shocked to realize how much money you spend eating out, buying coffee, or picking up small items at the grocery store. Just getting the facts on paper starts the process of improvement, and you may consciously decide to decrease spending in these areas. This is your opportunity to assess where you are and identify areas you would like to improve.

> See Worksheet 2-2

> "My problem lies in reconciling my gross habits with my net income."—Errol Flynn

> See Worksheet 2-3

2-2: Find It on the Web

SITES WITH HELPFUL CREDIT CARD, LOAN, AND INSURANCE INFORMATION

- CardTrak provides millions of consumers with timely information on credit cards and other payment cards via printed survey lists, newsletters, the national news media and the Internet: http://www.Cardtrak.com
- CardWeb.com is a comprehensive online database of payment card industry information: http://www.cardweb.com
- Compare mortgage loans, home equity loans, credit cards and CD rates: http://www.Bankrate.com
- SelectQuote pioneered an impartial, pressure-free way to buy individually underwritten term life insurance from competing insurance companies by phone: http://www.Selectquote.com

---

2-3: Find It on the Web

There are many worksheets online you can complete as well. Simply type "free budget form" or "free budget worksheet" into a search engine to find a digital worksheet.

In later chapters, you will revisit your finances as they pertain to your massage career. Each massage career path has its own level of financial need. If you do not use the forms in this book, keep your financial information somewhere you can easily access.

After you take the time to understand your financial behavior, take steps to assess your current situation, and make conscious decisions to map your financial path, you can launch into your massage career with a much better chance for success. To help you, Box 2.1 provides steps you can take now to secure a stronger financial future.

WHAT INCOME CAN YOU EXPECT AS A MASSAGE THERAPIST?

Before you read the following section on massage therapist income, take a moment to write down what you think you will make on an annual basis as a massage therapist, based on what you have heard or been told.

I will average $ _____ per hour as a massage therapist.

I will average $_____annually as a massage therapist.

Congratulations on doing the work to assess your current financial situation! Now, you begin the process of determining what you can expect to earn as a massage therapist. For some massage therapists, reality does not measure up to initial expectations. Many massage therapists earn a very good income, but you may be surprised at the facts that follow. To alleviate disappointment, this section explores various income possibilities and steps you can take to maximize your earning potential. As Abraham Lincoln said, "That some achieve great success is proof to all that others can achieve it as well."

Industry Estimates of Massage Income

In fields such as massage therapy, many therapists assume they will keep most of the money that clients are charged. Based on this, they may expect a better-than-average income. However, they often forget to consider all the factors that affect potential income, such as business expenses, the lower pay rates provided by employers, and the inability to work full-time.

Box 2.1 Success From the Start: Ten Steps to Financial Success

- Honestly assess your spending habits and find ways to save more money to improve your financial health.
- Consolidate debt with lower interest rates. Try to find 0% interest offers that allow you to live interest-free for a year. Stay aware of the expiration date and transfer fees so that you can transfer again if needed.
- Tackle your credit card debt. Vow to pay off your credit cards and discontinue their use unless you feel you can manage your balance responsibly.
- Save money with the goal to accumulate at least 6 months of living expenses.
- Protect yourself and those you love with insurance and a will.
- Simplify your bill-paying process by using online banking services.
- Once you are in your career, trade with or hire others to do the financial tasks you avoid, such as bookkeeping or end-of-year tax work.
- Write down the amounts of all late fees and due dates for your accounts. Post them to remind you to make payments on time. Many creditors will allow you one free pass per year, so make a quick call to them to see whether you can have a "free pass" if you slip up.
- Prepare for your future by making an appointment with a financial advisor.
- Give yourself a reward when you reach goals.

This section is intended to help calibrate your expectations to what is currently reported within the industry and through therapist interviews. The following information has been gathered from several sources, including U.S. government statistic data and surveys of massage therapists.

American Massage Therapy Association Reports on Income

The following information was gathered from the American Massage Therapy Association (AMTA), a professional, membership-driven organization dedicated to advancing the art, science, and practice of massage therapy (Box 2.2).

According to the AMTA data, there are more than 280,000 massage therapists. Most work part-time, earning an average of $40 per hour, and will practice massage therapy for just over 6 years. If you remember the statistics in Chapter 1 about practitioner attrition, this supports the ABMP's findings. To view the current *AMTA Massage Therapy Industry Fact Sheet*, visit http://www.amtamassage.org.

Bureau of Labor Statistics Facts on Income

Now, let us compare Bureau of Labor (BLS) reports on income for massage therapists. The BLS finds that employment for massage therapists is expected to increase 20% from 2010 to 2020, which is faster than average for all occupations. They also find that many therapists work part-time, often during evenings and weekends. They believe this means massage therapy can be a lucrative second income or a sustainable part-time job.[1]

According to the *BLS Occupational Employment and Wages Report,* May 2011 edition, the mean hourly wage for massage therapists was $19.19. The lowest 10% earned less than $8.80, and the highest 10% earned more than $33.21. Generally, massage therapists earn 15% to 20% of their income as gratuities. For those who work in a hospital or other clinical setting, however, tipping is not common. As is typical for most workers who are self-employed and work part-time, few benefits are provided.[2]

Box 2.2 Excerpts From the 2012 Massage Therapy Industry Fact Sheet

Todays massage therapists are . . .

- Most likely to be sole practitioners.
- Working an average of 15 hours a week providing massage. (Excludes time spent on other business tasks such as billing, bookkeeping, supplies, maintaining equipment, marketing, scheduling, etc.)
- Charging an average of $59 for one hour of massage.
- Earning an average wage of $47 an hour (including tips) for all massage-related work.

The fact sheet provides more details . . .
Massage therapy can be a rewarding and flexible career.

- In 2011, the average gross annual income for a massage therapist (including tips) was estimated to be $21,028.
- While massage therapists work in a variety of work environments, sole practitioners account for the largest percentage of practicing therapists (73 percent). Fifty percent work at least part of their time at a client's home/business/corporate setting, 29 percent in a spa setting, and 29 percent in a healthcare setting,
- Eighty-three percent of massage therapists started practicing massage therapy as a second career.
- Sixty percent of massage therapists say they would like to work more hours of massage than they presently do.
- More than half of massage therapists (53 percent) also earn income working in another profession.
- Of those massage therapists who earn income working in another profession, 23 percent work as a business/professional, 22 percent work in healthcare while 18 percent practice other forms of body work.

Excerpts from http://www.amtamassage.org/upload/cms/documents/amta2012_industryfactsheet.pdf.©American Massage Therapy Association 2012. Reprinted with permission.

The BLS data share many similarities with AMTA data and other sources. However, there are some differences in the amounts reported for hourly and annual wages. Keep in mind that AMTA reported the average income, and BLS reported the median income. The number differences might also reflect the probability that AMTA members have devoted more time and training to massage therapy and therefore earn higher wages.

Sorting Through the Facts to Determine Salary Range

Such a wide range of salaries makes it difficult to accurately assess your potential earnings. Statistically, you have a better chance of success in a larger city that is accepting of and open to massage. Self-employed massage therapists typically make more per hour than employees. However, self-employed massage therapists also have other expenses to consider, such as marketing, laundry, taxes, and overhead costs.

Practitioners employed at a salon, spa, resort, or similar location will usually receive tips on top of their hourly rate, whereas therapists in clinical settings such as hospitals and chiropractic offices will not always have this benefit. Additionally, working as a massage therapist can be both physically and emotionally taxing, so it is rare to find a massage therapist who works more than 35 hours a week.

Another factor that affects annual earnings is your amount of experience. The more time you have to develop your professional skills, the better your odds to succeed. New therapists face the challenge of loan repayment, start-up costs, and even a simple lack of confidence. As you gain experience, you improve your technique and build relationships with clients, both of which help you make more money (Box 2.3).

Types of Pay

On average, a 1-hour massage costs about $62. This rate can vary widely depending on the setting. A very exclusive spa might charge more than $200, whereas a sole practitioner in a small community might charge only $45. In most cases, you will receive only a portion of this amount in your pay. The following list provides you some insight into the pay you might be offered:

Base pay is regular income that is a fixed amount, such as a fee-per-service or hourly rate, which does not include additional incentives or variable pay.

Nonmassage pay is pay you earn while on duty, but not performing massage.

Salary is an established amount you receive in regular intervals and is not affected by the number of massages you provide.

Commission is usually a percentage you can earn by doing extra tasks such as selling products or extending service times (Fig. 2–4). Some employers pay you a base rate and commission for other work, including time doing massage.

Gross income is the total amount collected from clients. If you own your own business, you can keep the entire amount charged to the client, but some of this will go to pay for your business expenses.

Box 2.3 Factors That Contribute to a Higher Level of Financial Success

- Working as an independent contractor or entrepreneur
- Working in an environment that encourages tips
- Practicing in larger, more modern communities
- Improving skills and learning self-care techniques
- Having another job that reduces the potential of physical burnout
- Developing skills in modalities less demanding than Swedish and deep-tissue massage

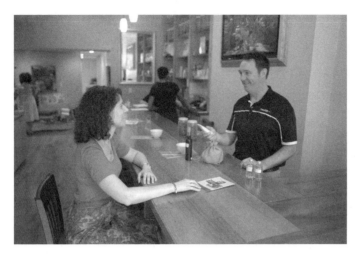

Figure 2–4 Massage thera-pists can increase their income through retail commissions.

Merit pay is an earned amount based on internal measures such as service length, client return rate, and financial performance.

Nonpay incentives are things that have value, but are not money. You might have access to free services, discounts, time off, continuing education, and benefits. You should factor these in if they are valuable to you personally.

Gratuities (Tips) are monetary gifts left by clients for the service performed. In some cases, you will keep all tips; in others, the entire tip total is shared among all employees.

Promotion pay is extra money earned by taking on a management role, such as lead therapist or department manager.

There are many factors to consider before accurately assessing how much you might make. Be sure to gather all this information before accepting a position or launching your own business.

Estimating Personal Income

Now, it is time to assess how your financial picture will look based on the work setting you choose. Most new massage therapy graduates do not immediately launch a successful private practice, but instead start work within an established business. From an experience perspective, this allows the therapist time to build confidence and skills without the immediate worries that come with launching an entrepreneurial business.

In later chapters, you will fully explore the career paths available. First, for the purpose of estimating potential income, let us briefly explore what you can expect when working in different scenarios.

Spas and Salons

Spas generally hire you either as an employee or an independent contractor. The 2006 International Spa Association's *Spa Goer Study* found that 70% of spa guests receive massage therapy, making it the most requested service. Their 2007 *Spa Industry Study* also revealed that there were about 24,000 massage therapist positions open. Based on these data, finding work and staying busy within a spa should not be too difficult.

Working at a spa, you can expect to make between $10 and $35 per session, depending on the spa type and location. For example, a hotel or resort spa usually pays more than a day spa, often because it charges more for the service (Fig. 2–5). Spas located in the central portions of the United States tend to pay more than in other areas.

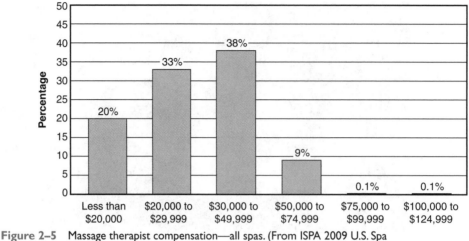

Figure 2–5   Massage therapist compensation—all spas. (From ISPA 2009 U.S. Spa Compensation Data.)

A spa also offers the opportunity to perform other services or cross-train for other departments, alleviating the physical demands of doing six to eight massages each day—a sure path to early burnout. Tipping is often mandatory at higher-end spas and optional at others, increasing your potential income.

Take a moment to write down one or two financial pros and cons of working at a spa.

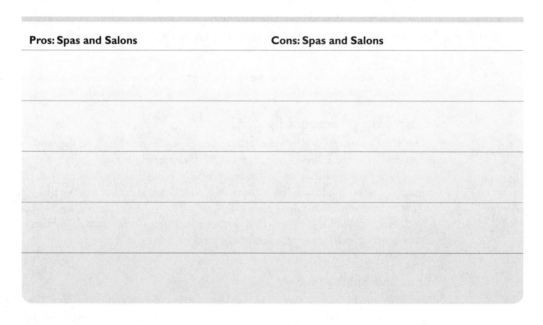

Pros: Spas and Salons	Cons: Spas and Salons

Massage Franchise

You are probably familiar with at least one or two massage clinics now being franchised. With the opening of franchises, more consumers have an opportunity for massage therapy at an affordable rate. As customers gain easier access to massage, the industry will continue to grow.

Because affordability is often part of the business model at a franchise, therapists will likely see this reflected in terms of the hourly wage. It is, therefore, important for therapists at high-volume clinics to fully understand the salary, tipping, and benefits offered in relation to the number of required

Peer Profile 2-1

Jessica, LMT
Missouri

Not long after I graduated from massage school, a massage franchise opened up near my house. I had heard different things about working for a franchise, but decided after I received my license to apply for a job there. I think what concerned me most were the stories I had heard about low pay and long hours. Surprisingly, I found that it really worked for me. Because I am an employee, I don't have to worry about saving up to pay taxes, and they have a program that helps pay for my continuing education. I like knowing I have a steady paycheck coming in. I do not have to worry about marketing and promoting myself to anyone outside the clinic. I try to build my clientele through educating the clients I see about the benefits of regular massage. I'm actually making more money than I did when I worked at a sandwich shop, and I enjoy this work more. I think about running my own business, but for now, I'm gaining experience that will make me a better therapist. To me, that makes it worthwhile.

work hours. Therapists' hourly wages can range widely. Often, as an employee, you are entitled to receive benefits such as training, health insurance, and free massage. For some, these benefits compensate for a potentially lower wage. For beginners, a franchise can be a good option, helping you quickly acclimate to giving regular massage and having a consistent income.

Take a moment to write down one or two financial pros and cons of working at a large franchise.

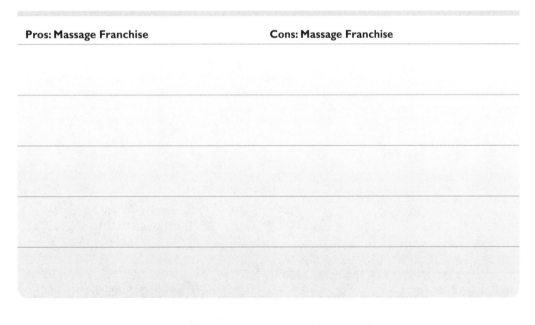

Pros: Massage Franchise	Cons: Massage Franchise

Hospitals, Chiropractic Offices, Nursing Homes, and Other Health-Care Settings

As the popularity and availability of massage grow, so does your opportunity to set up your practice within the structure of another established business. Generally, you either rent space or become an independent contractor. As more and more patients request preventive treatments, more hospitals and medical offices are adding massage therapy services. A national survey conducted by the Health Forum/American Hospital Association in 2006 found that:

- The number of hospitals offering massage therapy increased by 30% from 2004 to 2006
- Of the hospitals with massage therapy programs, 71% indicate they offer massage for patient stress management and comfort, whereas more than two thirds (67%) offer massage for pain management (Fig. 2–6)
- Sixty-seven percent of hospitals with massage therapy programs offer massage to their staff for stress management

This move toward an integrative approach to health and wellness bodes well for your clients' future health and your long-term career prospects.

When you work within established health facilities, you can follow the existing pricing guidelines established by the organization. If you are an independent contractor or a sole practitioner renting space, you might set your own rates. Fortunately, in these circumstances, you have a good chance of quickly building a practice based on regular referrals and the proximity to potential clients. More so than other avenues, medical offices accept insurance, which might affect your rate of pay. Some health facilities do not allow tipping, so check into this if you are interested in this work setting. There is much growth in the medical field, and it should continue to offer many positions for massage therapists drawn to this avenue.

Take a moment to write down one or two financial pros and cons of working in a medical environment.

Pros: Medical Setting	Cons: Medical Setting

2-4: Find It on the Web

RESOURCES FOR MASSAGE THERAPY CAREERS IN THE MEDICAL SETTING

- The Joint Commission (JCAHO): http://www.jcaho.org
- Hospital-Based Massage Network (HBMN): http://www.naturaltouchmarketing.com/HBMN-hospital-massage/HBMNHome.php
- National Association of Nurse Massage Therapists (NANMT): http://www.nanmt.org
- Planetree: http://www.planetree.org

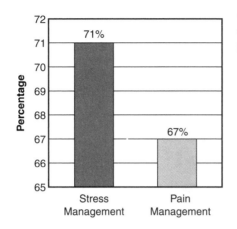

Figure 2–6 Reasons for hospitals to offer massage therapy programs to patients. (Source: 2006 Health Forum/American Hospital Association.)

Privately Owned Massage Clinic

Privately owned massage and wellness centers are plentiful and offer many employment options. These centers are likely to hire you as either an employee or independent contractor. The main factors affecting your pay are the going rate of massage in the area, how your pay is structured, and whether you are allowed to accept tips. Another factor to consider is that clinics usually reflect the personality of the owner. If the owner is very knowledgeable about massage, then you are more likely to receive good pay and benefits.

Take a moment to write down one or two financial pros and cons of working in a privately owned massage center.

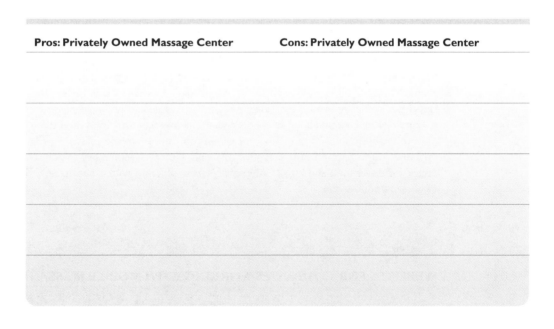

Pros: Privately Owned Massage Center	Cons: Privately Owned Massage Center

Corporate and Mobile Massage

As more businesses focus on employee welfare, many are offering onsite massage or bringing in mobile massage services. This trend began several years ago. Oxford Health Plans reported that 6% of employers offer massage, and when it is provided, 60% of employees relax with a massage (Fig. 2–7).[3]

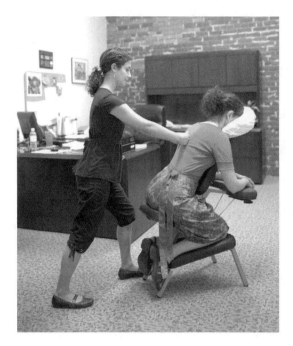

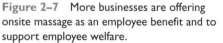

Figure 2–7   More businesses are offering onsite massage as an employee benefit and to support employee welfare.

According to the Society for Human Resources Management (SHRM) *2010 Benefits Survey*, at least 12% of businesses and organizations offer therapeutic massage as an employee perk, showing growth since the Oxford survey. SHRM believed companies are recognizing that massage reduces stress, increases employee productivity and morale, and reduces absenteeism. Several companies that have offered or used massage therapy as a job perk for workers are Google, SAS Software, Best Buy, and JC Penney.

The mobile massage concept accommodates corporate demand and carves out a unique niche. Some therapists want a full practice without all the overhead costs. Usually, out-call therapists are in business for themselves or are affiliated with a national mobile massage entity such as *GoMassage*, a therapist membership-based company that has a national presence. At *GoMassage*, potential clients can search for massage therapists by zip code and book an appointment for a massage therapist to meet them within a short time.

To establish yourself in this line of work, you can purchase a massage chair and portable table, enabling you to respond to requests for out-calls. However, remember to adjust your pricing to account for travel time and costs. Otherwise, you might find yourself running around a lot and not earning a good income.

2-5: Find It on the Web

WEBSITES FOR COMPANIES WORKING WITH MOBILE MASSAGE THERAPISTS

- Infinite Massage offers a network of chair massage therapists and mobile spa service providers: http://infinitemassage.com
- Ahh That's the Spot Massage offers chair massage programs for the workplace: http://www.ahhthatsthespotmassage.com/corporatemassage.asp
- Geared toward people on the go, GoMassage is the place to call when you just can't wait to relax: http://www.gomassage.com

Take a moment to write down one or two financial pros and cons of working at a corporation or having a mobile massage business.

Pros: Corporate and Mobile Massage	Cons: Corporate and Mobile Massage

Airports and Malls

It is no surprise to see massage popping up in unexpected places. Airports and malls are just the beginning. In these settings, service is most commonly provided as the client remains fully clothed during a chair massage. The focus is primarily on the head and feet. Services are usually shorter to accommodate impending flights or busy schedules. These 15- and 30-minute services usually cost between $15 and $40. One smaller company, *Destination Relaxation*, has a dedicated mall-based business at the Annapolis Mall in Maryland, as well as an airport location at the Baltimore-Washington International Airport. It offers quick, fully clothed massage, with a separate area for a full chair or table treatment.

Another, more national company, *Massage Bar®*, focuses solely on establishing massage businesses in airports. It is currently located at nine major airports and hires therapists as part-time employees.

There are special considerations when setting up in an airport. For example, clients need to hear announcements, and they require services that allow them to depart quickly.

Take a moment to write down one or two financial pros and cons of working at a public location such as a mall or airport.

Pros: Airport and Mall Massage	Cons: Airport and Mall Massage

Animal Massage

Interest in massage for animals has grown significantly, and several associations promote international recognition and regulation of animal massage. For animal lovers, there are exciting opportunities to work with both large and small animals.

You can attend a special school or take continuing education courses aimed at equipping you to deal with the special requirements of animals. Courses are available in animal massage, acupressure, Reiki, essential oils, and animal communication. Some states have regulations, so check with your state board about any special rules. Many therapists charge similar fees for animals as they do for humans. Most likely, you would perform this type massage on your own, and set your rates based on your own research. For large animals, you might have space considerations, or more likely would travel to where the animals are kept. Also, this type massage might act as a subsidy to your work with people. If you decide to pursue this avenue of massage, you will need to check with your state board to research any laws governing working with animals. Some states have very specific rules about working with animals, and it might even be illegal. Also, doing market research is very important because it might be hard to "break into" some industries, such as the equine industry.

Take a moment to write down one or two financial pros and cons of working with animals.

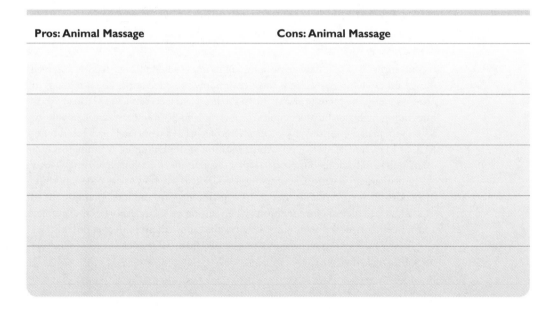

Pros: Animal Massage	Cons: Animal Massage

Entrepreneur

Becoming an entrepreneur, which the AMTA reports is the most common career path among its members, allows you to do and become whatever you wish, as long as you fully develop your business skills along with your massage skills. Most of the therapists who report the highest annual salaries own their own practice or business. The challenges, which will be explored fully in the entrepreneur

2-6: Find It on the Web

ANIMAL MASSAGE ASSOCIATIONS AND SCHOOLS

- International Association of Animal Massage & Bodywork: http://www.iaamb.org
- International Association of Animal Massage Therapists: http://www.iaamt.com
- Tallgrass Animal Acupressure Institute: http://www.animalacupressure.com
- Northwest School of Animal Massage: http://www.nwsam.com

Peer Profile 2-2

Harriet Ling, LMBT, NC
Dancing Horse Equine Massage Therapy

Yesterday, I used the hot stones in a horse massage for the first time, and was just blown away by the response I got. I expected to have to introduce them slowly and give the horse time to get used to the heat. That was **so** not the case with yesterday's "client"! I showed him the first stone before I got started, and that was all it took. I worked on him for a solid 90 minutes without him once getting fidgety. This in itself is huge because horses typically are ready to be done after about an hour (sometimes less). His eye was soft the whole time, he leaned into the work, and, of course, the tissue response was dramatic. This particular horse is permanently lame with several issues contributing to that, and so has chronic extreme muscle tension almost everywhere. On top of that, we had to miss his last appointment, so it had been 6 weeks since any bodywork had been done with him. After thoroughly warming up with the stones, I was able to work deeper than I ever had with him (subscapular work was amazing!), and some of the separating strokes that I use were absolutely effortless. It's **so** nice to be able to say, "I love my job!"

> Most of the therapists who report the highest annual salaries own their own practice or business.

chapter, are the upfront work required to build a solid business foundation and the ability to navigate all the job roles required to successfully run a business. Many find the extra duties too challenging and opt to continue working as an employee or an independent contractor.

Being in business for yourself requires special considerations, such as paying yourself, setting **profit margin** goals, understanding **cash flow**, managing costs, and handling tax implications.

It is also important to remember that many new businesses do not make a profit in the first few years, partly because of start-up costs.

Take a moment to write down one or two financial pros and cons of working as an entrepreneur.

Pros: Entrepreneurship	Cons: Entrepreneurship

Other Career Options

By now you have probably gathered that an extreme amount of dedication is required to have a higher income just by doing massage. If you wish to work only in the massage industry, there are many other ways you can add to your massage income. Massage therapists can teach, own a school, speak or present at conventions, write articles, publish books, and develop equipment. Some therapists have success in starting online businesses and blogs. You might be the massage therapist who carves out a new niche or explores a new idea that no one else has ever considered. When you set your goals and take action toward them, there are no limits.

> When you set your goals and take action toward them, there are no limits.

PERSONAL ASPECTS FOR FINANCIAL SUCCESS

As you consider your possible career paths, take account of personal areas that can affect your ability to earn a healthy income. These personal aspects are important because business analysis and wage assessment will not help if you cannot perform the work for personal reasons.

These basic elements require your ongoing attention. The following points offer insight into what you can do to ensure you stay healthy enough to earn a good income.

Building Stamina

One of the biggest surprises for new massage therapists is the level of stamina required to make a living with massage therapy. If you work at a spa or franchise and are scheduled for six to eight sessions per day, expect to be tired.

It is important not to deplete your personal stores of energy. To keep you healthy, creating a routine of physical activity is a great first step. Some ideas include yoga, Pilates, tai chi, martial arts, weight training, dancing, and walking (Fig. 2–8). You will know fairly quickly which part of your body tends to become sore or fatigued. Share these concerns with a fitness instructor, and ask for advice and recommendations on how to support and care for your body.

Skill Improvement

> "In the beginner's mind there are many possibilities, but in the expert's there are few."— Shunryu Suzuki

Always keep the heart and enthusiasm of a beginner who is willing to learn more skills. As you continue to learn new techniques and business savvy, you will begin to discover what really attracts you. Through this exploration, your passion will surface in specific areas. As you continue to grow in these areas, your skill level and enthusiasm will draw

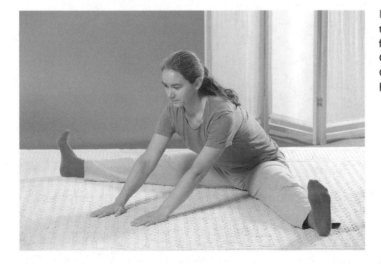

Figure 2–8   Create a routine of physical activity to keep healthy. (Reproduced with permission from Freeman, J.E., & Anderson, S.K. [2012], Career Longevity: The Bodywork Practitioner's Guide to Wellness and Body Mechanics. Philadelphia, PA: F.A. Davis.)

> Always keep the heart and enthusiasm of a beginner who is willing to learn more skills.

the clients you want the most. They will be more satisfied with your service, and you will be rewarded more as they pay more, visit you more frequently, and refer their friends and family to you.

During your continuing education classes, you will make new connections and network with your peers. They can be invaluable in answering questions you might have about finding a good job or deciding how much to charge for your services. If at all possible, find continuing education classes that excite you—not necessarily what is cheapest or most convenient. The excitement of doing something you love is worth the extra effort.

Self-Care

To earn client satisfaction, you have to be healthy. The engine cannot run when it is out of gas. Self-care comes in many forms, but at its essence is a focus on self. Allow space in your life for time dedicated just to your needs. You might consider actually scheduling your calendar for special time put aside just for you. If someone attempts to book or take up that time, let the person know that your schedule is full. This strategy ensures that you have the time you need.

Body mechanics is another aspect of self-care that you must address early in your career to avoid becoming a short-timer. For example, to avoid injury, you should learn to deliver deep-tissue massage without overusing your thumbs. Many therapists suffer and ache because they are not educated about techniques for preventing injury to themselves, especially during deep-tissue massage.

It is also highly recommended that you take additional classes soon after graduation. Reinforce what you learned in school, or address any gaps that were not covered.

CHAPTER SUMMARY

Taking time to do the work around finances can seem very laborious and boring. Not everyone is gifted with money management skills. To successfully plan your future in massage therapy, it helps to think through all the variances that may affect your career. Once you understand your past influences, your current behavior, and the opportunities that exist for you in the field of massage therapy, you are well on your way to beating the odds, avoiding the pitfalls, and successfully practicing massage for many years to come.

BIBLIOGRAPHY

1. http://www.bls.gov/oco/ocos295.htm.
2. http://www.bls.gov/oes/current/oes319011.htm.
3. http://www.prnewswire.com/cgi-bin/stories.pl?ACCT=104&STORY=/www/story/12-21-2000/0001391624&EDATE=).

REVIEW QUESTIONS

1. **When does money start having an impact on your life?**
   a. When you are old enough to pay bills
   b. The first time you go into debt
   c. At a very early age (childhood)
   d. When you open your first savings or checking account

2. **What is the most important step you can take to ensure a healthy financial future?**
   a. Understand your current financial status
   b. Understanding that your financial health is important to long-term success
   c. Receive a complete credit report and know your credit score
   d. Both a & c

3. **How is the information in a credit report used?**
   a. To calculate a numerical credit score
   b. To determine the likelihood of a debt being repaid
   c. To show payment history
   d. All of the above

4. **The higher your credit score, the:**
   a. Harder it is to borrow money
   b. Harder it is to acquire better loan rates
   c. Easier it is to borrow money
   d. Both a & b

5. **Which of the following information is *not* contained within a credit report?**
   a. Inquiries into your credit by outside parties
   b. Tax returns filed with the Internal Revenue Service
   c. Various creditor accounts
   d. Bankruptcies

6. **Requesting a credit report from all of the four major credit bureaus at the same time is a good idea.**
   a. True
   b. False

7. **Which of the following actions may improve your credit score?**
   a. Request a greater line of credit
   b. Stagger your credit report requests throughout several years
   c. Create an allocation of funds (a budget) and share it with the credit agency or collection agency
   d. Make arrangements to get caught up with companies you owe money and are behind in payments

8. **Even if you have a zero balance or cut up your credit card, your account is still considered active and is counted by firms when they decide whether or not to loan you money.**
   a. True
   b. False

9. **Which of the following is the best advice regarding credit cards?**
   a. Avoid putting charges on your credit card that you cannot pay off with short notice
   b. Never put regular expenses on your credit card
   c. Keep your credit card debt below the national average
   d. Both a & b

10. **Once a debt goes to collection, how long does it stay on your credit report?**
    a. 18 months
    b. 5 years
    c. 7 years
    d. 10 years

11. **Which of the following statements is most true?**
    a. Budgets help you become conscious of your financial processes
    b. Budgets give you insight to make sound decisions
    c. Budgets are guesstimates, but help you get organized
    d. Both a & b

12. **Which of the following will help you successfully launch your massage career?**
    a. Understand your behavior around money
    b. Assess your current financial situation
    c. Make conscious decisions to create a financial plan
    d. All of the above

13. **To help ensure financial success, which of the following actions should you take?**
    a. Avoid online banking because it makes it harder to control your expenses
    b. Save at least 6 months of living expenses
    c. Give yourself a reward when you reach goals
    d. Both b & c

14. **Most massage therapists work:**
    a. Full-time
    b. Part-time
    c. Comp-time
    d. All of the time

15. **How much income do massage therapists generally earn from gratuities?**
    a. 10% to 15%
    b. 15% to 20%
    c. 26%
    d. 50%

16. **Which of the following are *not* determining factors in a massage therapist's salary range?**
    a. Size of city or region
    b. Type of employer (spa, franchise, hospital, etc.)
    c. Amount of experience
    d. Credit score

17. **Access to free services, discounts, paid time off, and continuing education are examples of which type of pay?**
    a. Base pay
    b. Commission
    c. Nonpay incentives
    d. Merit pay

18. With the opening of _____, more consumers have an opportunity for massage therapy at an affordable rate.

    a. Spas
    b. Massage franchise
    c. Massage schools
    d. Hospitals

19. Every state allows massage therapy for animals.

    a. True
    b. False

20. More so than other avenues, medical offices accept _____, which might affect your rate of pay.

    a. Gratuities
    b. Complaints
    c. Insurance
    d. IOUs

21. Which of the following personal activities can positively affect your ability to earn a healthy income?

    a. Create a routine of physical activity
    b. Network with peers
    c. Continue to learn and take educational courses
    d. All of the above

Worksheet 2-1 My Past Relationship With Money

Place an X by the most appropriate answer and then draft some thoughts pertaining to your selection.

[   ] I grew up believing money was scarce

[   ] I grew up not really thinking about money

[   ] I grew up not feeling much constriction around money and thinking there would always be enough

[   ] I dreaded asking my parents for money because I knew it would result in some sort of tension

[   ] I had no problem asking my parents for money

[   ] I could ask one parent for money but not the other.

Write your thoughts on the above questions.

Were there many household conversations around money, the economy, financial woes, or gains? Explain.

Do you remember one parent having more financial power than the other? Was money used to control in some manner or was it shared without thought? Explain.

Did you have your own money or did you always have to get it from someone else?

Was money used as a reward for good behavior? Provide an example you remember.

Was money used to punish you when you misbehaved? Provide an example you remember.

You will see patterns emerge just by writing down your thoughts. Your answers will reflect constriction or ease. These patterns may very well have followed you into adulthood and may manifest in your current relationship with money as a mindset focused on either poverty or abundance.

Give yourself time away from your answers. Later, review your answers and write any thoughts you might have about how your early experiences with money might be affecting your current views.

If this type of financial exploration interests you, consider reading the book, *The Intersection of Joy and Money,* by Mackey Miriam McNeill. The book features similar work and further explores using introspection to create wealth.

Worksheet 2-2   Conscious Allocation Worksheet

Complete the worksheet below or one you have found on the Web. This will increase awareness of your financial transactions, as well as the income you will need to maintain your chosen lifestyle. If you are unsure of an amount, make a logical guess.

Conscious Allocation Worksheet

	Monthly	Annual
	Insert monthly amount	Insert annual amount (monthly × 12)
Income Categories		
Take-Home Pay #1		
Take-Home Pay #2		
Bonuses		
Dividends/Interest Income		
Other Income #1		
Other Income #2		
Other Income #3		
TOTAL INCOME	1A	1B
Expenses		
Alimony/Child Support		
Auto/Transportation		
Fuel		
Service		
Transportation		
Other		
Baby/Child		
Diapers/Formula		
Other		
Home Office Expenses		
Office Supplies		
Equipment		
Other Business Expenses		
Charitable Contributions		

Continued

Conscious Allocation Worksheet—cont'd

	Monthly	Annual
Clothing		
Clothes/Shoes		{
Laundry/Dry Cleaning		{
Other Clothing		
Daily Living		
Babysitting/Child Care		
Dining/Eating Out		
Groceries		
Personal Supplies		
Discretionary		
Name 1 Allowance		
Name 2 Allowance		
Dues/Subscriptions		
Club Memberships		
Print Subscriptions		
Child Sports		
Education		
Lessons		
School Lunch		
Tuition		
Other Education Expenses		
Entertainment		
CD/DVD/Books		
Dates		
Film/Photos		
Hobby		
Movie Rental		
Other Entertainment		
Gifts Given		
Health		
Medical Insurance		
Medicine/Drug		
Doctor/Dentist/Optometrist		
Hospital		
Other Health		

Conscious Allocation Worksheet—cont'd

	Monthly	Annual
Household		
Furnishings		
Appliances		
Improvements		
Maintenance		
Other Household		
Insurance		
Auto Insurance		
Homeowners Insurance		
Life Insurance		
Rental Insurance		
Other Insurance		
Lawn/Garden		
Lawn/Plants		
Tools/Equipment		
Other Lawn/Garden		
Loan Payments		
Auto Loan		
Credit Card Payments		
Educational Loan		
Installment Loan		
Personal Note		
Other Loan		
Miscellaneous		
Bank Fees		
Postage		
Other Miscellaneous		
Mortgage/Rent Expenses		
Rent Expense		
House Payment		
Savings Deposits		
Emergency Fund		
Transfer to Savings		
Investments		
Other Savings Expense		

Continued

Conscious Allocation Worksheet—cont'd

	Monthly	Annual
Utilities		
Electricity		
Gas		
Internet		
Telephone/Cell Phones		
Trash Pickup		
Water/Sewer		
Other Utility		
Vacation/Travel		
TOTAL EXPENSES	2A	2B
Income − Expenses		
(For each column, subtract your total expenses (1A & 2A from your total income 1B & 2B)		
1A − 2A = Monthly debt/income		
1B − 2B = Annual debt/income		

Worksheet 2-3 Income and Expense Observations and Plan

Take a few moments and write in the left column any significant observations from Worksheet 2–2 (Conscious Allocation Worksheet). In the right column, write any intentions you have to change.

Example:

I discovered the following about my income and expenses:	My intention around this discovery is:
I spend about $4 on coffee four times a week, which equals almost $70 each month	I will only have specialty coffees out twice weekly and will prepare more coffee at home instead
All my phone bills are adding up to almost $250 each month	I will shop for a less expensive family cell phone plan and cancel my land line
I spend a great deal of money at day spas	I will ask friends for references for more affordable choices and look for coupons
I am saving about $50 per paycheck	I feel good about this amount and will not change it
I spend $160 each month on a housekeeper	I will not reduce this because the investment is worth me not having to do these things

Now, you try it.

I discovered the following about my income and expenses:	My intention around this discovery is:

Chapter 3

What Every Therapist Must Know

"Details create the big picture."

—SANFORD I. WEILL

Outline

You will learn to...

- Define common licensure requirements to be a massage therapist
- Research various state licensure requirements
- Identify the importance of continuing education and the various forms of education available to massage therapists
- Analyze professional and trade associations in the massage therapy field

You will learn to...—cont'd

- Describe basic insurance needs as a massage therapist
- Describe the pros and cons of accepting health insurance from clients
- Identify key legal concerns related to massage therapy
- Describe basic personal safety considerations
- Build an efficient record-keeping system

Key Definitions

This chapter references several key terms, which are indicated in bold. For easy reference, these terms are briefly defined here:

Certification: Advanced or specialized education and recognition program, typically from a nongovernmental body.

Continuing education unit: A method of measurement used to quantify education received.

Disability insurance: This coverage insures your business against the disability of you or your business partners.

Insurance: Security that compensation will be received in the event of an unexpected loss.

License: Legal permission from a government entity to practice within a specific state, city, or county.

Modality: Different professions use the term "modality" in diverse ways, particularly within the health-care industry. Modality is used within massage therapy to describe the methods or techniques used for massage (i.e., Swedish massage, deep-tissue massage), whereas in physical therapy, the term may be used to describe treatments such as hot/cold packs or ultrasound.

Professional liability insurance: This insurance provides coverage against allegations of professional negligence or failure to perform professional duties.

Regulate: Requirements to control or supervise activities.

Sexual harassment: Unwelcome sexual advances, requests for sexual favors, and other verbal or physical harassment of a sexual nature.

Workers' compensation insurance: This insurance is paid for by an employer and covers medical and rehabilitation costs, as well as lost wages, if an employee is hurt on the job.

The professional work of a massage therapist is often an exciting adventure. You have chosen a career that offers you the potential to make a significant difference in the health and well-being of others. Over the span of your career, you might positively affect thousands of people. As a therapist, you are confronted with unique situations, new people and personalities, and diverse working conditions. Massage therapists also have the freedom to work in multiple settings and geographic regions throughout their career, which often adds to the adventure. The part many find not quite as exciting are the details involved in keeping your practice within legal requirements—things such as licensure, record-keeping, and insurance billing. Although some people love the details involved, most do not. Keeping up with all of the requirements to be a massage therapist is a different type of adventure. Luckily, there are resources and tools available to help navigate these requirements to stay in compliance and out of trouble.

LICENSURE REQUIREMENTS

Within the United States, licensure requirements for massage therapists are regulated at the state level, and each state has different requirements. In addition, some individual counties and cities also have requirements, which are not always the same as the state requirements. Therefore, licensure requirements depend on where a therapist plans to practice massage therapy.

As of May 2010, 43 states and the District of Columbia **regulate** massage therapy in their state by requiring therapists to go through a licensure, certification, or registration process. The other seven states may require licensure at the local level, but do not currently require a massage therapist to have a state license to practice. The list of states that require licensure is always changing; several unregulated states have legislation pending or in process. In addition, as the profession and industry continue to evolve, so do the state requirements.

It is important to point out the difference in the terms "**license**" and "**certification.**" These terms are commonly used in the profession and, although related, are distinctly different terms. It is important to understand the distinction. The two terms have become closely intertwined within the profession because many states require applicants to be nationally certified or to have successfully passed a nationally recognized exam in order to receive their license.

To add to the confusion, not all regulated states call their designation a "license." In the states that do, licensed therapists can use the designation Licensed Massage Therapist (LMT) in that state. There are, however, a few states that have a state "certification," which allows therapists to use the designation Certified Massage Therapist (CMT). And still, there are a handful that use "registered," making therapists Registered Massage Therapists (RMT) in those states. However, most regulated states use the term license, and for consistency, that is the term used throughout this text when referring to a government-granted authorization to practice massage therapy in a regulated state.

Massage License Versus Certification

Massage therapy is a regulated profession, and in most states, massage therapists are required to obtain a license from a government entity in order to practice massage therapy. This government-granted license provides legal permission for a massage therapist to practice within a specific state, city, or county. The licensure process helps regulate the profession by ensuring professionals meet minimal standards or competencies; thus, it is a tool the government uses to protect citizens and promote safe business and massage practices. A massage therapy license is usually granted based on a series of requirements, such as education, experience, examination results, and moral character. Licenses are usually valid for a limited time and must be renewed.

Certification is not typically a process conducted by the government but is a way for an industry or field to self-regulate. (In a few states, the designation they grant massage therapists is a state certification and not a license, but it is a government-granted certification.) Private organizations provide curriculum, training, and examinations in order to set professional standards within the field. Certifications may not be required, but they provide reassurance to clients, the community, and peers that an individual achieved, or had obtained, a certain level of knowledge or experience in order to become certified. Although certifications can recognize advanced or specialized knowledge, such as additional training in various modalities, in some industries certification has become the minimal bar that individuals must achieve in order to practice. This is becoming the case with the massage profession because most states require certification for licensure.

When a profession, like massage therapy, is regulated by the government, certification alone is not a legal pass to perform massage. Even individuals certified by a national accrediting body to perform massage must still have a license to practice in each state (or city or county) in which they perform massage, with the exception of the few unregulated states. You may hear the phrase "national licensure," but there is currently no license available that allows a therapist to practice massage in all

50 states. Therapists must have a license in most states and, in some cases, also in the city or county in which they perform massage.

> When a profession, like massage therapy, is regulated by the government, certification alone is not a legal pass to perform massage.

There are, however, "national certifications" and "national exams" that are recognized in most states. These certifications are minimal requirements that many in the profession would like to see become national standards, but not all states, companies, or individuals recognize them as such. Many proponents of standards and certifications support these initiatives because they advance the level of professionalism within the field, encourage self-regulation, and create more uniform requirements across the country.

Educational Requirements

For licensure, states require therapists to complete a certain number of educational hours. Most states require potential licensees to have a minimum of 500 education hours. However, some states have a higher requirement of 1,000 education hours, and those states that are unregulated have no state education requirements at all. The number of hours required for licensure has been a debate for many years, but most within the profession would agree that consistency across the country would be ideal. In recent history, state regulations have become more consistent, but are still a diverse patchwork of requirements.

The debate regarding the number of educational hours mainly centers on quality versus quantity. Some industry experts believe a high number of educational hours are necessary to obtain the appropriate level of knowledge and skills to be an efficient, effective, and safe massage therapist. Others believe it is more about quality than quantity—even with 1,000 hours of training, if the quality of the education isn't high, then the training is meaningless. Therefore, 500 hours of high-quality, effective training is more meaningful than 1,000 hours of low-quality education. The bottom line is how competent massage therapist are when they complete their education.

At the essence of this debate is the issue of quality education and curriculum, which has led to many states requiring students to graduate from an accredited or approved school before licensure is granted. Schools can be accredited by agencies recognized by the U.S. Department of Education or through specific massage therapy accrediting bodies, such as the Commission on Massage Therapy Accreditation. Just like individual certification, schools and educational institutions must reapply for accreditation to ensure continued quality. States may also outline requirements for "approved" schools, which can include total number of educational hours; required educational hours for specific subjects, such as anatomy, physiology, pathology, theory, professional standards, sanitation and safety; and clinic, practical, or apprentice hours. States differ on not just the required number of educational hours but also the subject matter hours, so it is important to find specific requirements for each state in which you intend to work.

Exam Requirements

In addition to educational requirements, most states require potential licensees to pass designated exams. A handful of states require license applicants to have passed an exam created and administered by the state. However, most require one of two nationally recognized exams: the National Certification Examination for Therapeutic Massage and Bodywork (NCETMB) and the Massage and Bodywork Licensing Examination (MBLEx).

The National Certification Board for Therapeutic Massage and Bodywork (NCBTMB) is a nationally accredited credentialing organization. NCBTMB has a nationally recognized certification program that evaluates core knowledge and skills expected of entry-level massage therapists. NCBTMB offers two examinations: the National Certification Examination for Therapeutic Massage (NCETM) and the NCETMB. The NCETMB is the exam administered by NCBTMB that is currently used by various states as a requirement for licensure. The exams have similar content, except as the name indicates, the NCETMB exam includes a bodywork assessment and application. The two exams also differ slightly in how the content areas are weighted.

NCBTMB also has requirements related to the type of education the candidate has received in order to take the exam. The school must meet minimal requirements determined by NCBTMB, such as a minimum of 500 hours of instruction, which includes 200 hours of in-person, hands-on instruction in a classroom. Other requirements include minimal number of hours related to specific content. Keep in mind that a state's requirement for education may be different from the NCBTMB requirement, even if the NCBTMB requires its examination for licensure. So, if you plan to practice in a state that requires the NCETMB exam, ensure your education meets both state and NCBTMB requirements.

The MBLEx is a second nationally recognized exam that was created and administered by the Federation of State Massage Therapy Boards (FSMTB) to test core knowledge and skills expected of entry-level massage therapists. FSMTB is a member organization of state massage boards. It also has requirements for testing, which include verification of education and training on core content areas and adherence to FSMTB policies.

See Worksheet 3-1

National Exams

Two organizations are widely known for their national massage therapy examinations, which are used in most states as a part of their licensure requirements.

National Certification Board for Therapeutic Massage and Bodywork (NCBTMB)
1901 South Meyers Road, Suite 240
Oakbrook Terrace, IL 60181
(630) 627-8000
http://www.ncbtmb.com
info@ncbtmb.com

Today, 37 states, plus the District of Columbia, use or recognize NCBTMB examinations (marked in green). Please note that these facts are current at the time of this book's printing. Visit the website given above for updated data.

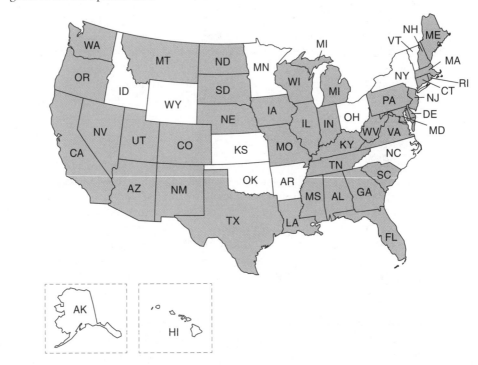

National Exams—cont'd

Federation of State Massage Therapy Boards
7111 W 151st Street, Suite 356
Overland Park, KS 66223
(913) 681-0380
http://www.fsmtb.org
info@fsmtb.org

Today, 25 states, plus the District of Columbia, use or recognize MBLEx examinations. Please note that these facts are current at the time of this book's printing. Visit the website given above for updated data.

For more information on the exams, including practice tests, visit http://www.massage-exam.com/. This website also provides information regarding each state's licensure and exam requirements.

Other Requirements

Not all state requirements have to do with education and examination scores. Some states have additional requirements, which include background checks, fingerprinting, physical examinations, tests for tuberculosis and other contagious diseases, cardiopulmonary resuscitation certification, first aid training, HIV-AIDS training, medical error prevention courses, and practical exams. In addition, some states require the applicant to have liability insurance before licensure. Again, states may have different requirements, so it is important to check with each state in which you intend to practice.

(Continued on page 77)

Peer Profile 3–1

Associated Bodywork & Massage Professionals
http://www.abmp.com*

■ **What are the key things a massage therapist must know about licensure?**

A massage therapist needs a license or some form of registration in 43 states, Washington DC, Puerto Rico, and the U.S. Virgin Islands. It is important for a massage therapist to investigate regulations before relocating because the portability of credentials has not yet been established among different states, although segments of the profession are working toward reciprocity. Some states have continuing education requirements for massage therapists to maintain their licensure. Although their philosophies are different, the two major massage therapy membership organizations often work together on regulatory and legislative issues. Associated Bodywork & Massage

---

*Associated Bodywork & Massage Professionals (ABMP) is a national membership association that provides comprehensive liability insurance and practice support for massage/bodywork practitioners and students. Founded in 1987, ABMP is now the largest massage therapy membership organization in the United States, with more than 70,000 members.

Professionals (ABMP), the largest such organization, does not support one-size-fits-all regulation, preferring to respect the readiness, needs, and unique characteristics of each state. For example, in densely populated areas, uniform licensing makes sense so that massage therapists working across several different counties can obtain a single state license, instead of coping with the regulations and fees of several jurisdictions. This duplication may not be a problem for massage therapists in other parts of the nation because of their geographical makeup. In some states, law enforcement welcomes massage therapy regulation as a tool in fighting prostitution and human trafficking disguised as legitimate massage.

■ **What are the key things a massage therapist must know about insurance?**

Insurance is absolutely critical for protecting massage and bodywork therapists from lawsuits that could be financially devastating to their practice and personal life. Massage therapists should have their own coverage even if they work in a spa, salon, or physician's office because employer coverage often does not protect massage therapists individually and may not cover all modalities and circumstances, such as when therapists practice massage in their homes or private offices. Even if employer coverage will pay a claim, therapists could be left holding the bag for their own legal defense costs, which could easily become a significant expense. There have been cases in which massage therapists assumed their employers covered them and learned too late the coverage was inadequate or nonexistent.

Occurrence-form policies are the best option for massage therapist liability insurance coverage. History shows that many claims aren't filed until just before the statute of limitations has run out (2 years after an incident in many states). If the therapist's occurrence-form insurance was effective in July 2010, but it lapsed a year later for whatever reason, the therapist would still be covered for any incidents occurring in July 2010. In the same situation, a claims-made policy would not cover that claim. Claims-made policies require that claims be made while the policy is still in effect. If the claims-made policy expires and a claim is filed, the therapist will have no coverage, even though he or she was insured at the time the incident took place. Claims-made policies are less expensive, but they provide considerably less coverage.

Although there are bare-bones insurance products on the market, the organizations offering them may not have the stability or track record that larger organizations can offer.

Customer service is another key issue; if a massage therapist gets into a claim situation, he or she will want sensible, compassionate advice and support. Some organizations simply refer members to the insurance company and aren't staffed to answer claims or everyday questions.

General liability is another important piece of the insurance portfolio and is often included as part of professional liability coverage. Whereas professional liability covers the actual work performed, general liability covers slip-and-fall scenarios and accidents that can happen in any business.

Beyond professional liability coverage, massage therapists would also be wise to consider business personal property insurance, which protects for loss of business equipment as the result of fire, theft, flooding, and so forth.

Therapists should ask if the association charges for additional insured endorsements (AIEs), which are often required by landlords or employers.

Massage therapists should make certain that coverage limits apply to members as individuals and are not aggregate (group) limits. Under aggregate coverage, the funds could run out by the end of the year if too many claims were filed by other members of a plan. If group limits are reached before a massage therapist files a claim later in the year, that later claim may not be paid. When therapists ask about coverage limits, they need to be sure the limits are per member, per year, and are not shared member aggregates.

Renewal Requirements

A periodic license renewal may also be required within the state or city you are working. Most states require a renewal fee to reissue a license, as well as a specific number of **continuing education unit** (CEU) hours. Depending on the state in which you practice, you may need to meet CEU requirements every year, every 2 years, or every 3 years. To illustrate the differences between even neighboring states, as of May 2010, North Dakota requires 32 CEU hours every 2 years, whereas South Dakota requires 8 CEU hours every 1 year.

Fee Requirements

Various fees are often required to process and issue a massage therapist license and other associated requirements. Most states have an application or license fee, or both, which can range from $25 to $300, as well as renewal fees, which range from $30 to $250, depending on the state. There may be other fees for duplicate licenses, fingerprinting, background checks, and exams. There are also different fees for different licenses, such as provisional, temporary, instructor, or student, which again vary by state. Be sure to check the state and city or county in which you are planning to work to determine fees associated with licensure and renewal.

Unregulated States

In May 2010, there were seven states that did not have statewide regulations for massage therapists; however, this does not necessarily mean therapists can hang their shingle and begin work. In these states, local requirements may apply at the city or county level. For example, at the time of this writing, the State of Alaska does not require massage therapists to obtain a state license to practice massage. However, there are local requirements within the state, such as the City of Anchorage, which requires a license fee but has no additional requirements. However, the City of Fairbanks requires a license fee, plus the following:

- Applicant must meet at least two of five minimum requirements: (1) complete at least 350 hours at a state-approved massage training school or program, (2) hold current professional class membership in a recognized national massage organization, (3) hold current certification by the NCBTMB or a similar organization, (4) have been licensed out of state within the past 3 years of application, or (5) have had 2 years' experience within the 5 years before application.
- Applicants must also be at least 18 years of age, not be addicted to drugs or narcotics, have no misdemeanor convictions for assault or dishonesty within 3 years of application, have no felony convictions within 5 years, and have never had a sexual misconduct conviction.
- Along with the application, applicants must submit copies of required certificates, drivers license, Alaska Business License, and Alaska criminal background report.
- Applicants must provide 5 years of criminal history. Applicants will need to provide a criminal history from each state of residency during the above-mentioned time period. The Alaska report must be dated the same date that the application is submitted.[1]

See Worksheet 3-2

Modalities

States and local governments may have differing definitions of what modalities fall within massage. Thus, for the protection of a massage therapist, it is important to research regulations related to the various modalities you practice within the state or local level to determine whether there are different regulations. For example, Utah recently issued a board opinion on Reiki and determined that "Reiki is defined as a 'spiritual healing art' that is performed on an individual by a Reiki Practitioner by 'transmitting healing life force energy' through the hands. It is the position of the Division that to the extent that Reiki is used as a 'spiritual healing art' and does not involve the methods outlined in the scope of practice of Massage Therapy, then Reiki is not a modality of massage. However, should a Reiki Practitioner while performing the 'spiritual healing art' involve the use of any of the methods outlined in the scope of practice of Massage Therapy, then the Reiki Practitioner must be licensed as a Massage Therapist."[2] (Fig. 3–1)

State Boards

States use massage therapy licensure boards to decide requirements and review applicants. Licensure boards may also review complaints made against licensed therapists. Board members are typically appointed for a specific number of terms and years. Boards may consist of massage therapists, professionals from related fields, and members of the general public and may vary in size. Members of a state's licensure board are typically listed on each state's website.

Staying in Compliance

A great resource regarding state requirements is your massage therapy school. The instructors and administrators should be knowledgeable about the requirements within the state. They may also have additional information concerning other state requirements as well.

Before practicing, check into local regulations that may apply to massage therapists because some cities and counties may have their own regulations. If this is the case, then massage therapists must comply with both the local and state regulations. If you are starting your own business and not going to work for an employer, then you will need to research requirements for a business license as well.

If you are a licensed therapist in one state and choose to move to another, you will need to obtain a new state license. To do this, you will have to determine whether you need to complete additional education hours, take another exam (e.g., state specific exam), or complete additional

---

3-1: Find It on the Web

Professional and trade associations are an excellent source of information regarding state boards and requirements. Two that monitor state massage therapy regulation are the American Massage Therapy Association and the Associated Bodywork and Massage Professionals. Both organizations produce an online listing of state requirements that is updated regularly:

- American Massage Therapy Association State Boards and Requirements listing:
  http://www.amtamassage.org/government/state_laws.html
- Associated Bodywork and Massage Professionals State Boards and Requirements listing:
  http://www.massagetherapy.com/careers/stateboards.php

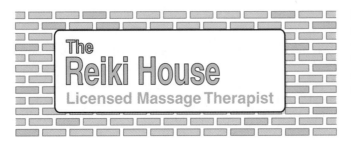

Figure 3–1 It is important to research regulations related to the various modalities you practice within state and local levels to determine whether licensure is necessary.

requirements (e.g., background check). You will also need to research whether there are specific requirements for the city and county to which you are moving. Contact city and state authorities, as well as local health departments, to gather information on massage therapy requirements (Fig. 3–2).

CONTINUING EDUCATION

Part of being a professional, particularly in a health and wellness field, is continued education. Continuing education is essential for the safety of clients but also serves to maintain and advance a therapist's level of knowledge. There are five primary reasons why continuing education is an integral part of a massage therapist's career:

1. CEUs are required by many states to renew a professional license.
2. The massage profession is a dynamic field in which to work, and continued education is imperative to stay knowledgeable about the latest research, legislation, news, and theories.

> ### 3-2: Find It on the Web
>
> For a sample of a state's requirements, visit the State of Utah Department of Commerce, Division of Occupational and Professional Licensing website Utah's massage therapy practice act: http://www.dopl.utah.gov/laws/R156-47b.pdf

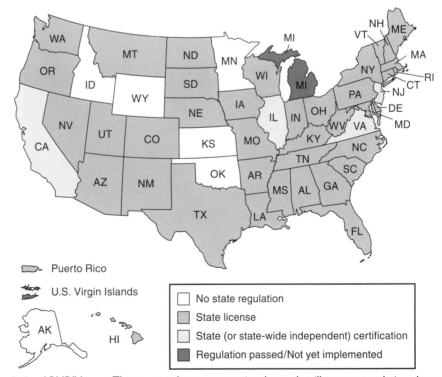

Figure 3–2   ABMP/MassageTherapy.com has a great national map that illustrates regulations by state. (Visit http://www.massagetherapy.com/careers/stateboards.php for a current updated map.).

3. A significant amount of efficacy research continues to be conducted surrounding the health benefits and concerns relative to massage therapy. As a professional, you must stay current on these benefits, as well as potential contraindications.

4. Throughout life, learning is important for both professional and personal growth. It keeps your thinking and discussions relevant, is fuel for your brain, and enhances other skills such as problem-solving and relationship building.

5. Continued education is a responsibility massage therapists have to their clients and themselves. To help ensure the safety and security of your clients, you must remain aware of the latest thinking, changes, and research relative to your interactions with clients and their health and well-being. Keeping informed of changes and developments also helps limit your professional liability and exposure. For example, if there are regulatory changes relative to protecting private client information, you need to be aware of these for a client's protection, but also for your own protection.

Continuing education comes in many forms and is not just limited to massage education. To be successful, it is also important to continually learn and receive training on other topics as well, such as the following:

- Business
- Client satisfaction
- Ethics and Professionalism
- Health and Wellness
- Legislative and Political Changes
- Products
- Research
- Trends (Consumer, Social, Workforce, Environmental, Economic)
- Technology

> Therapists who want to be successful must remain informed and knowledgeable about the world around them, specifically in regard to the many aspects that affect their practice.

This is just a partial list of very broad topic areas, which helps to illustrate the vast amount of information therapists need to collect and process. The world is moving very quickly, and change is continual. Therapists who want to be successful must remain informed and knowledgeable about the world around them, specifically in regard to the many aspects that affect their practice.

Sources of Continuing Education

Luckily there are many sources of continuing education. The hard part is often finding education that is best for you and obtaining it. We are naturally interested in some topics more than others, thus our educational focus is often on topics of interest. For many, legal and liability related topics, such as risk management, sanitation, safety procedures, tax laws, and other related issues, are not always at the top of the list for continuing education sessions. For a variety of reasons, they are not as attractive to many professionals. However, they are an essential part of continuing education. So, although a therapist may not be excited about seeking out these topics, the successful ones will include them in their education to ensure a successful future.

The other point to consider about finding education that is best for you is educational format. CEUs can come in various formats, such as e-learning, classroom education, and seminars at various conferences and events. To maximize learning, find a format that is best for your learning style, as well as your personal needs and budget.

For general education and information, a vast array of resources are available, including newspapers and magazines, local and national business organizations and conferences, specialized training and education courses, and colleges and universities. One of the simplest ways to stay informed is to get out of your practice and talk to people. Talk to those in and out of the massage profession about world events and changes going on within the community, state, country, and world (Fig. 3–3).

For massage-specific continuing education, there are also a wide variety of resources. In most cases, CEUs that need to be documented for licensure or certification renewal need to be approved or verified by the licensing or certifying body. However, general continuing education related to massage therapy can typically be found through:

- National and state association memberships, events, and publications
- Colleges, schools, and other specialized classroom training
- Certifications and certificates of completion from various massage and massage-related organizations
- Online courses available through schools and other private entities
- Industry-specific publications, websites and blogs

Certification

Certification is another formalized way to obtain continuing education. National certification, as previously discussed, can be a part of your licensure and initial credentialing as a massage therapist, but it can also be a tool used later in your career for advanced or specialized education. Many associations and membership groups offer certification, as do many specialized training programs. Certification provides a therapist with more than just additional education. It is also public recognition that a certain standard has been achieved. In most situations, certifications are not easily obtained; therefore, they are often coveted and prestigious credentials. These credentials establish practitioners as massage professionals with a high standard of excellence. They also serve as an excellent marketing tool, create a competitive edge, and provide additional reassurances to clients about skill, experience, and education. In addition, they give individual therapists something to be proud of and advance their opportunities in the field.

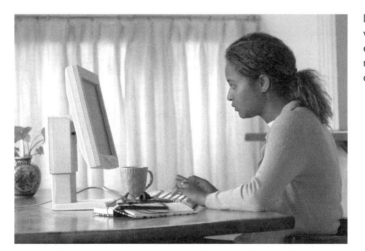

Figure 3–3   There are a wide variety of sources of continuing education, ranging from networking events to online courses, publications, and blogs.

3-3: Find It on the Web

NCBTMB publishes a searchable list of approved education providers on their website: http://www.ncbtmb.org/ceproviders_find_providers.php.

3-4: Find It on the Web

MASSAGE PUBLICATIONS

There are several massage magazines that are a wealth of information for industry professionals. Below is a list of some of the major publications:

- *Massage & Bodywork*
  Published bimonthly
  http://www.massageandbodywork.com
- *Different Strokes*
  ABMP's member newsletter, mailed as a supplement to *Massage & Bodywork*. Bimonthly publication
  http://www.massageandbodywork.com
- *Massage Magazine*
  Published six times per year
  http://www.massagemag.com
- *FutureLMT.com*
  Massage Magazine's free bimonthly newsletter for students and new practitioners
- *Massage Therapy Journal*
  Published quarterly
  http://www.amtamassage.org
- *Massage Today*
  Monthly publication
  http://www.massagetoday.com
- *Body Sense*
  Published two times a year
  www.bodysensemagazine.com
- *Journal of Bodywork and Movement Therapies*
  Published four times a year.
  http://www.bodyworkmovementtherapies.com

One of the most commonly referenced certifications in the massage field is the NCBTMB certification. Although there is no national licensure, most states recognize the NCBTMB certification, or the successful completion of its exam, as one of the licensure requirements. If you are not practicing in one of the states that requires this certification, obtaining it may still be in your best interest. This certification makes it easier for a therapist to move among the 37 states that do recognize this certification as a part of their licensure, and it is an additional credential that sets you apart from other therapists in your area.

PROFESSIONAL AND TRADE ASSOCIATIONS

To be successful in any field, you must stay abreast of the latest news, education, and research associated with your profession as well as related professions and industries. Associations keep you informed about recent developments in everything from industry regulations to labor market changes. The massage profession has several strong national and state associations that provide tremendous benefit to massage therapists. Associations host educational events, produce publications and research, provide education through a variety of opportunities, offer networking opportunities and job searches, connect therapists and suppliers, and provide insurance, marketing tools and resources, discounts, job and career services, and a host of other services and benefits. All of these services and benefits are a tremendous resource for helping a therapist to learn, network, and stay current and connected in the field. This is true whether you are an employee, independent contractor, or entrepreneur.

When evaluating associations, it is helpful to know there are two primary types. Professional associations represent individuals within a profession. Trade associations represent the businesses

(Continued on page 85)

National Massage Therapy Associations

Two prominent professional massage associations are the American Massage Therapy Association and the Associated Bodywork & Massage Professionals. These national associations are tremendous sources of massage information and education.

American Massage Therapy Association
500 Davis Street, Suite 900
Evanston, IL 60201–4695
(877) 905-2700
http://www.amtamassage.org
info@amtamassage.org

The American Massage Therapy Association (AMTA) represents more than 58,000 massage therapists. AMTA works to establish massage therapy as integral to the maintenance of good health and complementary to other therapeutic processes and to advance the profession through ethics and standards, continuing education, professional publications, legislative efforts, public education, and fostering the development of members.

There are specific qualifications for the various membership categories that must be met to apply for membership. AMTA holds an annual convention, hosts an annual massage therapy schools' summit, and has established a Council of Schools. AMTA also provides a variety of other benefits, including liability insurance coverage, state chapters, online job bank, directories, a professional magazine, and a variety of research and business/educational books. Visit their website for a full listing of benefits: http://www.amtamassage.org/membership/membership-chart.html.

Associated Bodywork & Massage Professionals
25188 Genesee Trail Road, Suite 200
Golden, CO 80401
(800) 458-2267
http://www.abmp.com
expectmore@abmp.com

Associated Bodywork & Massage Professionals (ABMP) is a national membership association that provides comprehensive liability insurance and practice support for massage/bodywork practitioners and students. Founded in 1987, ABMP is now the largest massage therapy membership organization in the country with more than 70,000 members.

There are specific qualifications for the various membership categories that must be met to apply for and renew membership. ABMP does not host conferences, but provides an extensive continuing education calendar. It also provides a variety of other benefits, including liability insurance coverage, directories, professional magazines, a variety of research, business/educational books and publications, customizeable brochures, websites and e-mails, and regulatory and legislative support. Visit their website for a full listing of benefits: http://www.abmp.com/membership/index.php#extensivebenefits.

State Massage Therapy Associations

Several large independent state massage therapy associations, as well as state chapters of AMTA, are options for more localized resources. A few of the more prominent state associations are highlighted below, but you can also visit http://www.amtamassage.org/chapters/index.html for a list of AMTA state chapters.

Florida State Massage Therapy Association
1870 Aloma Avenue, Suite 260
Winter Park, FL 32789
(877) 376-8248
http://www.fsmta.org
info@fsmta.org

The Florida State Massage Therapy Association (FSMTA) was founded in 1939. FSTMA works exclusively for therapists who practice in the State of Florida. Its mission is to unify the massage therapy profession while creating, representing, and promoting standards of excellence in health care. FSMTA hosts an annual convention and also offers liability insurance, a publication, and other benefits.

New York State Society of Medical Massage Therapists
PO Box 442
Bellmore, NY 11710-0442
(877)697-7668
http://www.NYSMassage.org
info@NYSMassage.org

The New York State Society of Medical Massage Therapists is a not-for-profit organization, incorporated in 1927, whose purpose is the education and advancement of the massage therapy profession. Its members live and work in New York, New Jersey, and Connecticut.

Oregon Massage Therapy Association
1710 Oakhurst Court
Eugene, OR 97402-8002
http://www.omta.net
info@bennouri.net

The Oregon Massage Therapists Association (OMTA) is an alternative grassroots professional organization. It includes a diverse, eclectic membership, dedicated to a collaborative, consensus process. OMTA serves its members, licensed massage therapists, massage students, massage schools, and others involved in health care by providing information, networking opportunities, and education to promote the growth of the massage profession.

Tennessee Massage Therapy Association
105 Jesse Drive
Byhalia, MS 38611
(662) 890-7783
http://www.tmtanews.org

The mission of the Tennessee Massage Therapy Association is to maintain the integrity of the profession, promote professional educational opportunities for members, promote community within the profession, and develop and improve membership benefits that prepare members to flourish.

State Massage Therapy Associations—cont'd

Texas Association of Massage Therapists
3801 Capital of Texas Highway N E240-156
Austin, TX 78746
(888) 778-9851
http://www.texasmassagetherapists.com
info@texasmassagetherapists.com

The Texas Association of Massage Therapists was founded in 1995 by a small group of therapists in San Antonio led by Richard Haslam. Its mission is to protect, maintain, and enhance the professional development, business success, and quality of life for all Texas licensed massage therapists.

within an industry. Other factors to take into account when evaluating associations include the following:

- Size of membership
- Diversity and scope of membership
- Membership fees
- Fees and costs for events, seminars, and publications
- Events and programs
- Publications
- Member benefits
- Return on investment
- Job and career services
- Networking opportunities
- Advocacy programs
- Consumer outreach
- Reputation
- Mission, vision, and core values
- Responsiveness

Gateway to Associations

The American Society of Association Executives (ASAE) is the membership organization and voice of the association profession. ASAE has more than 22,000 association CEOs, staff professionals, industry partners, and consultant members. They provide an online search tool of member associations that may help you in your search for massage and/or massage related associations (http://www.asaecenter.org/Directories/AssociationSearch.cfm).

Once you have found the right association for you, it is important to use your membership. Read the publications, attend key events that will have maximum benefit to you and your business, and consider volunteering for a committee or board service. There is no better way to keep your ear to the ground of potential changes and opportunities than networking with other leaders in your profession.

INSURANCE

Professional Insurance Needs for Massage

Predicting the future is something most of us are unable to do, at least with any accuracy. Because we cannot always predict when we will get sick, when someone will sue us, or when we will be at risk, we have insurance. Professional **insurance** is security that we will receive compensation in the event of an unexpected loss. Your needs will vary depending on whether or not you are an employee, independent contractor, or entrepreneur, which is covered later in the text.

Insurance can be complicated, so it is best to meet with an insurance professional to go through your options and what type of coverage is best for you. However, you still need a basic understanding of the various types of insurance, particularly liability insurance, workers' compensation, and disability insurance.

Liability Insurance

As of May 2010, six states required a massage therapist to have **professional liability insurance** before applying for a state massage license. Other states may require therapists, or a massage therapy practice, to have liability insurance in order to obtain a business license. Be sure to check state and local requirements regarding insurance. In states that do not require liability insurance, some therapists practice without it, but that is a risky gamble because any financial consequences of a legal suit would be the therapist's responsibility.

Liability insurance covers you or the business, or both, if sued for negligence. It typically covers (1) professional liability, such as malpractice; (2) general liability, such as accidents resulting from negligence; (3) product liability, such as allergic reactions to essential oils; and in some cases (4) legal expenses in the event of a lawsuit. Two of the largest massage associations provide members with professional liability insurance—the American Massage Therapy Association and Associated Bodywork and Massage Professionals.

It is also important to understand what your policy covers and does not cover and to remember this as you change and evolve with your practice. As you add, change, or stop practicing various **modalities** or treatments, or as the operations of your business change, discuss these changes with your insurance agent to ensure you have the appropriate coverage. It is a good practice to meet with your agent on an annual basis to review your business and any changes.

State Liability Insurance Requirements

Below is a list of the seven states that require proof of liability insurance before licensure is granted. Also included are the specific state requirements as of May 2010.

Alabama: Professional liability insurance policy of $1,000,000 personal liability coverage.

Colorado: Professional liability insurance policy of $50,000 per claim and an aggregate liability limit for all claims during a year of $300,000.

Indiana: Professional liability insurance, with no set financial coverage stated, that lists the state as an additional insured.

Massachusetts: Professional liability insurance policy of at least $1,000,000 per occurrence and at least $1,000,000 aggregate required.

Missouri: Professional liability insurance required, but no set financial coverage stated.

South Dakota: Professional liability insurance policy of a minimum of $250,000.

Wisconsin: Malpractice liability insurance not less than $1,000,000 per occurrence and $1,000,000 for all occurrences in 1 year.

Workers' Compensation Insurance

Workers' compensation insurance covers medical and rehabilitation costs, as well as lost wages, if you are hurt on the job. This coverage is regulated at the state level. It can be complicated, and there are insurance agents and attorneys who specialize in this type of insurance, but as an employee, or an employer, you need to understand the basics of workers' compensation and what is required of you as a business owner or your rights as an employee. If you are an employee, this information should be included in your employee orientation or available through the owner, management, or human resources department.

Disability Insurance

Short- and long-term **disability insurance** coverage is also available and provides either short-term or long-term financial relief if you are disabled, depending on your coverage. Unlike workers' compensation insurance, you do not have to be hurt on the job to receive benefits. Benefits typically include a portion of your salary for the time you are unable to work. This coverage is available to business owners, and some employers provide it to their employees.

For more information about risk management and the various types of insurance, talk with an insurance agent who is knowledgeable about the massage therapy industry and profession. You can also contact one of the national massage therapy associations that provide liability insurance.

Accepting Health Insurance

"Do you accept my health insurance?" It is a common question in today's environment, but might not be one you've considered from the other side of the health care window. As a massage therapist, will you accept insurance? Determining whether or not to accept health insurance as part of a practice has many implications. Independent contractors and entrepreneurs will face and likely struggle with this decision. Although employed massage therapists will not have to make that decision, they can be affected by it if their employer does accept insurance. Employees may need to learn the operations of managed care, such as how to handle billing and the associated paperwork. Also, as an employee, you might receive a lower fee-per-service if you provide therapy to a client who is using health insurance benefits.

A growing number of major health insurance providers cover complementary and alternative therapies, and massage is one of the most often covered therapies in this category. Although insurance companies are starting to cover massage therapy services, they still often restrict coverage, usually limiting the number of covered visits per year.

There are several ways coverage can work, but it typically involves the practitioner offering discounted rates. Fee-per-service rates are negotiated and contracted between the health insurance company and the massage therapy business. In some cases, the client pays the entire discounted rate at the time of service and then files a claim with the health insurance company to be reimbursed. In other cases, the client pays the practitioner a copayment, and the practitioner files a claim with the health insurance provider for reimbursement of the remaining contracted fee. It is also a popular option for insurance carriers to have a contracted network of providers that offer discounted rates to their members. In this case, a group of massage therapists would agree to offer services at a lower rate to insurance company members than to nonmembers. In exchange for the discount, the insurance provider markets and promotes your services to its clients. The client receives a discount, but payment comes from the client and is received at the time service. This way, neither the therapist nor the insured client has to deal with additional billing procedures, but the therapist or business still agrees to accept a lower fee.

Consider these pros and cons of accepting health insurance payments:

PROS

- There is the potential for increased customers because their out-of-pocket expense is lower.
- The insurance company can help promote and market your services to its clients.

- Practitioners may be able to serve individuals who are in great need but who might not have been able to afford therapy without the insurance.

CONS

- Insurance companies determine the "value" of your services by contracting agreed-on reimbursement payments.
- Learning the health-care system and proper coding to get reimbursement can be challenging.

See Worksheet 3-3

- Reimbursement payments from insurance companies can be slow.

KEY LEGAL CONCERNS

As a massage professional, you must be aware of key legal matters that may affect you and your career. Professional advisers can help you navigate this complex arena and hopefully avoid legal concerns altogether. It is imperative to do your homework and select someone knowledgeable, respected, and responsive who has an excellent reputation among the people you trust. It is helpful, but not critical, that these advisers be familiar with the massage profession. It is more important that they are knowledgeable in their area of expertise.

Three key advisers you should consider are:

1. Attorney
2. Accountant
3. Insurance agent

These three advisers can help you with drafting and interpreting contracts, setting up accounting and financial systems, completing accurate tax returns, interpreting tax law, and getting the appropriate insurance coverage to keep you protected.

From a business and risk management perspective, you need to be aware of a few of the key legal concerns within the massage profession, which include the following:

Sexual harassment: Claims against the therapist (and also against clients) can be devastating to a therapist, business, and other involved parties. Even when falsely accused and found innocent, a claim alone can ruin a massage therapist's career. To help prevent this, ensure you follow proper protocols, such as draping, and know how to handle potential or real inappropriate situations. In addition, report any situation immediately to a supervisor if you believe something may have been misinterpreted or even if your intuition tells you something isn't exactly right.

Client safety and privacy: Always follow an employer's standard operating procedures, especially in regard to client safety. These include things like proper sanitation, keeping floors dry and clear, protecting confidential client information, and monitoring client safety, client reactions, and equipment. If you are an entrepreneur, then develop your own operating procedures to follow regarding client safety (Fig. 3–4).

Medical/health disclosures: Some companies and attorneys differ on their opinions regarding whether or not medical/health information should be disclosed by a client to the therapist or business and, if disclosed, whether it should be provided in writing or verbally. Either way, if a client discloses medical information to you, it must be kept private and confidential and must be factored into whether or not it is safe to perform a massage. If you have any concerns or questions about the safety of a massage given a client's medical condition, then it is best to cancel the massage until you know for certain it is safe.

Tax reporting: Create systems that help you track your income and business-related expenses to ensure you have an accurate account of your financial affairs for tax reporting. This includes gratuities and commissions, which may be provided through paychecks, separate income checks, or cash.

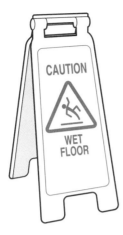

Figure 3–4   To protect both you and your client, ensure you follow standard operating procedures, including maintaining proper sanitation, keeping floors dry and clear, protecting confidential information, and monitoring client safety.

Code of Ethics

For other considerations regarding legal issues, review these partial Code of Ethics from these three established massage-related organizations:

ASSOCIATED BODYWORK & MASSAGE PROFESSIONALS
(Partial Code)

- I shall maintain the highest standards of professional conduct, providing services in an ethical and professional manner in relation to my clientele, business associates, other health-care professionals, and the general public.
- I shall respect the rights of all ethical practitioners and will cooperate with all health-care professionals in a friendly and professional manner.
- I shall refrain from the use of any mind-altering drugs, alcohol, or intoxicants before or during professional sessions.
- I shall always dress in a professional manner, proper dress being defined as attire suitable and consistent with accepted business and professional practice.
- I shall not be affiliated with or employed by any business that uses any form of sexual suggestiveness or explicit sexuality in its advertising or promotion of services, or in the actual practice of its services.

For the full Code of Ethics, visit: http://www.abmp.com/about/code_of_ethics.php.

AMERICAN MASSAGE THERAPY ASSOCIATION
(Partial Code)

Massage therapists/practitioners shall:

- Demonstrate commitment to provide the highest-quality massage therapy/bodywork to those who seek their professional service.
- Acknowledge the inherent worth and individuality of each person by not discriminating or behaving in any prejudicial manner with clients and/or colleagues.
- Demonstrate professional excellence through regular self-assessment of strengths, limitations, and effectiveness by continued education and training.
- Acknowledge the confidential nature of the professional relationship with clients and respect each client's right to privacy within the constraints of the law.

Continued

Code of Ethics—cont'd

- Project a professional image and uphold the highest standards of professionalism.
- Accept responsibility to do no harm to the physical, mental, and emotional well-being of self, clients, and associates.

For the full Code of Ethics, visit: http://www.amtamassage.org/about/codeofethics.html.

INTERNATIONAL SPA ASSOCIATION CODE OF CONDUCT FOR SPA GUESTS: (Partial Code)

As a spa guest, you have the right to:

- A clean, safe, and comfortable environment
- Stop a treatment at any time, for any reason
- Be treated with consideration, dignity, and respect
- Confidential treatment of your disclosed health information
- Trained staff who respectfully conduct treatments according to treatment protocols and the spa's policies and procedures
- Ask questions about your spa experience
- Information regarding staff training, licensing, and certification

For the full Code of Conduct, visit: http://www.experienceispa.com/about-ispa/ethics-and-standards/code-of-conduct/.

PERSONAL SAFETY

Your personal safety is also an area of critical importance. When considering your personal safety, keep these tips in mind:

- Listen to your body. If your hands, arms, or other parts of your body are telling you they are tired or overworked, listen and give them a rest.
- Listen to your intuition. If you find yourself in an uncomfortable situation, then leave the room immediately and report the situation to a supervisor.
- Protect your feet. Not only are your hands and arms actively involved in the field of massage therapy, so too are your feet. You stand on them for most of the day, and they also need to be properly taken care of by ensuring you have appropriate footwear.
- Perform massage according to appropriate protocols. If massage is performed incorrectly, it can cause damage to not only the client but also the therapist, so be sure to follow appropriate procedures and techniques.

There are also increased risks associated with outcalls, or performing massage services outside of the practice. Many therapists will go to a client's home or perform in-room massages at hotels. For outcalls, following are a few safety pointers to keep in mind.

Communicate your schedule with others and make sure they know your schedule. For example, tell a peer you are going to perform a massage at a new client's house at noon and will call at 1:30 to say you are finished. Also make sure you give your peer the address. If for some reason you don't call at 1:30, he or she will know there may be cause for alarm and can take appropriate action.

For in-room hotel massages, take a partner. If it's not realistic to have someone go with you to set up and meet you at the conclusion of an in-room hotel massage, then communicate to the front desk manager your appointment times and what times you will be finished. Make arrangements to let them know when you have safely left the guest's room (Fig. 3–5).

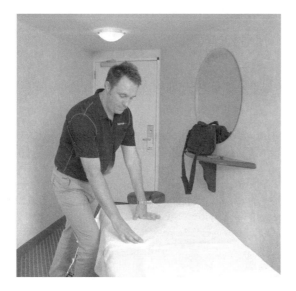

Figure 3–5 For outcall massages, there are important personal safety precautions to keep in mind.

> *Personal Security Tips From AMTA*
>
> Below are five security tips from the American Massage Therapy Association:
>
> 1. Screen first-time clients to verify that they clearly understand the nature of massage.
> 2. Ask clients to read and sign an information form that explains what to expect during the massage.
> 3. Set office policies regarding personal property, loss, restricted access, and personal privacy.
> 4. Install an emergency buzzer in case you need to call for assistance.
> 5. Have a plan for handling inappropriate comments or behavior by clients.[3]

See Worksheet 3-4

Another practical tip to help ensure your safety is to carefully review articles and educational sessions regarding risk management and personal safety and to talk with other massage therapists about tips and tricks they've used.

RECORD-KEEPING

As a massage therapist, you deal with the health and well-being of the clients you serve. You are also a part of the business community. Both of these facts make record-keeping an essential part of your professional career.

It is important to establish and maintain a reliable record-keeping system for client data, business information and records, and financial information. Keeping track of key information, whether an entrepreneur or an employee, is an important part of each individual's responsibility. This includes insurance papers and proof of insurance, licenses, certifications, tips, tax records, compensation, and expenses. If you are an employee, the company you work for may have established policies and procedures for record-keeping, and you should become familiar with these. If the company's policies are not in writing or published, then talk with the management and owner to find out how they want you to handle various types of records.

In addition to maintaining reliable records, you also have a responsibility to ensure that you capture complete and accurate information and that data and records are properly documented, saved, and accessible for as long as they have value. For example, the Internal Revenue Service requires a

3-5: Find It on the Web

The Internal Revenue Service provides guidelines and helpful information regarding what tax records to keep and how long to keep them: http://www.irs.gov/publications/p552/ar02.html#en_US_publink10008614.

company or individual to keep the back-up documentation (e.g., receipts, check stubs, W-2 forms) related to their tax information for a specified number of years, depending on the circumstances. After that time has expired, the documents no longer have a value and may be properly destroyed, unless you have other personal or professional reasons to keep the back-up documentation.

How you manage and store client records is both an ethical and legal issue because there may be personal client information contained within the records. Personal information can include payment details and contact information as well as client health information, medical conditions, and treatment notes. Ensuring a client's private information is protected at all times is an important part of your role as a massage therapist, and this applies to electronic, digital, and paper versions as well as any verbal communication.

HIPAA

In 2003, the U.S. Department of Health and Human Services issued regulations under the Health Insurance Portability and Accountability Act of 1996 (HIPAA). HIPAA protects an individual's right to privacy in matters involving their health care. This act helps ensure the protection and security of medical records and other personal health information by creating extensive health information privacy rules. In addition to HIPAA, there state privacy laws and regulations that may apply to personal health information that should also be reviewed in regard to appropriate documentation and sharing of health information.

The U.S. Department of Health and Human Services provides a helpful online summary of the HIPAA Privacy Rule and the Security Rule, including requirements for protecting information: http://www.hhs.gov/ocr/privacy/hipaa/understanding/summary/index.html and http://www.hhs.gov/ocr/privacy/hipaa/understanding/srsummary.html.

From High Maintenance to VIP

A massage therapy practice had an internal system that noted when a repeat client had high expectations, made many demands, and was generally difficult to please. The owners felt it was important that therapists knew this about the client beforehand so that they could be prepared and better cater to their needs, just by knowing a little about them upfront. For repeat clients who fell into this category, staff was instructed to type "high maintenance" in their private electronic file because only staff working with that client would have access to the information. The system worked well until one day a therapist printed out the client's electronic chart and it contained the phrase "high maintenance." The client saw it and was furious. She never returned. The owners were very upset that the therapist allowed this to happen, but still believed it was good business to notify employees of high-maintenance clients. So, the owners decided to change their coding system and instead of noting "high maintenance" on these clients' file, they began noting them as "VIPs." Client information was still carefully protected, but in the unfortunate event that clients did see their file, all they would see was how special they were to the business.

If private information is not protected, such as health information, you could be held legally responsible. Here are some basic things to keep in mind:

- Keep private paper documents in a secure location that can be accessed only by authorized individuals.
- Keep electronic data secure using passwords, encryptions, and other protective means. Also, if data are stored on an external hard drive, laptop, jump drive, or other easily transported device, make sure this hardware is also well protected and use every effort to ensure it is not stolen or lost.
- Private records that are no longer needed should be properly destroyed using a shredder or professional service.
- Do not discuss a client's private information with other employees or clients.
- If there is anything that would financially affect a client, such as banking or credit card information, ensure it is protected. There are federal laws in place to protect consumers against negligence and misuse of their financial information.
- If there is anything that could emotionally damage a client, such as notes or information on the client's treatment or emotional condition, ensure it is kept private.

See Worksheet 3-5
- Clients are not the only individuals entitled to protection of their private information. This protection also applies to employees.

Getting Your Records Started

Using the earlier activities and topics covered, pull together information you've already researched and conduct additional research to begin organizing your reference material. Organize your information into folders, where you can easily access and add to it. This will be a treasure trove of valuable information as you continue along your career path. Files that will be helpful include:

- Associations
- Educational opportunities/sources
- Financial records
  - Revenue
  - Expenses
  - Credit cards
- Insurance
- Legal issues/case studies
- National exams
- Publications/websites
- Record-keeping tips/tools for professionals
- Safety tips
- State/local licensure requirements
- Tax returns

CHAPTER SUMMARY

While still fragmented, industry regulations are beginning to have more consistency and uniformity than ever before. In addition, there are many more resources and communication vehicles available to navigate the diverse requirements, which makes entering the profession much easier than in recent history. With these changes and additional resources, the massage industry continues to professionalize and increase opportunities for both massage therapists and the clients they serve.

As a new massage therapist, keeping up with licensure requirements will be an important responsibility, and one that you will likely have to continue throughout your career. As state regulations change and evolve, you'll need to keep up with these changes.

A professional career begins with education, and education should continue throughout your career. Lifelong learning is a key to success for most professionals, and particularly for massage therapists, to ensure safe and effective professional services. A dedication to continual learning will also help keep you prepared and knowledgeable about the risks associated with practicing massage. There are risk-management tools you can use, such as appropriate insurance and proper record-keeping, as well as some common-sense safety protocols, which will also be helpful in safeguarding yourself and your practice.

An easy way to keep up with all of the things you need to know as a professional is through education, networking, and membership in professional organizations. Because of the private and personal nature of the profession, therapists tend to become removed from social interactions, especially in group settings. Try to avoid this pitfall by talking with your peers and other health and wellness professionals in your community, in addition to networking in a variety of settings. It is a fantastic way to market your business and services at a grassroots level, and it also helps you stay informed of all those things you need to know.

BIBLIOGRAPHY

1. Alaska Department of Labor and Workforce Development. (2010, Feb.) Licensed Occupations: Massage Practitioner. Retrieved May 8, 2010, from http://www.labor.state.ak.us/research/dlo/fmassage.htm.
2. State of Utah Department of Commerce, Division of Occupational and Professional Licensing. (n.d.) Utah Board Opinion on Reiki. Retrieved May 5, 2010, from http://www.dopl.utah.gov/licensing/massage_therapy.html.
3. American Massage Therapy Association. (n.d.) Safety and Security—Risk Management. Retrieved February 12, 2011, from http://www.amtamassage.org/career_guidance/detail/162.

REVIEW QUESTIONS

1. **Licensure requirements:**
   a. Are the same in all states
   b. Are the same as a national certification
   c. Vary depending on where a therapist plans to practice
   d. Vary by state, unless a therapist has a national license

2. **Even if a state doesn't have a licensure requirement for massage therapists, the town, city, or county may have licensure requirements.**
   a. True
   b. False

3. **Why is licensure required by some states?**
   a. To regulate the profession
   b. To promote safe businesses
   c. To promote safe massage practices
   d. All of the above

4. Licenses are usually valid for:
    a. A limited amount of time
    b. The life of the therapist
    c. An indefinite amount of time
    d. 15 to 20 years

5. National certifications and exams:
    a. Are recognized by a minority of states
    b. Are recognized by a majority of states
    c. Are recognized by all states
    d. Are recognized by no states, only local cities or counties

6. There is a national license that allows a therapist to legally practice in all 50 states.
    a. True
    b. False

7. Most states require license applicants to have a minimum of how many education hours?
    a. 100
    b. 250
    c. 500
    d. Most states don't require education hours for licensure

8. Which of the following is *not* typically required for state licensure:
    a. Minimum amount of education hours
    b. Graduation from an approved school
    c. Successfully passing a designated exam
    d. Professional or trade association membership

9. Before practicing massage, you should ensure you meet which of the following requirements:
    a. State requirements
    b. City/county requirements
    c. Exam requirements
    d. All of the above

10. Continuing education is:
    a. Often required by states to renew a professional license
    b. Only required for an instructor's license
    c. A responsibility massage therapists have to their clients and themselves
    d. Both a & c

11. Which of the following do successful massage therapists include in their continuing education?
    a. Risk Management, Sanitation, and Safety Procedures
    b. Trends, Technology, and Legislation
    c. Massage Benefits and Contraindications
    d. All of the above

12. **Which of the following keeps massage therapists informed about everything from industry regulations to labor market changes?**
    a. National and state certifications
    b. National and state associations
    c. State credentialing boards
    d. Clients

13. **Which of the following is a common type of massage insurance?**
    a. Liability insurance
    b. Auto/property insurance
    c. Identity theft insurance
    d. Both a & c

14. **Which of the following is a key legal concern within the massage profession?**
    a. Product recalls
    b. Personal safety and health
    c. Client safety and privacy
    d. Certifications

15. **When it comes to personal safety, listen to your _____ and _____.**
    a. Body; intuition
    b. Feet; hands
    c. Manager; colleagues
    d. None of the above

16. **Why is it important to perform massage according to appropriate protocols?**
    a. For your personal safety
    b. For client safety
    c. To help avoid legal issues
    d. All of the above

17. **In record-keeping, you must maintain reliable records and:**
    a. Ensure data are documented, saved, and accessible for as long as they have value
    b. Keep your sanity by hiring someone to help you when needed
    c. Publish them regularly
    d. Purge them monthly

18. **Which of the following is *not* a basic way to protect private information?**
    a. Do not discuss a client's private information with other employees or clients
    b. Recycle private records
    c. Keep electronic data secure using passwords and other protective means
    d. Keep client financial information in a secure location

Worksheet 3–1   Preparing for the National Exams

Before taking the national massage therapy exams, research the content and details for the two major exams so that you can be fully prepared for these important tests. Research length, format, content, locations, time limits, and application requirements to ensure you are prepared. Also document handbooks, study guides, or practice tests are available and their costs.

NATIONAL CERTIFICATION EXAMINATION FOR THERAPEUTIC MASSAGE AND BODYWORK (NCETMB)

Length:

Format:

Specific content and weighting:

Locations exam given:

Dates exam given:

Time limits:

Application requirements:

Cost:

Key states exam is accepted:

Handbooks/study guides/practice exams:

MASSAGE AND BODYWORK LICENSING EXAMINATION (MBLEx)

Length:

Format:

Specific content and weighting:

Locations exam given:

Dates exam given:

Time limits:

Application requirements:

Cost:

Key states exam is accepted:

Handbooks/study guides/practice exams:

Worksheet 3-2   Put It in the File

Research at least three different state licensure requirements, including those states in which you intend, or hope, to work. Complete the following information for each state and start your file for state licensure requirements:

State:

State board contact information:

Required number of education hours:

Education/school requirements (e.g., number of specific content hours, instruction requirements):

Examination requirements:

Other requirements:

Renewal requirements:

Licensure and renewal fees:

Insurance requirements:

Note: If a desired state is unregulated, look for local requirements in the major cities.

Worksheet 3-3 The Pros and Cons of Accepting Health
Insurance

Contact a massage therapist who accepts insurance and one who does not. Use the following questions to interview them and record the pros and cons of accepting health insurance.

THERAPISTS WHO ACCEPT INSURANCE

- Please describe how health insurance billing is handled.

- What are the benefits of accepting health insurance?

- What are the drawbacks of accepting health insurance?

- What advice would you give someone considering accepting health insurance at their practice?

THERAPISTS WHO DO NOT ACCEPT INSURANCE

- Why have you chosen not to accept health insurance?

- Have you ever accepted health insurance? If yes, what was that experience like?

- What are the benefits of not accepting insurance?

- What are the drawbacks of not accepting insurance?

- What advice would you give someone considering accepting health insurance at their practice?

Worksheet 3–4   Safety Worksheet

Develop a list of tips on staying healthy and safe. Gather information by talking with other massage therapists and instructors, reading publications, or doing Internet research.

1.

2.

3.

4.

5.

6.

7.

8.

9.

10.

Worksheet 3-5   Managing Client Records

Imagine the following scenario and write your response in the space provided.

Cindy had done a great job in filling her practice. She is so busy; in fact, she rarely dedicates time to filing and keeping her client's credit card information secure and stored in a safe place. Her home office was broken into one day while she was out running errands. When she returned, she was faced with the fact that a pile of credit card forms was taken from her office area.

She was devastated when she realized she could not be sure whose information had been taken, what the legal ramifications were, and how to go about warning her clients of the risk.

Draft your thoughts on how you will manage client records and avoid Cindy's (and now her clients') problem.

Chapter 4

Navigating the Ethics of Business

"Ethics is firmly based in the understanding that one's own happiness can never be had at the expense of someone else's."

–His Holiness the Dalai Lama

Outline

You will learn to...

- Understand the function of your moral compass
- Define and communicate boundaries
- Understand the three categories of business ethics
- Maintain the integrity of your practice

Key Definitions

This chapter references several key terms, which are indicated in bold. For easy reference, these terms are briefly defined here:

Brand: A person or company's identity, which implies a promise of what the client can expect when doing business with that particular company.

Boundary: Clearly established rule or guideline that can either be kept or broken, which is usually established to protect something.

Diffused boundary: A boundary that is unclear, undefined, or an established boundary that is not enforced.

Ethics: A set of moral principles that allows an individual or company to distinguish right from wrong.

External perceptions: The beliefs held by others about your business, which are based on how your business interacts with them.

Foundational ethics: Primary, internal values and beliefs that govern the creation and maintenance of a business.

Policy: Written statements that outline corporate and management intentions associated with various internal and external operations.

Rigid boundary: A sharply defined, objective boundary with distinct parameters.

Semi-permeable boundary: A boundary that factors in circumstances before making a decision. This type of boundary functions as a flexible guideline that can change based on circumstances.

Social media: Online technology tools that allow people and businesses to easily communicate and share information and resources. The trademark of social media sites is the ability for users to actively interact.

Unconscious representation: Nonverbal communication and behavior of which you are likely unaware.

Values: The timeless principles or ideals that define who you are and your actions.

INTRODUCTION TO ETHICS

Ethics is broadly defined as a set of moral principles that allows you to distinguish right from wrong. Your actions are considered ethical when they conform to a prescribed set of **values** and unethical when you do not adhere to those values. Because you are not born with a guidebook clearly defining what is right and wrong, you learn to base your decisions on internal and external guidance. When you are an infant, your parents' voices help you begin the process of cementing what will become your own, unique set of principles. Outside people and events are external influencers of your behavior, but you also have a finely tuned internal guide that can awaken to offer you assistance through life's dilemmas.

Your Moral Compass

The internal voice of conscience is like your moral compass. When you are faced with situations that cause you to assess what is right or wrong, your compass awakens and helps guide your analytical process. You weigh and examine the issues and then make the decision you believe is right; or, you ignore the results of your analysis and still decide to act amorally. Although you may strive for moral behavior, the appropriate action is not always clear. Your behaviors are continually being shaped by inner guidance, external circumstances, and the results of your actions (Fig. 4–1).

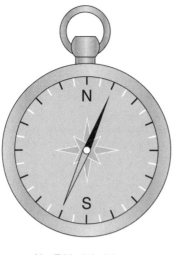

Figure 4–1 When faced with challenging or uncertain situations, your moral compass helps guide your analytical process.

N = Ethical decision

S = Unethical decision

For example, your moral compass may activate in the following scenario. You are unpacking your groceries from the shopping cart and realize there are some items on the bottom rack that you inadvertently did not pay for. The second you notice these items, there is a good chance that your moral compass will activate as you take a moment to weigh your next action. Do you take the items back and pay for them, or do you toss them in your trunk, reasoning that the store has likely over-charged you many times? For some, the answer may come effortlessly. For others, an internal dialogue may rage as they waver back and forth about what should be done. This example is more easily defined and solved than many others you will face in your lifetime and career as a massage therapist. Technically, you would be stealing if you threw the items in your trunk. The law is clear on that. However, people can be skillful at rationalizing when they want to.

You may have found that the more you must think about a decision, the closer you edge toward an action out of alignment with your moral compass. This may be especially true if you feel the need to engage in self-talk, justifying the action you are about to take.

Some believe people are born with a defined sense of what is right and wrong. For most, this innate sense of right and wrong is further developed by what is reinforced externally. As a young child, if you become frustrated with a playmate, your first instinct may be to bite. You may continue to think this behavior is fine until your perception is changed by external reactions. If the bitten child screams and breaks into tears, you may realize quickly that your action resulted in pain to some-one else. Your moral compass adjusts as you recognize there will be a negative reaction to this behavior. This initial impression of wrongness may be further reinforced when an adult explains to you that hurting someone else is not the best way to handle anger, and offers other solutions for you to con-sider. Later, if you have the urge to respond in a similar fashion, you may remember the experience and respond differently, or you may not. Regardless of your decision, you have a more defined sense of whether that behavior is right or wrong for you. As of today, a lifetime of situations have entrenched within you a moral framework from which you make decisions. You are constantly referencing this framework for guidance to help you navigate the daily ethical situations that arise.

In a profession such as massage therapy, ethical situations surface often. The ethical boundaries existing between practitioner and client are often uncertain. Most people do not have careers that require their clients to disrobe and lay face down, mostly naked and vulnerable, to be touched. While acceptable and professional for our field, this creates the potential for many misperceptions and unclear ethical boundaries. Just as ethical situations will arise from this aspect of your career, working in massage therapy will also bring up business ethical situations. This chapter focuses only on the ethical situations arising from business scenarios.

Code of Ethics

Most professional organizations have a code of ethics that includes guidelines meant to define acceptable behaviors for members of the group, association, or profession. Besides establishing ethical parameters, this code can encourage trust that the organization is committed to the highest standard of behavior. You can easily reference the codes of ethics already established by organizations within the massage industry by visiting their websites (Box 4.1).

The Ethics of Business

> "The purpose of ethics in business is to direct business men and women to abide by a code of conduct that facilitates, if not encourages, public confidence in their products and services."
> —From an article written by Dr. Katherine T. Smith and Dr. L. Murphy Smith, CPA.

> Your ethical decisions reflect who you are and what you and your business practice stand for.

> "The reputation of a thousand years may be determined by the conduct of one hour."
> —Japanese Proverb

See Worksheet 4-1

Your ethical decisions reflect who you are and what you and your business practice stand for. When it comes to business ethics and morals, everything is important, including the day-to-day, smaller things (Box 4.2).

Some are quick to assume that the success of a business is measured by its financial gain. Profitability is often a result of good business practices, but not always. Many profitable companies have fallen when ethical scandals surface about illegal information trades, overstating assets, or not reporting income. Who can forget the news stories about companies using their bailout tax dollars to pay huge bonuses to top executives, or the photos that emerged after the oil leak in the Gulf? In the aftermath, the public does not care whether the incident was purposeful or accidental. Never underestimate the importance of careful analysis as you create the structural values of your business or personal practice.

Financial success is much more rewarding when it springs from a business with integrity and values. When your daily work is aligned with your moral fiber, you experience peace of mind, noticed by your patrons and employees.

A nice summary of ethics can be found in the book, *Ethical Issues in the Practice of Accounting*. Michael Josephson defines the "Ten Universal Values" of business ethics as honesty, integrity, promise-keeping, fidelity, fairness, caring, respect for others, responsible citizenship, pursuit of excellence, and accountability.

BOUNDARIES

A **boundary** is a clearly established rule that can either be kept or broken. A boundary is usually put into place to protect something. People spend their lives defining and enforcing boundaries. A literal-world example is a fence around a chicken coop to keep the chickens in and other animals out. In the figurative world, a boundary is an invisible line drawn to protect oneself. A personal boundary may be that you will not borrow my jewelry without asking permission; a business boundary may be that if you are 10 minutes late for your session, you will forfeit 10 minutes of bodywork so as to not make others late for their sessions. For now, our primary focus is the importance of establishing and enforcing boundaries to keep the business side of your practice within the ethical framework you define (Fig. 4–2).

Others can be taught to honor the boundaries you establish. Their behavior is usually a response to whether you enforce the lines you have drawn or allow others to cross them.

Types of Boundaries

Boundaries fall into three areas: diffused, semi-permeable, and rigid.

Diffused Boundary

A **diffused boundary** is unclear or still undefined. Often, you learn of the need for a boundary through experience. An example may occur when you have a person in their late 80s come in for

Box 4.1 Code of Ethics Examples

The following are examples of the code of ethics established by two professional organizations within the massage industry.

The **American Massage Therapy Association Code of Ethics** is a summary statement of the standards by which massage therapists agree to conduct their practices and is a declaration of the general principles of acceptable, ethical, professional behavior.

Massage therapists shall:

1. Demonstrate commitment to provide the highest-quality massage therapy/bodywork to those who seek their professional service.
2. Acknowledge the inherent worth and individuality of each person by not discriminating or behaving in any prejudicial manner with clients and/or colleagues.
3. Demonstrate professional excellence through regular self-assessment of strengths, limitations, and effectiveness by continued education and training.
4. Acknowledge the confidential nature of the professional relationship with clients and respect each client's right to privacy.
5. Conduct all business and professional activities within their scope of practice, the law of the land, and project a professional image.
6. Refrain from engaging in any sexual conduct or sexual activities involving their clients.
7. Accept responsibility to do no harm to the physical, mental, and emotional well-being of self, clients, and associates.

The following has been taken from the code of ethics established by the **Associated Body Work and Massage Professionals** for image and advertising.

- I shall strive to project a professional image for myself, my business or place of employment, and the profession in general.
- I shall actively participate in educating the public regarding the actual benefits of massage, bodywork, somatic therapies, and skin care.
- I shall practice honesty in advertising, promote my services ethically and in good taste, and practice and/or advertise only those techniques for which I have received adequate training and/or certification. I shall not make false claims regarding the potential benefits of the techniques rendered.

Box 4.2 Examples of Ethical Business Situations

To start your thinking in the right direction, below are some examples of ethical business situations:

- Exaggerating your skill set to book an appointment
- The way you talk about other massage therapists
- Tone and type of e-mails you write and forward to others
- How you handle client complaints
- Privately working with clients who are also your clients at your place of employment
- What you put on your billing sheets, time sheets, and expense reports
- Office supplies you consider taking home
- Allowing sessions to run long, disrupting your schedule
- "Unimportant" work policies you think are fine to break
- Avoiding conversations with clients who owe you money
- Credit you appropriately share (or don't share) with others
- Not delivering on what your marketing message offers
- Allowing some clients to break your policies, but not others

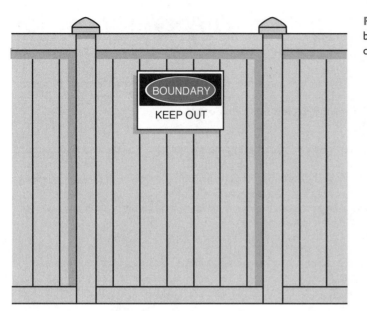

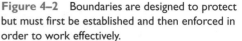

Figure 4–2   Boundaries are designed to protect but must first be established and then enforced in order to work effectively.

massage work. Throughout the session, you notice that you feel uncomfortable working with the person because you fear hurting him. You may decide to not work on older clients in the future, or you may decide to take classes to build your confidence with this population. A previously diffused or unclear boundary is now more defined for you.

A diffused boundary can also be the inability to enforce established rules. Some people have a hard time speaking up for themselves, or confronting others who attempt to cross a line. So, although the boundary may be clearly drawn, it becomes diffused and leaky when it is not enforced.

Semi-Permeable Boundary

A **semi-permeable boundary** considers the circumstances before making a decision. Let us say you have a clear **policy** that payments for service are due immediately at the end of each session. You have a client who has been seeing you for several years and has never missed a payment. For the first time, she walks out without paying you. Because of your long-term relationship, you may postpone addressing this until she arrives for her next appointment. For a first-time client, you may use a different approach, such as quickly trying to collect payment or simply not rescheduling her. This type of boundary can function as a guideline that is usually intact but can change based on circumstance.

Starbucks is a great example of a company that encourages the use of semi-permeable boundaries. Their strongly infused company culture allows employees some latitude and creativity in correcting service problems and dealing with unsatisfied customers. Employees are authorized to give immediate discounts, free drinks, and other small items to rectify service problems. A more rigid boundary comes into play if their semi-permeable boundaries cannot satisfy the customer. In these situations, a manager becomes involved. The employees' freedom to work within a loose framework of rules is beneficial because it keeps the service flowing and eliminates the need to halt the service process to call management for minor mishaps. This smart move clearly indicates that Starbucks trusts its employees to make the best decisions for the well-being of the customer and the company.

Rigid Boundary

A **rigid boundary** is sharply defined, and there is no subjective analysis. It is a clearly defined edge that others are not allowed to cross. If this boundary is crossed, analysis is usually not required to make a decision. When broken, rigid boundaries often cause the most havoc.

Most written company policies are rigid in nature. A massage clinic may have very strict draping guidelines that result in immediate termination if broken. Not enforcing such boundaries can result in severe repercussions such as lawsuits. Other, less obvious examples are a massage clinic's posted hours. If posted hours are from 9:00 a.m. until 5:00 p.m. and appointments are scheduled accordingly, then any delays or extensions are crossing a clearly communicated boundary. The repercussions that result from crossing these boundaries, although not legal in nature, can still negatively affect the business. The clients are affected if the clinic opens late, causing their sessions to start late. The employees can be affected if the clinic closes late, especially if a front-desk person must wait for the final session to conclude before locking up and departing. What is supposed to be a rigid boundary becomes diffused if not enforced properly. If it happens regularly, either situation can negatively affect the clinic's finances and reputation.

Within every business, there is a mixture of boundaries. Some will become flexible; others will stay firm. As lines are crossed, you will learn which boundaries have room to flex and which ones cannot change (Fig. 4–3).

For massage professionals, establishing and reinforcing boundaries can be a challenge, especially when you are in business for yourself. When you work so closely with your clients, it can be difficult to navigate all the feelings that arise when enforcing rules. Until a specific situation crosses a line, you may not even realize a boundary is needed.

Gina's story in Peer Profile 4-1 demonstrates how an expected, rigid boundary is allowed to become diffused by management's lack of enforcement, leading to a decision that may backfire if an employee decides to file sexual harassment charges.

As you encounter situations that require you to set or reset boundaries, you will fine-tune the process that works best for you. The clearer the rules you expect yourself and others to follow, the more you can prevent future problems (Box 4.3).

DEVELOPING AND MANAGING PERCEPTIONS OF ETHICS

Ethics is a broad topic that influences all aspects of your life. Professional ethics require building and continually managing ethical business structures and processes. Establishing and maintaining this core foundation requires focus in key areas:

1. Developing **foundational ethics.** Foundational ethics are the primary internal values and beliefs that govern the creation and maintenance of the business. Developing and identifying these values and beliefs is the first area of focus because they become the foundation from which a business will grow.

Types of Boundaries

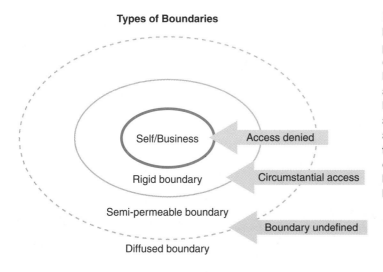

Figure 4–3   This illustration demonstrates the boundaries you establish around yourself and your practice. The farther the boundary is from the core (self), the more permeable the boundary becomes. The clearer you are about how a boundary affects yourself and others, the more rigid it becomes. Rigid boundaries are black and white, and if crossed, they require immediate protective action. The outer layers, semi-permeable and diffused boundaries, allow circumstantial access and, often as a result of actions awakening these boundaries, aid in the creation of more rigid boundaries.

Peer Profile 4–1

Real-Life Scenario

Gina, LMT
West Virginia

I live in a fairly small town, so massage jobs are hard to come by. I began working for a well-established country club that offered massage to its members. Most of the members were affluent and had well-established cliques within the community. A certain older gentleman continually broke the policies established by the country club. He would ask for what I felt was inappropriate touch and he would make comments that were mildly sexual in nature. It wasn't completely off the charts, but I didn't feel comfortable with him. This was happening to several of the therapists on staff. When we reported this to the club management, they just laughed it off and said that not only was he harmless, but also he was a long-time member of the club. I continued to work there, but I never feel safe when I know he is on my calendar. He continues to do as he pleases even to this day.

Box 4.3 Model for Communicating Boundaries

You can follow steps that make it easier to communicate boundaries. These are useful immediately after there has been an infraction.

The moment you realize a boundary is being crossed, do the following;

1. **Stop and become present.** Take a few moments before you react. Become aware of all the circumstances involved in the immediate situation. Notice whether you are getting upset or are calm enough to handle the situation in the moment. Try to find neutral ground mentally to assess the broken boundary.
2. **State the obvious.** Bring attention to the situation in a way that is nonjudgmental. This will diffuse potential conflict. An example of this may be, "I have noticed you have arrived late for our last two appointments."
3. **Gather more information.** Before determining action, sometimes it is important to allow the other person to give his side of the story. Often, there is confusion about the existence of a boundary. If it is a repeat situation or involves a rigid boundary, such as a sexual one, you can skip this step and go right to number five. You can say something like this: "I have noticed you have arrived late for our last two appointments. Is everything fine with this appointment time?"
4. **State the defined rule.** After hearing all the facts, you must restate the rule. You have either allowed it to change based on the information you gathered, or you have kept the original boundary intact. Regardless, in most situations, it helps to remind others of the rule. You can say something like this: "I know traffic is really tough at this time, and we can make your appointment at a different time if you like. It is important that my clients arrive on time so that I can provide them the full service promised. I cannot allow my next client's session to start late, so I will provide you only with the remaining time based on your arrival."
5. **Decide next steps.** The final step is to determine your next move. Either the situation will work itself out and you will continue on, or you will decide not to interact with this person any further. In some coworker situations, you may have to modify your behavior in order to interact peacefully with someone you have to see regularly. In the example of the tardy client, if he continues to be late, you must either accept the shorter massage time or possibly ask him not to return.

2. Guiding **external perceptions.** Guided by the foundational ethics, external perceptions are the beliefs that others hold about your business because of how your business interacts with them. There are ways to develop an ethical structure that helps guide, and even control, external perceptions of your business to ensure they are in harmony with your values and beliefs.

Once key ethical structures are developed, they require constant navigation to ensure the continued integrity of the ethical structure.

Foundational Ethics

The first category, foundational ethics, contains the beliefs and values that you bring to your business and that guide the internal design of your practice. From these, you will build the foundation of the business you plan to operate. You will integrate your own values to build a business that matches who you are. Regardless of whether you plan to be in practice by yourself or to someday own a large massage clinic, the foundational ethics established now will become the fundamental core and personality of your business. If you plan to work for someone else, it is beneficial to find an organization that has values similar to your own.

Many companies lay their foundation on the early ethical guidance of its founder. For example, each of the following companies has a unique core personality mostly resulting from the ethics and morals established by its founder. Herb Kelleher, the founder of the fun and interactive Southwest Airlines, allowed many of his personality traits to shine through during the early development of the successful company. He established an employee-centric culture that, like himself, moves fast, finds humor in all situations, celebrates at every opportunity, and is responsive to feedback. He built his company with a strong focus on empowering and rewarding employees. He often stated frankly that his employees came before customers. He believed that if he built a company focused on employees, they in turn would deliver success by exceeding customer expectations. To reinforce the values he put in place, he exemplified fun, arriving to work on his motorcycle and donning funny costumes for press interviews. Although he is no longer at the helm, his sense of playfulness is still a fundamental aspect of the airline's culture. History shows that these values have led to one of the most successful airlines in existence.

Another company that took on the ethical traits of its founder is Chick-fil-A, the restaurant known for its black-and-white bovines encouraging us to "EAT MOR CHIKIN." S. Truett Cathy, a devout Southern Baptist, made many business decisions founded in his religious beliefs. One of his most notable choices was closing the restaurants on Sundays to honor his religion. This was a bold move when you consider that Sunday is a very profitable day for restaurants, especially those primarily located in shopping malls. The people-oriented company invests heavily in community services and scholarships that support Cathy's foundational values. Building a company strong in values has proved very profitable for Chick-fil-A as well. As long and hard as Chick-fil-A worked to promote a positive brand and image, a few comments made by its founder caused great damage in 2012. This is another example of how one unethical misstep can derail all your good intentions and years of hard work.

These two examples demonstrate how the early moral decisions made by decision makers can affect how the business operates and how it is perceived by others. So, too, will your decisions define the core of your business and determine the course of your career.

Your ethical structure cannot be communicated during a quick introduction to someone. You must establish processes and policies that uphold and build your ethical foundation. Building a solid, ethical foundation takes time and requires thought, documentation, and constant management. Others will learn about your ethics through word of mouth, through impressions, or because of their history with you.

Your internal structure is the foundation on which all aspects of your future business will rest. It can be solidly built with integrity and values that weather the storms, or it can be hurriedly built and weak, developing cracks that create a precarious perch when the winds of challenge come to visit. When you look at it this way, it is unlikely you would dream of using poor-quality material for a structure you expect to keep you safe for a long time—potentially your whole career. Your chosen career as a massage therapist will bring you challenges. You can never predict all the situations that may arise, but you can begin by having a well-run, well-thought-out practice.

Even if you never plan to own and operate a large company, the energy you put into thoughtfully building your practice is well worth the effort. The rules and policies you draft for yourself in the beginning are the basis for many future decisions. As we move through this chapter, you will be provided scenarios pertaining to business ethics. You will be asked to write down your thoughts as they relate to the chosen topic. When you are ready to build your client and employee policy forms, you can reference your work in this book, which will greatly assist with the finalization of your forms.

Creating Internal Policies

Keeping in mind your personal belief systems, you will establish rules that govern how you run your practice. Or, as an employee, you will be expected to behave in accordance with the policies set in place by your employer. As you build your policies, some will be drawn from your vision and values, creating a personality for your business. Others are required by law, providing safety and protection for yourself and others. Even if you plan to employ just yourself, it is a good idea to draft the conduct rules to which you plan to adhere. These can be a good reminder about what is important to you. If you hire employees later, you will have these beliefs in writing, and you can model the behavior you expect (Box 4.4).

See Worksheet 4-2

Not included in the checklist, but well worth thinking through, are the values you plan to integrate into your culture, such as team building, "me" time, fun, and creativity. What kind of personality do you want your practice to have? Figure this out, and then build in aspects that support your vision.

Maintaining the Integrity of Internal Communication

All of your communications should reflect and support your values and policies. Avenues of internal communication can include memos, meetings, employee newsletters, e-mail, and bulletin board materials. Internal communication is no less important than external messages in determining how

---

Box 4.4 Checklist for Creating Policies for Your Practice

The following is a checklist for you to reference as you begin creating policies for your practice. These primarily are aimed at governing you and your employees.

- Personnel record storage
- Disability accommodation
- Equal employment
- Sexual harassment
- Drug and alcohol use
- Gift and tip policies
- Personal use of business space and items
- Parking and exterior building rules
- Breaks and smoking
- Payroll details
- Timeliness
- Closing process
- Phone use
- Emergency plan
- Community involvement
- Donations
- Dress code

> Internal communication is no less important than external messages in determining how your business is perceived by others.

your business is perceived by others. Remember to communicate with your employees in the same professional manner you use for your most important guests. Before distributing any internal communication, reread it to ensure it represents the values established for your practice or by your employer.

A good rule of thumb is to assume that all internal communication will be viewed by the press. If you would not want the local television station to report the information you are ready to disseminate internally, then do not put it in writing. Sensitive internal forms and e-mails have the potential to be quite inflammatory. Setting up a separate e-mail account for your business ensures the separation of business from personal communication, thus avoiding accidental forwards and replies. A solid, ethical communication process will ensure that the internal integrity of the business stays solid.

Maintaining the Integrity of Work Space

Maintaining the integrity of your work space is important, especially it if is shared with others. Often at work, the area where you or your employees spend time is out of the clients' sight. Even so, before you post anything within a business, ask yourself if you would feel comfortable with clients seeing these items. Remove any inappropriate materials that other viewers may find disturbing. It is fine to allow your personality to shine in your personal area, but never post anything that may offend others.

> See Worksheet 4-3

External Perceptions

The next area of ethics includes externally disseminated information, which affects how your business is represented to others, and the ensuing public perception. When you and your business distribute information, the resulting impression can have a lasting effect on your career success, which is something you should strongly protect. It only takes a couple of missteps to damage your reputation, possibly permanently. Always put yourself in the place of the perceiver when preparing to communicate or represent yourself publicly. It is harder to correct poor perception than to prevent it from the start.

As an extreme example, if Bill Clinton's name is brought up during a discussion of great presidents, often people think first of the poor ethical decisions he made with a certain intern. Regardless of how many great things he accomplished during his presidency, such as balancing the budget and creating 6 million jobs within the first 2 years of his term, he will forever be linked to his poor ethical decision-making. In the massage industry, you do not have to look hard to find cases when massage therapists made poor decisions and found themselves in personal or legal trouble. Unfortunately, when a therapist crosses these boundaries, it can have a negative impact on the entire industry. Visit any Internet search engine and type in "massage arrest." You will find numerous stories about your peers making poor decisions. Sometimes these are technically not your peers, meaning licensed professionals, but people using false advertising or posing as massage therapists. Unfortunately, media scandals involving those claiming to be massage therapists taint the entire industry.

Another caution to remember is that the public still perceives a close association between massage therapy and the sex industry. For an uneducated portion of the public, just knowing you are a massage therapist can evoke various internal beliefs and perceptions. You have no control over their thoughts, so it is even more important that everything you do to promote yourself and your business clearly delineates you from sketchier areas sometimes associated with massage. This will help prevent some of the ethical situations you can find yourself in, outside of business ethics.

It is your responsibility to manage to the best of your ability how others perceive your business or the business you work for. You can accomplish this with some simple attention to detail. We will walk through areas that can be managed to ensure you maintain a stellar and professional reputation.

Professional Organizations

Most industries have organizations that help to convey the professionalism of their business. Generally, for a nominal fee, they offer you the ability to make new connections, access educational resources, and stay current with industry news and events. This alone can be well worth the cost of membership. On another note, being a member of a professional group states to the public that you take your profession seriously and are willing to invest in this commitment. Once you become a member, you are usually provided with logos to display in windows, on advertisements, and your printed forms.

Some associations can be joined only after you've completed a certain level of education and testing. National certification, for example, can be acquired only through completing a certain number of hours of primary and continuing education, and then passing a national exam. These certifications can also go a long way in ensuring that the public views your business favorably.

Marketing and Advertising

The most obvious representations of you and your business are the materials that promote and advertise your services. These can be advertisements, brochures, signage, business cards, stationary, and your website. From an ethical standpoint, all materials referring to your business should be completely honest and professional in nature and should represent your skill set accurately. Ideally, they all have a similar look and a consistent message. These materials, followed by the experience your client has with you, begin the process of creating your **brand**. Your brand is the promise of what the client can expect when doing business with you. A brand takes time to develop and should be managed carefully.

All marketing materials should be reviewed for clarity as well. Never put into print anything that is not completely true. If you do not plan to refund all of a client's sessions, do not state that satisfaction is guaranteed. If you are willing to give refunds, then definitely say it. If you have only taken a 1-day class in hot stone massage, do not advertise that you are certified or an expert in this modality. However, if you do hold certifications or advanced training, by all means communicate these skills. Verify that any promotional materials accurately reflect the reality of the experience you can deliver.

Printed Forms

The printed forms you hand to a client are another, often overlooked avenue of external perception. Take the extra time to make them professional in appearance and content. Go out of your way to use this avenue as a way to reinforce the ethical structure of your practice. Consider addressing draping, tipping, and anything else that may lead to confusion if not addressed. Any item you hand to a client, such as intake and policy forms, will influence the client's perception of who you are and the ethics that govern your practice. Just as you review your marketing materials with an eye for how you are representing yourself, you should review your client forms in the same way. Avoid producing forms that are copied crookedly or contain typos. Take the time to create professional forms that communicate your policies, values, and basic business information. Remember, too, that these items once completed by the client are confidential and should be maintained following the policies of client record-keeping (Fig. 4–4).

Waiting and Treatment Rooms

Your waiting and treatment areas are observed by your clients on a regular basis. It is important to keep them neat, tidy, and free of any offensive materials. If you have a front-desk area, ensure that conversation is kept purely professional. Discourage employees from hanging out in these areas because personal conversations can be disruptive to waiting guests. You can purposefully use these areas in subtle ways to encourage positive thoughts about your values and services. You can post certifications, your code of ethics, and any items that may improve their confidence in your work. Remove anything that may erode this positive perception.

| See Worksheet 4-4 |

Pricing and Fees

When it comes to the hard-earned dollar, people become very sensitive about the perceived value and the amount they actually end up paying. Be very clear when communicating fees. Discounting your services can confuse and anger clients if it is not handled how they expected. Make sure offers

My Massage Business

All information shared will remain confidential

Name_____ Date of Birth_____ Referred by_____

Phone _____ (c) _____ (h) E-mail _____

Address _____

What brings you here today and what results would you like from your session?

How do you relax?

Please circle below to indicate any parts of your body that you **do NOT** want your therapist to work with:
Scalp   Face   Neck   Shoulders   Arms   Hands   Abdomen   Upper Torso   Back   Buttocks   Legs   Feet

Medical History
Are you under the care of a medical professional or other heath-care provider?   YES   NO
If yes, for what?

Have you had any accidents or injuries, been hospitalized or had surgeries?   YES   NO
If yes, please list:

What medications have you taken in the past 6 months?

Have you had professional massage therapy before?   YES   NO

List and describe any chronic bodily discomfort:

Do you have or have you ever had any of the following conditions/illnesses/problems?

☐ Arthritis	☐ Elimination problems	☐ Muscular Injuries/Disease
☐ Cancer	☐ Allergies/Asthma	☐ Neurological problems
☐ Circulatory problems	☐ Headaches	☐ Kidney problems
☐ Diabetes	☐ Depression	☐ Liver problems
☐ Heart condition	☐ Anxiety	☐ Reproductive problems
☐ High/Low blood pressure	☐ Fatigue	☐ Respiratory problems
☐ Spinal/Skeletal problems	☐ Insomnia	☐ AIDS/HIV
☐ Respiratory problems	☐ Dizziness	☐ Stroke history
	☐ Skin disorders	☐ Pregnancy (list due date)

Because a Massage Therapist must be aware of any existing conditions that I have, I have listed all of my known medical conditions and physical limitations, and I will inform my Massage Therapist of any changes in my physical health. I understand that a Massage Therapist does not diagnose any medical, physical or mental disorder, prescribe medication or perform any spinal manipulations. In general, I understand that massage therapy is for the purpose of stress reduction, relief from muscular tension/spasm, improving circulation, and/or facilitating greater bodily awareness for optimal mind, body, spirit functioning. I am responsible for consulting a qualified physician for any physical ailments that I might have. I freely assume any and all risks of treatment whether presently contemplated or hereinafter discovered.

Signature _____ Date _____

Figure 4–4   This form appears very professional and will reflect positively on your business.

are communicated very clearly and offered equally to all. Subjective discounting causes trouble and is not worth the energy required to resolve the problem. Never sell yourself short, but also never argue over a few dollars if the price was not communicated very well.

Tipping is another aspect of pricing that needs established rules. Although you do not want to overtly ask your clients for tips, you can communicate whether you accept tips or not. Clear communication will often alleviate any discomfort clients may be feeling about this topic. You can have signs that indicate tips are welcome or have tipping envelopes available for client use (Box 4.5).

See Worksheet 4-5

Social Media and Websites

Social media is another avenue of external communication that can influence perception. An Internet-based avenue of communicating with others, social media sites can house text, video, pictures, and links. They offer an exciting way to quickly get in touch and stay up to date. This form of modern interaction allows many people to easily expand their networks of friends, associates, and followers. Take your first steps into social media by understanding how to set up your social site so that it communicates to your audience in the right way.

Just as you put thought into building a foundation for your business, put the same early effort into planning your online platform. By designing an online presence that promotes your values, you can have a successful foray into the digital world. Sometimes you may need more than one site or account to support your personal and professional needs. Although not always necessary, this separation can save you from future headaches.

Too often people learn the hard way to be careful about what they say and post for the world to see. Blogs are generally universal, so you can assume that anything you post on a blog is read by everyone. Also, if you would not feel comfortable having certain pictures in a photo album in your waiting room, then do not post these pictures to sites your clients may visit. Also, use caution with language, images, and sexual references. You may attract the wrong type of clients to your practice. That is not to say you cannot have a fun and active social site—just think about who may visit the sites or pages you set up.

Once the site is active, you usually have the ability to decline or block followers. This categorization feature gives you some control and allows you to refer others to places you feel are more appropriate.

Caution aside, social media can be a growth opportunity for you. In the marketing chapter, we will discuss more about using social media to engage and promote your practice.

Conversely, social sites can be used by others to post information about you and your business. With many service seekers visiting the Web to read reviews and comments about others, it is good to remember that comments about your business can find a home on someone's blog, personal page, or website. If you visit an online search engine and type in the words "great massage" or "horrible massage," you can find many comments posted about people's experiences. Usually, people have no qualms about listing the name of the person or business that provided the service they are reviewing.

See Worksheet 4-6

Box 4.5 Fee Structure Considerations

The following is a checklist of items to consider when defining and communicating your fee structure:

- What type of payments you accept
- If you will invoice or expect payment at time of service
- If you have structured fee increases
- If you have different prices in different situations
- If you offer discounts or referral incentives and how they work
- Your tipping policy

4-1: Find It on the Web

Here is a short list of social media sites. The company descriptions were obtained from their websites.

- Facebook helps you connect and share with the people in your life— http://www.facebook.com.
- Twitter is a service for friends, family, and coworkers to communicate and stay connected through the exchange of quick, frequent answers to one simple question: What are you doing? —http://www.twitter.com
- More than 40 million professionals use LinkedIn to exchange information, ideas, and opportunities—http://www.linkedin.com
- YouTube is the leader in online video and the premier destination to watch and share original videos worldwide through a Web experience—http://www.youtube.com
- Your blog. Share your thoughts, photos, and more with your friends and the world— http://www.blogspot.com

Unconscious Representation

You communicate with others in ways of which you are likely unaware. Everything about you sends a message without saying a word. You and the environment you work in speak volumes to those who spend time with you. This form of quiet communication can be called **unconscious representation**. Personally, this can include your tone of voice, eye contact, nervous habits, or crowding people's personal space. Professionally, this can be the tidiness of your work space, cobwebs on the ceiling, the condition of the product you use, and the linens on the table. You can easily overlook these things if you deal with them every day, but a new client pays attention to everything. You can have the best marketing materials in the world, but if you deliver an experience that is inconsistent with your message, your clients are in for a letdown.

> Everything about you sends a message without saying a word.

Another way you can unconsciously represent yourself is by the people you surround yourself with. When hiring employees or choosing others to work with, remember that there will be assumptions made because of your relationships. The suppliers and vendors you choose also represent who you are. If a company has a bad reputation, it may not be best to showcase its products or services in association with your business. Choose wisely when selecting the associates and service providers who can affect the perception of your business. People are continually assessing their environment to ensure their safety in the world. By paying attention to these small details, you can go a long way in maintaining a professional, ethical atmosphere.

> See Worksheet 4-7

Personal Appearance

If you are employed by a company, it most likely has a dress policy outlining its requirements for your appearance. You may be required to wear a uniform and have your hair a certain way. The company will let you know whether piercings or tattoos are allowed to be seen by clients.

If you are making these decisions on your own, it is important to assess how your appearance may affect your clients' impression of you ethically. Consider the following items, and strategically decide how you will represent yourself: clothing, shoes, hairstyle, hair color, body piercing, tattoos, makeup, and scents. Examine more subtle things like the condition of your nails, body odor, stains on clothing, visible cleavage, tightness of clothing, smoking odor, and breath. Everything about you will either enforce or erode the image you are trying to establish (Fig. 4–5).

> See Worksheet 4-8

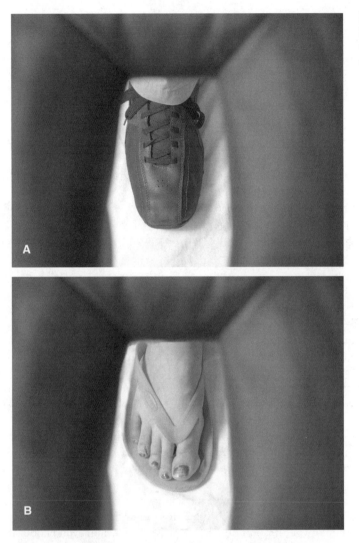

Figure 4–5   When your client is lying facedown, this is the view. Choose wisely when deciding how your feet look.

Peer Profile 4–2

Real-Life Scenario

Debra, Author
Florida

I am the type of person who goes into every business constantly analyzing how the business is delivering its customer experience. I have found that you do not have to look too hard to find people unconsciously representing the company they work for, and often not in a good way. In fact, I am sitting in a coffee shop as I write this chapter's draft. As I looked for examples of how unconscious representation can affect a customer's perception, I did not have to wait long. Only one employee was behind the counter. Apparently, the other one who was supposed to be there did not show up for work. One of the regulars asked the employee how his coworker was doing by saying, "So, how is your new side-kick doing?" The frazzled employee said, loud enough for everyone to hear, "She's more like a kick in my side, not a side-kick." After bashing her for a while, he then started to grumble about how the customers must have sensed he was alone because they bombarded him as soon as the door opened. There's nothing quite like blaming those who make your paycheck possible! He failed to positively acknowledge those waiting in line, choosing to ignore them. This was another indication of lack of care for the customer. From my perspective, it was a horrible way to represent not only himself but also the shop he worked for. Now, this probably is not enough to deter customers from coming in, but it is an unconscious representation of the shop owners and managers. When representing a business, it is wise to always act in a way that clearly reflects the established ethical foundation. I left feeling that this shop was a poorly run small business. If it had not been the only coffee shop in town, I would not have returned.

Managing the Ethical Structure

The first two steps of building and guiding perception of your ethical framework are important because they build the core of who you are professionally and ensure that others see you this way. The next area of focus involves the strategies and processes you will draw on to manage and reinforce the structures and perceptions you have put in place.

Once you have established guidelines for your internal and external ethics, there are plenty of opportunities to put them to the test. In fact, you have future clients and coworkers just waiting for you to show up so that they can begin to test your boundaries. Managing your ethical structure entails the constant assessment and refinement of the ethical beliefs you hold. Whenever you choose a career in which you work closely with people, you must constantly assess your ethical choices and how they will affect you or your client long-term. You learn to be flexible and open to change as you find where your true boundaries lie. Your diffused boundaries may become more solid. You also quickly learn where you are inflexible and your boundaries are clear and rigid. Everyone has different levels of tolerance and acceptance of what is right and wrong. What is most important is making decisions that are based on what you believe is right for you and that do not harm others.

Creating Client Policies

Legally and personally, it is important to have a set of policies explaining the structure you have established for your practice. These policies are the basis from which you establish and manage client relationships. If you work for yourself, you must create the policies yourself. Many therapists before you have already done this, so search the Web for some great examples to model. If you are an employee, your employer most likely has policy forms for you (Fig. 4–6) (Box 4.6).

Informed Consent

Often therapists take for granted that clients understand everything about massage and what to expect during a session. As professionals, it is important to remember that clients have a right to agree to all aspects of the treatment and also have the right to refuse any aspect of the service. These client rights are called informed consent. We agree to inform, and they agree or disagree to what we have educated them on. This sounds simple, but it can be challenging to communicate, especially to new clients. Your perception of massage may be totally different than theirs. The higher your level of modality training and the more you use items other than your hands, the more important this becomes. Imagine for a second that a client has asked for a Swedish massage, and halfway through the session, the therapist grabs a bamboo roller and starts working on the client's back. Although not harmful, the client did not have the opportunity to learn about the roller and consent to its use. This simple lack of communication and consent could ruin the session for them, thus losing you a client.

My Massage Business

Your first session: Please arrive for your appointment(s) 15 minutes prior to the scheduled starting time. This allows you time to complete a confidential health history and client information form (if you would like this to be e-mailed to you in advance, please contact me at my e-mail address).

Health information: It is important to make me aware of any health conditions, change of medications, or recent injuries and surgeries you may have had. There are some contraindications to massage so receiving this information in advance at each appointment is crucial.

Arrival: Please plan on arriving a few minutes early for your session. If you arrive late, your session will be shortened in order to accommodate others whose appointments follow yours, with payment being expected for the full reserved session time.

Cancellation: We understand that unanticipated events happen occasionally in everyone's life that might impact your ability to keep your appointment. In our desire to be effective and fair to all of our clients and out of consideration for our therapists' time, we have adopted the following policies:

- 24 hour advance notice is required when cancelling an appointment.
  This allows the opportunity for someone else to schedule an appointment.
- If you are unable to give us 24 hours advance notice, you will be charged in full for the missed appointment.

Session length, rates, and payment: I accept cash, credit cards, and checks for payment for your session. Payment is due at time of service. My rates and session lengths are outlined below:

1 hour (50 minutes of actual massage time): $xx
1 and 1/2 hour (80 minutes actual massage time): $xxx
Additional service (hot stone massage, aromatherapy): Add $xx

Sexual misconduct: Sexual behavior by the client toward the therapist is always unethical and inappropriate. Such behavior will result in immediate termination of the session with payment due in full.

Confidentiality: The massage and bodywork profession has a code of ethics and respects clients' rights of confidentiality. Consent must always be given for any massage procedure.

Tipping: I do accept gratuities with much gratitude. However, gratuities are not expected and remain your decision. There is an envelope in the massage room in which to place tips or you may add one at the time of your payment.

Communication around pressure: I will check in with you every session within the first 5 minutes of your session to ensure I am delivering the level of pressure you prefer. If at any time you would like more or less pressure, please communicate this. My goal is to leave you highly satisfied with your session.

Draping: At all times your modesty will be protected with professional draping. I have extensive training in draping procedures and will use these techniques during your session.

I appreciate your business and if you have any questions about these policies, please let me know.

Debra Koerner

Figure 4–6   A client policy form should look professional, as this example illustrates.

Box 4.6 Items to Include in Your Practice Policies

Below is a list of items to consider including in your policies. Some of these are for your own personal reference, and others should be placed into written form for your clients. After you complete the work in this chapter, you will have already drafted many of the guidelines and rules you plan to establish. You can quickly reference this work when drafting forms for your business.

- Process for scheduling appointments
- Cancellation policy
- Payment process
- Tipping
- Minimum age
- Privacy of records
- Arrival procedures
- Late arrival repercussions
- Refund policy
- Insurance acceptance or not
- Office and phone hours
- Draping guidelines
- Gift certificate purchase and redemption
- Sexual harassment

Plan on clearly communicating your intention for each session and acquire consent. Most importantly, deliver what you promise. If midway through a session your find yourself wanting to go outside the parameters of the agreement, you can always ask for permission during the session. Once you have consent, then you can move forward with your plan.

The "You Are Not Important" Client

Managing clients is a continual process. Some clients fall into a pattern of not respecting your time or policies. When you have a client who often oversteps your business boundaries, you may be facing someone who believes his world is more important than yours. These clients, hopefully few in number, can affect your entire practice if you let their actions go unchecked. These people are the ones who miss appointments, run late, decide that paying you is optional, and generally ignore many of the rules and policies you have communicated. Once your business ethical boundaries are established, you must dedicate time to reinforcing the standards you have in place and ensuring consistency in client management. Word travels fast if you have leaky boundaries that can be pushed. Poorly enforced boundaries can negatively affect those you work with—or, most importantly, yourself.

See Worksheet 4-9

The "You Are So Important to Me" Client

On the other hand, you may have clients who think you are the greatest thing that ever happened to them. They may bring you gifts, leave large tips, or expect special treatment because of their perception of your relationship. The boundaries they push may include asking for special favors, allowing personal affection to overshadow guidelines you have established around fraternization, and generally bending the rules because, after all, they are such great clients. This situation too can lead to complications if not handled properly and fairly. If you find yourself making exceptions or bending the rules for particular clients, it is probably time to assess your true relationship with them and determine whether it is still within the ethical framework you wish to have with your clients.

See Worksheet 4-10

CHAPTER SUMMARY

Ethics will never be an easily defined process. There will never be a guidebook that offers solutions for every situation. Fortunately, some issues are black and white, and you can easily establish rules on how to respond when they are broken. For situations that rest more in the gray areas, you must rely on your own set of personal values to continually mold and help solidify your guidelines. Your life circumstances, advice from others, and lessons from your future mistakes all help you with this process. The best you can ever do is make decisions that feel right for you and that do not cause purposeful, malicious harm to others or yourself. The following story is said to come from Native American legend and sums it up nicely.

A Cherokee Legend

An old Cherokee was teaching his grandson about what is right and wrong. "A fight is going on inside me," he said to the boy.

"It is a terrible fight and it is between two wolves. One is evil—he is anger, envy, sorrow, regret, greed, arrogance, self-pity, guilt, resentment, inferiority, lies, false pride, superiority, and ego." He continued, "The other is good—he is joy, peace, love, hope, serenity, humility, kindness, benevolence, empathy, generosity, truth, compassion, and faith. The same fight is going on inside you—and inside every other person, too."

The grandson thought about it for a minute and then asked his grandfather, "Which wolf will win?"

The old Cherokee simply replied, "The one you feed."

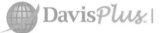 For additional resources visit Davis*Plus* at **http://davisplus.fadavis.com.** Keyword, Koerner.

REVIEW QUESTIONS

1. Behaviors are continually being shaped by which of the following factors?
    a. External guidance and consequences
    b. Lawmakers and law enforcement
    c. Inner guidance and external circumstances
    d. None of the above

2. The more you have to think about a decision, _____.
    a. The more likely it is a rigid boundary
    b. The closer you move toward a misalignment with your moral compass
    c. The more thoughtful you are becoming
    d. The more ethical the results

3. A lifetime of situations have entrenched within you a moral framework from which you _____.
    a. Make decisions
    b. Consciously allocate money
    c. Deal with your emotions
    d. Create initial impressions

4. The ethical boundaries that exist between massage practitioners and clients is often _____.

    a. Very clear if you are willing to be nonjudgmental
    b. Uncertain
    c. Certain
    d. Obvious

5. Financial success is much more rewarding when it springs from a business with _____.

    a. Caring and respect for others
    b. Responsible citizenship and accountability
    c. Pursuit of excellence and purity of values
    d. Integrity and values

6. Which of the following is a way to teach others to honor your established boundaries?

    a. Enforce your personal boundaries
    b. Be tolerant of others
    c. Model the "Ten Universal Values" by Michael Josephson
    d. React positively and calmly when boundaries are crossed

7. Boundaries fall into which three areas?

    a. Defined, semi-defined, and undefined
    b. Strong, permeable, and weak
    c. Flexible, semi-flexible, and rigid
    d. Diffused, semi-permeable, and rigid

8. The draping procedures for a massage practice is an example of a:

    a. Semi-permeable boundary
    b. Semi-flexible boundary
    c. Rigid boundary
    d. Defined boundary

9. Until a specific situation crosses a line, you may not even realize a boundary is needed.

    a. True
    b. False

10. The _____ the rules you expect yourself and others to follow, the more you can prevent future problems.

    a. Clearer
    b. Tougher
    c. Simpler
    d. More ethical

11. The following is an example of building and guiding perception of your ethical framework:

    a. Establishing processes to manage policies
    b. Maintaining the integrity of work space
    c. Pricing and fees
    d. Both b & c

12. Once strong ethical structures are developed and part of your core foundation, they require little attention.

    a. True
    b. False

13. Which of the following is *not* an example of foundational ethics?

    a. Maintaining the integrity of internal communication
    b. Unconscious representation
    c. Maintaining the integrity of work space
    d. Creating internal policies

14. **What builds the base of a business?**

    a. Foundational ethics
    b. External perceptions
    c. Management of the ethical structure
    d. All of the above

15. **Building a solid, ethical foundation requires which of the following?**

    a. Tolerance and the pursuit of excellence
    b. Money and other financial support
    c. Thought, documentation, and constant management
    d. A strong support network

16. **Internal policies are made up of both your personal belief system and those required by law.**

    a. True
    b. False

17. **Which of the following is a good rule of thumb to follow regarding internal communications?**

    a. Reread internal communication to ensure it represents your values and/or the company's values
    b. Assume that all internal communications will be viewed by the press
    c. Speak from the heart, where your core values can guide you
    d. Both a & b

18. **Use of professional organizations, honest marketing materials, responsible social media behavior, and unconscious representation are all examples of _____.**

    a. Developing foundational ethics
    b. Diffused boundaries
    c. Guiding external perceptions
    d. Managing the ethical structure

19. **It is an effective method of guiding external perceptions when you post certifications and code of ethics in your internal work space.**

    a. True
    b. False

20. Which of the following is *not* an example of unconscious representation?

    a. Tone of voice

    b. The vendors and suppliers you select

    c. Cobwebs on the ceiling

    d. Marketing materials and advertisements

21. Managing your ethical structure requires which of the following?

    a. Constantly assessing and refining the ethical beliefs you hold

    b. Never compromising your ethical beliefs

    c. Establishing rigid boundaries and communicating them effectively

    d. Both b & c

Worksheet 4–1   Values for Your Practice

In the following space, write down phrases that reflect the ethical values you wish to integrate into your practice. Consider writing these on a separate paper and posting them somewhere you can see often.

Examples:

I will be **on time** for every appointment

I will always **professionally drape** my clients

Worksheet 4–2   The Framework for a Practice

Scenario:

John has been practicing massage for quite some time. More than half of his clients are repeat clients who have been with him long-term, and they are extremely loyal to him. Knowing their personalities so well, he has learned which clients will allow sessions to start a bit late without getting upset. He has been scheduling these clients on the days he drops his kids off at school. Most of the time he is timely, but occasionally, because of traffic, he arrives a couple of minutes late.

The above scenario demonstrates how John is building the framework for his practice. Do you think John is making a wise decision to schedule clients according to their acceptance of lateness? If he ever has employees, how can this influence how they build their practices?

Worksheet 4–3   **Private Areas of Shared Office Space**

Scenario:

Josh has been sharing office space with several other therapists. There are two treatment rooms, a private break area, and two restrooms. One restroom is located in the employee break area, and the other is in the main area and designated for client use. When Josh came in to work, he noticed a sign hanging on the client restroom indicating it was out of order and asking clients to use the one in the break room. Not thinking anything about this, he referred his next client to this area before the session. Unbeknownst to him, the other therapists had started posting a list on the bulletin board of clients they did not recommend working with, for various reasons, some of which were due to sexual advances. His client never said a word about this and maybe did not even notice the list. It wasn't until Josh went on break that he saw the list and viewed it through the eyes of his client. He quickly removed the list and locked it up with the other client records.

Write out a list of items that should be kept secure and out of view at all times.

1.

2.

3.

4.

5.

6.

Worksheet 4–4   Room Details Promote Ethics

Draft your thoughts on what you may add to your rooms to professionally promote the ethics you have established for your practice and to build credibility.

Worksheet 4–5   Payment Policies

Draft some details on the types of payments you will accept and when you expect your clients to pay for your products and services.

Write your thoughts on what types of discounts and incentives you may offer. Draft the words exactly how they would be written for your clients to read. Have someone else read them to see if they are clear.

Worksheet 4-6 Social Media in Business Practices

Scenario:

After much encouragement, Pat finally decided to start his own Facebook account. It was quite exciting. He quickly connected with school friends he had not talked to in years, members of his family, coworkers, and also his clients. He was very quick to log in every day and post comments about his activities. Problems began to surface when some of his old high school buddies started using good-natured but inappropriate language and posting embarrassing pictures Pat was tagged in. Because he hadn't created a structure when he built his account, these landed on his home page. The energy he had been putting into conversation quickly diverted to deleting tags, removing friends from his list, and managing content to ensure it was not offensive or embarrassing. He has since started a business page that his coworkers and clients can join. It takes Pat a little more effort to keep everyone updated, but he is able to control and select the content that posts to each site.

Share any stories on social media sites as they relate to managing a business and protecting personal information. You can use examples of good process and of mishaps you have noticed.

Worksheet 4–7   Ethics in Practice

Scenario:

Mary, a new therapist, signed up for an outcall massage company. The company was very well established and had a professional website and quality marketing materials. It marketed primarily to large companies that often scheduled therapists for on-site employee sessions or events. Mary became a contractor for them and received an hourly wage for her time. The company contacted her about once every other week to show up and do chair massage. They provided her with a logo T-shirt and business cards that promoted their company. Quickly realizing she could be making more money if she worked with these clients privately, she began to carry her own business cards and pass these out while she was working for the company. On some level, she thought this was probably wrong, but she justified it by thinking that they were her clients too, in a way. She acquired several new clients in this manner.

Write your thoughts on this situation, specifically on how Mary is representing herself ethically and how this may influence the perception of the clients she gets from these events.

Worksheet 4–8   Workplace Appearance

Draft your thoughts on what type of attire you think is fine to wear during a massage and what is not appropriate. How will you handle tattoos and piercings?

Worksheet 4–9   Balancing Ethics and Nonpayment

Scenario:

Jessica has been working with a client named Mary for a while now. During this time, Mary has opened up to Jessica and shared some personal stories of abuse that occurred during her childhood. Jessica maintains her professional boundaries and allows Mary to share without interjecting advice or counsel. Being kind-hearted, she feels for Mary and silently mourns for her trauma. She finds herself feeling sorry for Mary quite often. Recently divorced, Mary has fallen into some financial difficulty. She is already behind two payments. Tearfully, she asks for Jessica to continue working with her, promising that she will catch up her payments as soon as she can. Jessica has a policy in place stating that if clients should fall behind by two payments, she can no longer work with them until they bring their accounts current.

How would you handle a situation like this one? How would your decision affect other clients?

Draft your policy on nonpayment.

Draft your policy on how you would handle clients arriving late for their appointments.

Draft your policy on cancellations, including amount of notice required, avenues of communication, and rescheduling.

Worksheet 4-10   Ethics, Gifts, and Tips

Scenario:

Rob has been working with Janice for just a short while. Janice is new to massage and has made a couple of inappropriate comments about her personal life. After every session, she leaves Rob very generous tips, and schedules with him regularly. Recently, she has begun to bake cookies for Rob and brings these in to him. When she begins making comments that make him feel uncomfortable, he finds himself having internal dialogue that sounds something like, "Well, here she goes again. I guess maybe she doesn't know any better. I really should let her know that I feel uncomfortable, but I do not want to lose her as a client because she tips really well and comes so often. Maybe next time I will say something to her." As time passes, Rob begins to notice that she is getting even bolder, and he has even felt at times that she is hitting on him. He finally addresses his concerns with Janice. Unfortunately, enough time has passed that she has misread his failure to react to her previous comments and believes that their relationship may go to another level. She personalizes the discussion as a rejection. She does not return to Rob for more sessions.

Write your thoughts about this situation.

Write some thoughts on how you may feel if you have to let go of a client who is bringing you substantial income.

Draft your thoughts on receiving gifts from clients.

Write about how you plan to handle tipping and the communication you will have around this topic.

CAREER OPTIONS IN MASSAGE THERAPY

THREE CAREER PATHS

Most likely, you have heard both positive and negative stories about life as a massage therapist. You may have also had discussions about the pros and cons of working for others or being your own boss. As a massage therapist, you have several professional options available to you. There are numerous resources available to help you, but the key place to start is by fortifying yourself with knowledge. Ultimately, your professional success depends on a combination of knowledge, preparation, and luck.

Your professional journey begins with a thorough understanding of the three career paths available to you in the massage therapy field:

- The path of the **employee**
- The path of the **independent contractor**
- The path of the **entrepreneur**

After graduating and, if required, receiving your license, you may choose to become a full- or part-time employee of a company, such as a spa or massage therapy center. You may also choose to become an independent contractor, whereby you may work for one or several different companies and have more autonomy than an employee. The third opportunity is the entrepreneurial path, in which you would open your own massage business. Over the course of your career, you may journey down one of these paths—or all three—and you may even explore more than one path at once. For example, you may become a part-time employee at a day spa while running a mobile massage business on your own. No path is better than another—each has benefits and challenges that appeal to or dissuade different people.

The next few chapters will help you choose the path that is right for you at this stage in your life. Once you know which path you'd like to start with—employee, independent contractor, or entrepreneur—you can then narrow down your choices, begin gathering knowledge, and start preparing for your career.

By now, you may realize that all three paths can be both fulfilling and challenging. It is important to understand that each step in your career path has the potential to bring you closer to personal fulfillment, but each step also offers its own set of unique challenges and rewards. The road to personal fulfillment and a successful career is smoother if it is planned out, leading you to the fulfilling career you desire. Knowing the challenges you will likely face helps you to prevent the most common pitfalls. It also helps to remember that every work situation we find ourselves in is in effect preparing us for the next level of our career, if we choose to learn from our situations. Often, we learn as much from our discomfort with career choices as we do from the ideal job. As John Joyce put it, "A man's errors are his portals of discovery." So, if you find yourself on a path that isn't providing the expected experiences or results, then learn from your experiences and take these lessons with you on your next journey.

> "One thing is sure. We have to do something. We have to do the best we know how at the moment ... If it doesn't turn out right, we can modify it as we go along."
> —Franklin D. Roosevelt

Chapter 5

Your Path as an Employee

"In order that people may be happy in their work, these three things are needed: They must be fit for it. They must not do too much of it. And they must have a sense of success in it."

–John Ruskin

Outline

Continued

Outline—cont'd

You will learn to...

- Define what a massage therapist's career looks like as an employee
- Identify desirable employee qualities, including those that are your strengths and those that need improvement
- Define employer expectations, including those for scheduling, teamwork, appearance, policies, and the guest experience
- Build a strong resume
- Successfully interview with prospective employers
- Identify types of companies that hire massage therapists
- Analyze employee compensation and benefits

Key Definitions

This chapter references several key terms, which are indicated in bold. For easy reference, these terms are briefly defined here:

Ability: The power to perform an activity, which is evidenced by the performance of an activity or work. It is an action that can usually be taught.

Adaptive skill: Self-management skills such as dependability, being a team player, and self-direction.

Base pay: Regular income that is a fixed amount, such as a fee-per-service or hourly rate, which does not include additional incentives or variable pay.

Compensation: Total value of base and variable wages, as well as benefits, such as insurance and paid time off.

Employee: A person hired to provide services to a company in exchange for compensation, who does not provide these services as part of an independent business.

Entrepreneur: A person who begins a business and assumes all related risks and rewards.

Functional skill: Transferable skills used with people, information, or things, such as organizational and management skills.

Independent contractor: A person who is hired to provide services but is not hired as an employee of that person or company. The terms and specifications of work provided are outlined in a contract or agreement for short- or long-term engagement. They are sometimes called "contractors" or "freelancers."

Knowledge: Information and understanding that can be taught and is typically factual or procedural in nature.

Personal characteristics: Personal traits innate to an individual, such as attitude, patience, and creativity. These characteristics can be worked on and improved, but for the most part, one is either born with them or not.

Policy: Written statements that outline corporate and management intentions associated with various internal and external operations.

Practical massage: Providing a massage to potential employers as a part of the interview and hiring process so that they can evaluate a potential employee's skill.

Procedure: Written step-by-step outline regarding how to handle various situations or perform certain key functions. They are sometimes called Standard Operating Procedures (SOPs).

Skills: Combination of both knowledge and ability, which is observable, measurable, and quantifiable and can be taught.

Values: The timeless principles or ideals that define who you are and your actions.

Variable pay: Irregular income that fluctuates with a variety of factors. This pay can include bonuses, gratuities, and commissions, such as retail sales commissions.

EMPLOYEES

An employee is a person hired to provide services to a company in exchange for **compensation**, and does not provide these services as part of an independent business. Employment is a contract between two parties, one being the employer and the other being the employee. *Black's Law Dictionary* defines an employee as, "A person in the service of another under any contract of hire, express or implied, oral or written, where the employer has the power or right to control and direct the employee in the material details of how the work is to be performed." Going beyond this definition, let us explore the areas that help ensure success and happiness while in the employment of a company (Fig. 5–1).

Employment is the most common early career path because it is easy to step into after graduation, compared with immediately launching your own business. The benefit to becoming an employee first is that you build your physical stamina and your professional and business skills and hopefully further your education by participating in various training opportunities provided by your new employer. Even if you desire to become an entrepreneur and open your own business one day, you

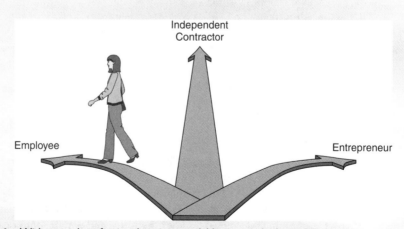

Figure 5–1   With several professional options available to you, the best place to start your journey is fortifying yourself with knowledge.

may still start your career path as an employee, knowing you are building the skills and resources to eventually launch your own business.

Employees Versus Independent Contractors

The most confusion seems to revolve around the differences between employees and independent contractors. Independent contractors will be explored fully in the next chapter. There are some nuances between the two paths that help employers decide which way to work with massage therapists. Managers who prefer employees over independent contractors generally do so because their top priority is to build a strong team of engaged workers dedicated to achieving the company's vision. Employers indicate it is much harder to get a group of independent contractors to engage in the business' vision when they are potentially not as vested because of other career obligations. Another reason that companies prefer hiring employees is the greater ease of creating a consistent level of service excellence. Managers can include training and resources as part of their employees' work requirement. It is much harder to enforce these consistently if they must coordinate with numerous nonemployee schedules. It is more expensive on the front end for companies to hire employees. When you apply for an organization that hires employees, they are more invested in creating a compliant workforce that will deliver the experience they have defined.

Standards of Employment

Every employer has different policies, procedures, and expectations as well as different types of compensation and benefits. Here are some broad categories that outline some of the realities of employment standards for massage therapists.

Policies and Procedures

As an employee, you are expected to follow certain **policies** and **procedures**. These are likely tied in with your job duties and are determining factors in receiving your compensation. In most well-established companies, these policies and procedures are written and provided to employees. However, in some companies, these policies are not formalized but implied or they may have written policies that are no longer reflective of what management desires. Policies are written statements that outline corporate and management intentions associated with various internal and external operations. These policies can range from the corporate policy regarding appearance and personal phone calls to smoking and job performance evaluations. Procedures are typically a written step-by-step outline regarding how to handle various situations or perform certain key functions. They are sometimes called Standard Operating Procedures, or SOPs. These can range from how to set up and clean a massage room to how to handle guest complaints or accidents. These policies and procedures are created for risk management and insurance reasons, but also for general business reasons. For example, policies are a way to help ensure consistency of the guest experience and services as well as reinforce the image of the company. Also, from a human resource perspective, documented employee policies pave a clear path for expected behavior and allow room for proper enforcement. For an employee, there are almost always consequences if policies and procedures are violated (Box 5.1).

Set Wages

Company compensation packages differ, depending on the organization and its compensation goals. Most massage therapists are paid per service or hour, but some are paid with an annual salary. The pay mix may also include a **base pay** or **variable pay**. Base pay is a guaranteed and agreed-on fixed wage, such as $25 per hour. Variable pay is not guaranteed and fluctuates with a variety of factors. Variable pay can include annual bonuses, gratuities, and commissions on services or products, such as retail sales commissions. So, although you may earn a lower base wage, you may have the opportunity to earn a high commission from the variable pay options. It is important to completely understand

Box 5.1 Sample Checklist of Policies and Procedures

Policies and procedures vary a great deal from facility to facility, but the below sample checklist will provide you with an idea of the range of policies companies may have.

Appearance

- General appearance
- Hygiene
- Jewelry
- Name tag
- Piercings/tattoos
- Uniforms

Behavior and Conduct

- Customer service standards/protocols (e.g., greeting/receiving guests, handling complaints)
- Internet use
- Personal e-mails
- Personal phone calls
- Smoking policy

Employment Policies

- Counseling and disciplinary procedures
- Customer disputes
- Drug/alcohol policies
- Inspections (personal items, such as packages, backpacks, and purses)
- Insurance/benefit procedures
- Leave of absence (paid and unpaid)
- Pay period
- Paid time off
- Sexual harassment
- Transfer policy
- Wage discrepancies

Facility and Equipment

- Accidents
- Computer/technology use
- Emergencies
- Parking
- Staff use of facilities/services
- Supplies

Job Duties and Performance

- Booking policies
- Close-of-shift procedures
- Evaluation/review process
- Gratuity/tip reporting
- Refund policies
- Safety procedures
- Staff recognition program
- Start-of-shift procedures
- Treatment room departure procedures
- Treatment room sanitation/cleanliness
- Treatment room setup

a company's base and variable wages and how your compensation is structured. Tips are another factor to consider. By law, employers require you to report tips as part of your income. For those not used to doing so, this sometimes comes as a surprise.

Benefits

Most companies will offer an employee benefits package; however, the depth of benefits can range dramatically. Benefits can include health and life insurance, paid time off (e.g., holidays and vacations), disability plans, retirement savings plans, and discounted services. Workers' compensation, often required by state law, can be viewed as a benefit when considering the chance of injury during your massage career. Find out what policies are in place if you were to become unable to work. Self-employed practitioners are required to purchase these policies on their own.

Some of the most common benefits offered to therapists are paid time off, liability insurance, and the opportunity for additional training. However, some companies may offer their employees only discounts on products and services. Take the entire package into consideration when deciding on a job offer. When being offered an hourly rate, factor in the benefits being offered as part of your assessment of total compensation. These benefits can be of great value if you are hurt on the job, when you are saving for retirement, or if you like the security of being paid even when you are not working, such as on vacation and holidays.

Scheduling

When you work for a company, your employer sets your work hours. Some employers offer flexible schedules and may allow you to have input about your hours, but you will still have to follow a set schedule. The synergy of the team and the delivery of a great experience rely on employees being there as scheduled. This includes arriving and leaving on time because other employees may be depending on you to show up so that they can leave. As an employee, you have a limited number of days off and must give notice within an agreed-on amount of time. You will be expected to plan accordingly.

For many companies that employ massage therapists, scheduling can be tricky. In some situations, massage therapists may not know their exact schedule until the day before they are scheduled to work. Or, therapists may be "on-call" certain days and will go in if enough appointments are booked, or perhaps not at all. Also, if heavy bookings are expected, but appointments are not booked as anticipated, then therapists may be let go early. Or, vice versa—therapists may not be scheduled to work, or even on-call, but are called in anyway because of an increased number of bookings. For massage therapists, all available appointment times may not always be booked. Companies want to have availability for guests who decide to book a massage at the last minute. However, most companies don't like to pay employees to sit and wait for appointments, so they are sent home early or assigned other duties for the day.

Massage therapists sometimes get pulled in several different scheduling directions, and as an employee, you must be flexible and understand the needs of the clients and the company.

Uniforms

As an employee, you may be expected to wear a certain uniform (Fig. 5–2). Most employers want to balance fashion with function. They want employees to look well groomed, be recognizable, and portray the image of the company. Organizations vary regarding whether or not they pay for uniforms and their upkeep, so it's important to find this out. Also, your uniform may not be limited to clothing. Employers have individual policies about jewelry and visible tattoos. Often they will ask employees working closely with customers to be odor-neutral, which means no strong colognes or scented products. These policies may not always reflect your personal beliefs or style, but you will have to compromise as part of your agreement as an employee. You agree to abide by the defined uniform rules to achieve the image your employer wishes to project to customers.

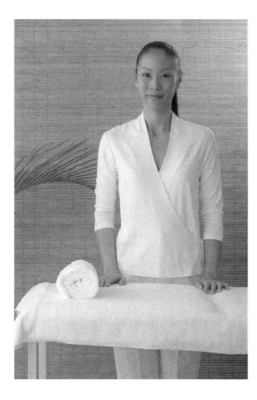

Figure 5–2   Employers often require employees to wear a uniform so that they look well groomed, are easily recognizable as staff, and portray the image of the company.

Treatment Rooms

Treatment rooms come in many different shapes, sizes, and forms. Some can be adequately sized, whereas others are cramped for space. As you will be spending much of your time in the massage rooms, it is important to ensure you have adequate room to perform the work in a way that takes care of your body. A too-small room can lead to problems with body mechanics, ultimately leading to physical problems. If the space is too small and the employer is not willing to change it, you may choose another place to work. The short-term paycheck is not worth the long-term physical ailments you may acquire as a result of a poor work space.

Temperature, equipment, flooring, and room amenities (e.g., sink, towel stands, robe hooks, music) can all vary greatly. As an employee, you often have little control over these things. You may be responsible for cleaning the room after each use and changing the linens on the tables, or there could be an attendant assigned to this task.

In some facilities, you may be assigned one room for the day or every day. However, in most facilities, particularly spas, you will more than likely share multiple rooms with other massage thera-pists. Everyone is different, with unique quirks, likes, and dislikes. You may have to share space with someone who leaves behind a messy room, adjusts the temperature too high, turns the lighting down too low, or leaves the table at a height you constantly need to adjust. These are all things to consider when working for and with others. As a rule, most employers want you to leave the room in excellent condition and ready for the next client.

Training

Training is an essential component of your success as an employee. It can also be a valuable benefit. When you are hired by a company, you should be properly trained regarding policies, procedures, and how to perform your job duties as expected. You were hired because of your knowledge, skills, ability, and talent, or your potential in these areas. The company is responsible for providing you with the proper training so that you can perform the job as agreed.

As an employee, you may be offered the opportunity to receive additional career-related training, which can range from learning new massage techniques to management training. Training of this nature can bolster your career and professional experience. However, it is important to know and understand any "strings" attached to training. Some organizations may provide free training, partially paid training, or incentives for additional certifications or for memberships in professional organizations. Others may not provide any compensation but still expect you to maintain licensure and stay on top of trends and techniques within your industry. If companies do provide compensation for training, they may also require that you stay with the company for a certain amount of time so that they do not lose their investment in you. In most facilities, if you leave before the agreed-on amount of time, you will be required to reimburse the company.

Varied Job Duties

Often, you will be cross-trained in other areas. For example, there may be times when you are expected to answer the phone, book appointments, sell retail products, or assist with cleaning the facility (Fig. 5–3). As discussed under "Scheduling," if you are scheduled to work a 6-hour shift but only have three appointments scheduled, employers may ask you to assist in other departments between your appointments. This makes good business sense, allowing you to provide value to the company even between appointments. You may be asked to perform a wide variety of tasks, such as running inventory, picking up towels, and cleaning the changing or relaxation rooms. Ideally, these duties are communicated early on to prevent any surprises, but in most job descriptions, you will find an expectation that states "perform other duties as assigned," which means you can be asked to perform a variety of tasks.

On the other hand, these varied job duties can break up the monotony of your day and expose you to other professional areas that increase your skills and knowledge. You may find that you like the

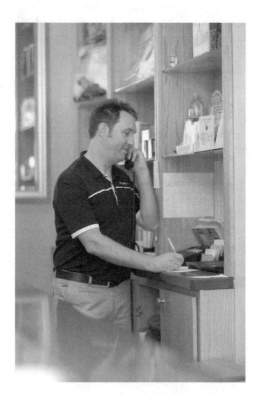

Figure 5–3 Massage employees may be expected to answer phones, book appointments, sell retail products, or assist with cleaning the facility.

balance of working both at the front desk and performing massage therapy. Or, you may become interested in esthetics and seek out additional training so that you have two sets of technical skills. This kind of cross-training can set you up for a promotion if you are interested in doing more than massage.

Learning different aspects of how the business works can prepare you for a management position. Management is another area that employees can grow into at many facilities. Many spas will hire "lead therapists" who perform massage but also supervise other therapists. Another opportunity you may wish to explore is being placed in the role of educator or trainer. In this role, you would train other staff on various techniques and customer service skills, and perhaps handle new hire orientations. Using spas as an example again, you may be interested in being assistant spa director or spa director, two common leadership positions within spas. Knowledge of all spa areas is essential for these positions. If you have the desire to move into a management position, seek out more job duties to help you learn all aspects of the company you work for.

> Learning different aspects of how the business works can prepare you for a management position.

Teamwork

As an employee, you can expect to work with other people on a regular basis. Depending on the type of business, it can be a relatively small, intimate group or a large, multidepartment group. This team environment can create camaraderie and make the day go by quickly and enjoyably, or it can be challenging if the team doesn't get along. You can create long-lasting friendships through working with a team, but if you don't like those you work with, it can be stressful and uncomfortable. As an employee, you will be expected to do what you can to foster a sense of teamwork within your group.

Performance Evaluations

Most companies provide performance evaluations, at least on an annual basis. Your performance ratings may or may not be tied to a salary increase. In most companies, raises depend on the performance of the individual and the company. Good managers who are cultivating a positive environment will provide frequent ongoing feedback on employee performance, rather than just annually. They let you know throughout the year where you are performing well and about areas needing improvement. During formal evaluations, you can expect to review your job description, define performance objectives and expectations, and discuss whether or not they are being met. If handled correctly, these sessions offer great opportunities to evaluate yourself as well as review and set goals. Goal setting can include discussions about training and service goals, and you may even bring up your interest in career advancement or new techniques.

Less Paperwork

One feature many people find attractive about being an employee is the reduced amount of record-keeping and paperwork. As an employee, you will complete tax and financial forms when you are first hired—and that is about it. Some companies may require you to sign a noncompete clause. This form means you agree not to pursue a similar profession or disclose company information to another organization in direct competition with your current employer. You may also have to agree not to take clients with you if you decide to leave your employment. When it comes to your pay, most companies will remove your taxes, benefits, and other items from your check so that you do not have to keep track of all the details. At the end of the year, you receive a W-2 form with all your information, and you submit this with your taxes. If you are an independent contractor or entrepreneur, you can expect to spend much more time on bookkeeping and saving receipts.

In your day-to-day job, the amount of paperwork may be similar to other career paths. You will most likely be keeping treatment records, managing intake forms, and acquiring health history forms. You will receive training after you are hired on what paperwork you will be responsible for on an ongoing basis.

Security

One of the greatest benefits of being an employee is the level of security. Employers provide security in several forms. First, you can expect steady work and a regular paycheck. In general, you know what you can depend on each week as far as income and work hours, so you can plan accordingly. There is also an added layer of financial protection when it comes to clients who write bad checks, are not able to pay, or simply do not show up. The employer handles these situations and collects the fees. Facilities vary in their policies regarding how therapists are paid when clients do not show or have insufficient funds, so be sure to check on this so that you know in advance.

Second, as an employee, you enjoy the security of having someone else look out for your well-being. The company that employs you has the responsibility to provide a safe working environment. It provides things like workers' compensation insurance, which protects you if you get hurt while on the job. Companies also add a layer of security to help reduce the risk for personal harm or injury. As an independent contractor, you may perform treatments in a wide variety of potentially unsafe venues, such as a hotel room or private home. In a corporate environment, you are working in a business with security procedures and others around to assist you. Even if you work in a resort or hotel spa where massages are provided in hotel rooms, there are safety protocols to help ensure the safety of employees. So, although employment comes with many policies and procedures to follow, it also comes with extra layers of safety and security.

Lastly, being an employee frees you to focus most of your energy on doing massage, rather than on marketing and promoting your practice. The business is responsible for attracting, scheduling, and providing guests with a place to come for massage. As an employee, however, it is still your job to ensure you are rebooking and building clientele for the employer. A returning client is more economical for everyone, in contrast to continually needing to advertise to gain new ones.

See Worksheet 5-1

Ensuring a Great Start as an Employee

Most employees would agree they want to work for a great place around great people. Every year, *Fortune* Magazine publishes the "Best 100 Companies to Work for" list. The list almost always contains companies that hire massage therapists—places such as hospitals, resorts, and clinics. It is a good idea to review this list and see if any look interesting to you. These companies made the list because they understand the importance of creating a great employee culture, which helps them to deliver profitability.

If you are not in a position to go to work for one of these companies, never fear—many great places to work never make the list. You can perform some due diligence during your job search by evaluating potential companies and what they are looking for. This helps ensure that your career as an employee gets off to a great start.

EVALUATIONS

To find a job that you can enjoy, thrive, and grow in, you first need to evaluate both yourself and potential employers.

Self-Evaluation

Before you actively seek employment, there are certain things you should know about yourself. Knowing who you are, your values, and your personal goals will help you grow personally and professionally.

5-1: Find It on the Web

● *Fortune Magazine* Top 100 Companies to Work for:
http://greatplacetowork.com

Self-evaluation, as demonstrated in Chapter 1, helps you develop priorities in your life and know what you want to do, and not do, with your time and energy during your professional career.

You want to clearly know your own core **values**, which are the timeless principles that define who you are and your actions. They help you identify what is most important to you, so that you can align with the core principles of the company you are seeking employment with. This is important for many reasons, including the fact that most companies would report they are seeking alignment from employees. Alignment means employees understand what their employer is seeking to deliver, and they deliver it. For a massage therapist working in a spa environment, this may look like, "Our mission is to ensure that all our guests completely relax and forget about their busy schedules while they visit." If therapists at this spa talk during the entire session or go beyond the client's threshold for pain, they are demonstrating behaviors out of alignment with the spa's vision for guests.

Knowing who you are is a challenge some people struggle with their entire lives, but for the purposes of finding a job and a good match in an employer, you at least need to know your **knowledge**, **skills** and **abilities**, and **personal characteristics**. Making a list of core features of your personality—both good and bad—helps you think through how you will be as an employee. These traits can help or hinder you in your job search and career, and it is best to recognize them so that you can work with them.

You should also compile a list of your professional or educational accomplishments. This will bolster your confidence, remind you of all the things you do know, and help you with developing your resume and during the interview process. It's never too early to start tracking your accomplishments because sometimes with time and circumstances, it's easy to forget the things we have done.

See Worksheet 5-2

It's also a good idea to visualize your dream job. In your dream job, are you managing others? What is the work environment like? What type of people are you surrounded by? Which of your skills and abilities are you using most often?

Employer Evaluation

Finding a company that fits you is a very important part of your job search. To be successful, you must find a company you will truly enjoy working for. This means knowing what is most important to you—the things that came out of your self-evaluation such as working with an enjoyable team, alone, or a mix of both, and structured versus flexible work schedules. When evaluating employers, look for corporate traits and environments in alignment with the things that are important to you and were discovered in your self-evaluation. Just as you have your own unique traits and values, so do companies. In advance of sending in an application, you can research the hiring company. Now that you have a better idea of your values, goals, and dream job, ensure these match with the companies you are interested in to ensure proper alignment and a successful fit.

There are several variables to consider when evaluating companies: company principles, age, and size, and who you would be reporting to (i.e., an owner or another employee).

Company Principles

When considering who you would like to work for, it is good to know more about a company's principles. A company's principles are the backbone of the organization—their mission, vision, and core values. Their mission is a statement and belief about what they provide and why. Their vision is where they want to go, and their core values are the timeless principles the company stands by. A founder may have a great passion for taking the company's product or service to the greater public, and behind that are a vision, mission, and core values. These may not be formalized; however, a good company will have these formally developed and written and will use and operate by them. Usually, you can find a company's mission, vision, and values on their website.

Company Age

For employees, the experience with a relatively new company can be significantly different from that with a company that has been in business for a long time. Both situations bring unique opportunities and challenges. Many times, entrepreneurs in the creative or growth stages of their business focus all of their energy on just getting their business off the ground. Sometimes, they are so focused on this that they don't realize they aren't prepared to handle all the other aspects of running a business, such as managing employees. If the owner has not strategically planned for growth, then the operations of the business can be quite messy. With these companies, you may have a lot of freedom and opportunity because the rules, policies, and procedures may not have been clearly established yet. With older companies, it's easier for the departments to become compartmentalized and not work collectively, and employees may begin to do certain things for the simple reason of having always done them that way.

Company Size

Size is another variable when considering potential employers. For example, in a large Fortune 500 company, there may be a very large reporting and operational chain within the organization. One person may be responsible for all of the different business units. Then, within each unit, there may be a president, who also has an extensive reporting channel and responsibilities. She may be responsible for hundreds or even thousands of employees in different departments, such as marketing, operations, customer service, and product development, as well as be accountable for the arduous task of ensuring that both employees and customers are happy. Each of these departments may be made up of a variety of vice presidents, directors, managers, and front-line employees. The other end of the spectrum is a company with just two employees. An example would be a chiropractic office in which the employee reports directly to the chiropractor. This is a very short operating and communication structure, requiring less time and effort to share information. Each business structure presents its own set of challenges and benefits.

The Boss

Work experiences can be very different depending on whom you report to. Most companies begin because someone had a passion for something. This passion, when working directly with the founders, can become contagious and inspire action and behavior. In some cases, it can also make it nearly impossible to present new ideas or ways of operating because the founders are so engrained in their vision. In most businesses, the visionaries will have to relinquish to others what they created—a task that may sound easy—but it can be difficult for some visionaries and can lead to disharmony and failure if not properly planned and handled. For example, savvy owners must learn to entrust their beloved product or service to employees and trust that their vision will be implemented. In return, they financially compensate employees to help them fulfill their vision and passion. But not all employees are working to grow and nurture someone else's vision. They may be working just to have a job and get a paycheck. Their core values and interests may not be in harmony with the owner's.

Not all employees will have an opportunity to work directly with a company's founders. In many cases, you may work for another employee of the company, such as a manager. In fact, the original founders of the business may no longer be involved with the company, leaving other employees to carry out their vision and run the business. Whether the founder is still involved or not, a strategic business will have appropriately planned for carrying out their founders' passion through all the ranks of employees. Smart companies will often look to their employees for guidance when manifesting change or trying new things.

The managers you work with on a daily basis may not have the same passion as a founder. They also have their own drivers and motivators for working for the company and various beliefs about themselves and their position within the company. They have varied responsibilities and their own set of challenges and rewards (Fig. 5–4).

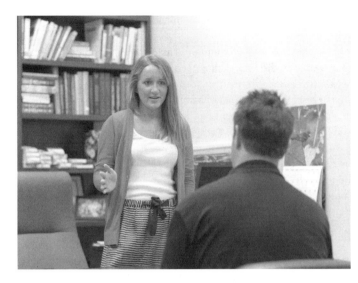

Figure 5–4 Your professional experiences can vary greatly depending on whom you report to. In fact, the main reason many individuals leave a company is a difficult relationship with their boss.

No matter whom employees report to, the principle of developing a foundation of care and trust between employee and employer is vitally important as well as clearly defined roles and expectations.

What Employers Are Looking for

To remain competitive in today's labor market, companies must continually seek talent with the knowledge, abilities, skills, and personal characteristics to move their organization forward (Box 5.2). According to an American Massage Therapy Association (AMTA) article, "Massage is a healing art

---

Box 5.2 Fifteen Tips for Being a Fabulous Employee

Being a fabulous employee is easier when you do your homework before looking for the best job. It requires diligence and engagement on your part after you are hired. Any job is what you put into it. When you have the job, you must be willing to make an effort to excel. Being an excellent employee is something to be proud of and can happen if you focus on the following 15 tips:

1. Clarify your goals with your boss early on.
2. Follow the rules, but don't be afraid to recommend improvements in a nonconfrontational way.
3. Go above and beyond what is outlined in your job duties. Always look for areas you can help with during slow times.
4. Take initiative in finding ways to help your boss accomplish her goals if she is open to it.
5. Share with your boss important customer insights you gather while working.
6. Memorize the values of the company and live them every work day.
7. Make connections across departments, do not fall into the "my department–your department" mentality.
8. Stay on top of what competitors are doing and share this information with your boss or the marketing person.
9. Subscribe to online blogs within your company's industry and stay current with trends.
10. Take responsibility for your education and improve in opportunity areas.
11. Become an expert in the massage industry field and offer to provide departmental updates.
12. Offer to mentor new employees.
13. Do not engage in negative conversations about your employer or coworkers.
14. Stay open to change and recognize it is the only thing that stays constant.
15. Take care of yourself and practice what you preach.

as well as a science. It requires a balance of academic and technical knowledge, clinical skills, manual dexterity, sensitivity, and awareness."[1]

Knowledge plays a key role when being hired as a massage therapist, and it is typically factual or procedural in nature—that is, the knowledge needed to adequately perform the job. An example for massage therapists is knowledge of human anatomy. Ability is the power to perform an activity. Ability is evidenced by the performance of an activity or work. Ability is about the "doing" or performance of the knowledge. There is a big difference in knowing how to do something and actually having the ability to do it. Someone may have a great deal of knowledge about human anatomy, but not have the ability to perform a massage that relieves tension in tight muscles. On the other hand, someone may have the ability to massage muscles in a way that relieves tension, but not an in-depth knowledge of the musculoskeletal system.

Skill is in some ways a combination of both knowledge and ability. It is something you can observe, measure, and quantify. Demonstrated skill typically implies that you possess the required knowledge and aptitude to perform the job. For massage therapists, part of the interview process is often **practical**, which entails providing a massage to the potential employer so that the employer can evaluate your skill, that is, your knowledge and ability to perform a satisfactory massage. However, skill is deeper than just an ability to perform duties directly related to your job. It also encompasses **functional skills**, which are transferable skills used with people, information, or things, such as organizational and management skills as well as development and communication. There are also **adaptive skills**, which are self-management skills, such as dependability, being a team player, self-direction, and punctuality.

Employers look for all of these categories in employees, but which specific knowledge, skills, and ability they hire vary greatly depending on their specific needs and goals. Knowing up front what an employer's needs are for the position, the geographical area, and the company is important. It lets you determine whether your knowledge, skill, and ability would be a good fit within the company.

Although employers look for core skills, knowledge, and ability, they also know these things can be taught. What can't be taught are personal traits and characteristics, such as attitude. That is why if employers can't find a person with everything they want, they will often hire for personal characteristics and train for the skill set. Personal traits and characteristics include attitude, patience, work ethic, and creativity. Teamwork was previously mentioned as a component of being an employee. One of the unquantifiable factors employers are considering when evaluating a potential new employee is team chemistry. There is a certain chemistry among a well-working team, which is made up of many factors, especially personalities. This does not mean employers will look for another employee exactly like the ones they have because good employers strive for diversity. Employers will weigh personalities, traits, and perspectives and seek out those that will complement those of their existing team.

> "Do not hire a man who does your work for money, but him who does it for love of it."
> —Henry David Thoreau

Lastly, most employers will be seeking to hire those who demonstrate enthusiasm and passion. Henry David Thoreau said, "Do not hire a man who does your work for money, but him who does it for love of it." Employers want someone who comes into work each day looking forward to the activities and tasks at hand and not just their paycheck.

Walking in an Employer's Shoes

To be a great employee, it is important to mentally wear the proverbial "other shoe" and understand what it is like to be an employer. Visualizing and understanding what it is like to own or manage a business provide helpful insights into the expectations and intentions behind your employer's behavior and decisions. Consider what employers are looking for in their employees. If you owned a business and were paying individuals for their services, what would you be looking for when making the decision to hire someone? Some of the attributes that come to mind are commitment, engagement, honesty, and willingness to go beyond what is expected. These are great words, but simply writing them in a job description and telling an employee this is what is expected of them doesn't ensure they happen. Good employers understand that a foundation of care and trust must be established before they can elicit these types of behaviors. Success for both the business and the employee depends on a positive relationship between the employee and employer.

See Worksheet 5-3

Once you know more about the company (Box 5.3), you can more accurately answer the question, "Why should I apply for this particular job, with this specific company?" Knowing the answer to that question will help you draft your resume and ace the interview.

GETTING THE JOB

As previously covered, getting the job right for you depends on knowledge, preparation, and luck. Now is the time to use your new knowledge to find a successful employer match, prepare your resume and cover letter, and get ready for the interview. This is also where luck comes into play because getting the job sometimes has a lot to do with timing, and even who you know.

A Resume to Get You Noticed

A resume is a brief document highlighting your skills, experience, and education. It is the first indicator of what type employee you will be. In short, its intent is to get you noticed and to secure an interview. Although many companies have moved to online applications and resume submissions, it is still valuable to take the time to collect your basic career information into a written format. Many employers still ask for a written version of a resume. If a prospective employer has an online process, you can use your document to copy and paste, simplifying your work down the road. It is recommended to create a general resume but then customize it to specifically fit the job you are seeking.

Often, employers receive numerous resumes for one position. You want your resume to stand out from the rest. Successfully landing an interview from a resume submission depends on two things. First, it depends on how effectively you state your knowledge, abilities, skills, traits, accomplishments, and experience. Second, you must quickly and easily establish why you would be the best fit for the job, by highlighting how your abilities and experience fit their needs.

There are some specific things you can do to ensure yours floats to the top:

1. A resume should be brief and to the point and should highlight the most relevant experience as it pertains to the job being sought. A good rule of thumb is one letter-size page for every 10 years or less of work experience.
2. Your resume should stress what you have to offer employers and, whenever possible, quantify your accomplishments and results. When writing about your job experiences, focus more on the positive results you achieved than on the actual work duties.

Box 5.3 Company Research

There are several ways you can find out about a company, including the following:

- Explore the company's website.
- Call the human resources department and ask for information or to schedule an appointment to talk more about the company.
- Ask your friends and colleagues about the company.
- Type the company's name in an Internet search engine and see what it turns up, keeping an eye out for media articles.
- Post a request for information on your Facebook or MySpace page and ask your friends to pass it along, to see if you can get a personal connection to the company.
- Do an online search to read consumer reviews of personal experiences. For example, type in "[company name] reviews."

3. Craft a visually neat, clean, and easy-to-scan resume with ample white space around the margins and between lines. Limit formatting options and graphics to strategic use only, such as one simple graphic to make your resume stand out. Bold your name and the critical points you most want an employer to notice.

4. Everything must be grammatically correct. Use spell check on your computer, and also manually check for spelling and grammatical errors. You should also let others proofread your work before you send your resume out. Typos in resumes often cause applicants to be removed from further consideration.

5. Customize your resume to meet the objectives sought by each job and company for which you apply.

6. Your language use should include short sentences that are hard-hitting and have an impact. Start most sentences with action verbs, such as achieved, led, created, established, and assisted. Avoid using the word "I" as well as passive verbs.

7. Carefully consider placement of your experience within your resume. You want to place your best experience first—not necessarily in chronological order. For example, where you list education and training or prior work experience depends on which is the most qualifying experience. If you don't have a lot of work experience, but a great deal of education and training, then that will get more positive attention at the top.

8. Avoid simply listing job functions you have performed and instead focus on the accomplishments you achieved while doing those job functions. For example, instead of listing, "I held a management position for 5 years" state instead, "During my five years as a shift manager, my department achieved three customer service awards."

9. When creating lists, place your most powerful work experience or sentences first, second, and last. These positions are the most memorable.

10. Avoid submitting partial pages and, if possible, fit your resume on one page (Fig. 5–5).

As you add new skills and experiences to your tool box, plan on adding these to your existing resume. When you are ready to seek another job, you will be reminded of the things you accomplished since the last resume. Resumes are like personalities; there are many styles and layouts. Fortunately, with today's resources, there are many ways to access great resume templates. You can choose any style that you like as long as it contains the right information.

Cover Letter

If the resume's main purpose is to get you an interview, the main purpose of the cover letter is to get the potential employer to actually read your resume. Your cover letter should grab the potential employer's attention. This is not an easy task because employers typically scan the cover letter, giving it just a few seconds of their time. Therefore, just like your resume, the cover letter must be customized for each employer, concisely stating your experience and accomplishments as they relate to the job

---

5-2: Find It on the Web

Resume templates and guidelines are easy to find with a quick Internet search, but here are five options to get you started:

- About.com/Job Searching: http://www.about.com
- Massage-Certification/Massage Jobs: http://www.massage-certification.com
- Resume-Resource: http://www.resume-resource.com
- Resume Templates: http://www.resumetemplates.org
- Sample Resume Templates: http://www.sampleresumetemplates.com

Your Name Here
Address • Phone • E-mail

"When the body gets working appropriately, the forces of gravity can flow through. Then, spontaneously, the body heals itself." ~ Ida Rolf

Professional Profile

I am a licensed massage therapist highly skilled in several modalities with a deep understanding of the softer client skills required to deliver an amazing massage experience. The massage modalities I have the highest level of skill and passion for are deep-tissue and Thai massage. I have over 6 years of hands-on experience in spas and massage clinics. I truly understand what it takes to deliver a great massage for each client and my rebook rate is evidence of that.

Abilities and Qualifications

Massage Therapy
- Specialization and advanced certification in deep-tissue and Thai massage
- Utilize the intake to ensure I understand what type of massage each client is looking to receive and then deliver to their requests
- High level of understanding for anatomy and soft tissue allowing me to educate my clients in a professional manner
- Communicate as needed throughout a session to ensure the client is having a great massage and to educate at timely stages

Customer Service
- Understand the nuances of what allows a client to relax and enjoy their massage, such as draping, delivering the type of massage the client has asked for, checking in on pressure, and maintaining a healthy therapeutic environment
- Comfortable with educating the client on their personal experience and how regular massage can benefit them
- Confident with asking for return visits in a professional, educational, and authentic way

Education and Associations

- Graduated from (school name) a 600-hour program
- Advanced certification in (deep-tissue training) and (Thai training). xx hrs.
- Additional training in sports massage and hot stone work
- Member of the American Massage Therapy Association
- CPR certified

Work History

Employer Name, Location   Dates of employment

Figure 5–5   A resume's job is to get you an interview and therefore should be neat, clean, easy-to-scan, and yet stand out from the rest.

you are seeking. Just like in sales, emphasize the benefits of hiring you by highlighting the important contributions you can make. Also explain why you want to work at that specific company and do that specific job, and state why you are the best choice for the position. Let your personality and interest come through in the cover letter.

Interviewing

Hopefully your fabulous cover letter and resume land you the all-important job interview. It can be nerve-wracking preparing for an interview, but knowing what is expected of a good interviewee can help ease discomfort. How you interact with the interviewer is probably more important than how many deep-tissue techniques you know. Knowing this, the more prepared you are, the more relaxed and natural you can be. Interpersonal "chemistry" is vital, which is why interviews are so critical (Fig. 5–6). As an employee, you will always represent the company you work for. If you have difficulty interacting, communicating, and answering questions, your interviewer can assume you will be the same with their clients.

Timeliness

Arrive for your interview 10 to 15 minutes before the scheduled time. If you are unsure of how to get there, take time in advance to plan your route or even test-drive it. Being tardy on your first interview is a kiss of death for a future with the company. It never fails that when you need to be somewhere at an exact time, every stoplight is red.

The other end of the spectrum regarding timing is making sure you have scheduled enough time for the interview. Although it does not demonstrate good professional etiquette on the part of the interviewer, sometimes situations arise that cause interviews to start late. There are a variety of reasons you may stay later than expected for an interview, so carefully plan any personal commitments following the interview. You do not want to rush off before the interview is over to pick up children, go to another job, or leave to make a client appointment.

First Impressions

There are a couple of facts to consider as you prepare for your interview. First, you have exactly 2 seconds to make a first physical impression. Go ahead and count it out: one ... pause ... two ... pause. You have just cemented a prospective employer with a lasting impression. Hopefully you have taken care with your appearance, which counts for a lot.

Imagine yourself being greeted by your interviewer, and your cell phone rings just as she walks up with her hand extended. Or, as you are shaking hands, you realize your hands are wet from

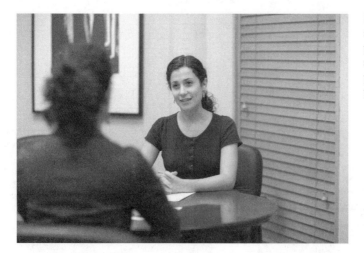

Figure 5–6 Remember to arrive a few minutes early to your interview, pay close attention to how you present yourself, and be prepared for your interview.

See Worksheet 5-4 a recent washing. Take care of all these details in advance, and make sure to practice introducing yourself.

Appearance

Consider the type of employer and purpose of the interview as you plan what to wear. For a practical interview, you will want to wear professional clothing that lets you comfortably perform a massage. If you are interviewing with a high-end spa, consider taking your dress style up. Employers rarely complain about prospective employees showing up too well dressed. As an employee, you will most likely wear a uniform, so choose practicality over creativity when you dress for your interview. Use your spare time to show the world what a creative, expressive person you are. To make a great first impression at an interview, think moderation (Box 5.4).

Body Language

Stay aware of what your body is communicating during the entire interview process. Studies show that more than 80% of communication is nonverbal. People constantly form opinions based on what they see the body doing, regardless of what the mouth is saying. Here are some quick ways to avoid nonverbal disasters:

1. Keep your arms open and loose. Crossed arms indicate defensiveness or resistance.
2. Avoid rubbing your nose. This can imply deception or poor hygiene.
3. Honor personal space. Do not move in too closely or touch someone or their things (e.g., papers, photos, books) without permission.
4. Point your feet away from a door. Pointing feet toward the door may communicate a desire to escape.
5. Avoid slumping or slouching. This may communicate laziness or lack of interest.
6. Pay attention to head nodding. Nodding your head up and down too much may indicate you are a pushover, whereas complete lack of nodding indicates skepticism.
7. Be aware of your facial expressions to ensure you present an open and positive image. Avoid frowning or crunching your eyebrows together. Instead, keep your eyes soft, with a very slight upward curve to the corners of your lips.

Questions to Expect

During the initial interview, the prospective employer assesses whether you are a fit for the open position. This means assessing not only your experience but also how you respond to questions in the moment. Employers want to observe how you communicate and get a feel for your presence

---

Box 5.4 Interview Appearance Tips

Do have:

- Clean, well-fitted clothing
- Minimal piercings and tattoos
- Closed-toed shoes or nice sandals
- Tidy, well-groomed hair
- Nails that are short, clean, and free of nail polish

Don't wear:

- Heavy, overpowering perfume or cologne
- Clothing that shows excessive cleavage
- Miniskirts or shorts
- A lot of accessories

and your ability to connect. Pay close attention to what the interviewer is saying. If you are constantly thinking about what you are going to say next, you miss what they are saying now.

There is no limit to the number or types of questions you may be asked in an interview. The experience can be nerve-wracking, but you can keep your nerves from getting the best of you. Remember that you are also there to find out information. You are both deciding whether or not you would be a good fit for the position. Essentially, both you and the employer are aiming for the same goal during the interview, although from different angles. Although you don't know the specific questions you may be asked, there are ways to prepare for a successful interview.

First, as you have read, knowing who you are, your values, and your goals can go a long way in helping you have a successful interview. Be prepared to tell the employer who you are as a person, including areas of strength and areas needing improvement and how you plan to improve them. You should also be able to demonstrate your positive personality traits that will be important to this position. Know why you want this particular job. Be familiar with the specific and special knowledge, experience, or abilities you bring to the table. Going into the interview, you should also be prepared to articulate a few things about yourself that set you apart from the rest.

Second, pick out some potential questions and practice answering them (Box 5.5). You will probably be asked at least some version of the most popular interview questions. Consider how to answer the questions in a positive manner, especially those about your areas of improvement. Another way to select potential questions is to put yourself in the shoes of the interviewer. What would you like to know about a potential employee and what would be most important? Think of responses that tie in your best experiences and achievements.

Box 5.5 Potential Interview Questions

- Tell me why you have chosen massage therapy as a profession.
- Why do you think you want to work in a [spa, chiropractic, medical] environment?
- What additional training have you taken to stay current with massage techniques?
- What aspects of massage are you most passionate about?
- What traits do you possess that would make you a good fit for our massage team?
- What do you think clients would say are the most important aspects of a massage therapy session?
- What do you find challenging about being a massage therapist?
- Professionally, what has been your most significant achievement? Why was it so significant to you?
- What is your greatest success?
- How do you define success?
- What is the most difficult work-related situation you have ever faced? How did you handle it?
- Give me an example of a situation in which things were not going well. What role did you play? Why did it happen?
- Give me an example of a time when your work was criticized. How did you deal with it? Have you received this type of criticism more than once?
- What has been your greatest obstacle? How did you overcome it?
- Can you give me an example of when you went the "extra mile?"
- What have you done to show that you are qualified for this job?
- Thinking about your last position, what was your favorite thing to do? What was your least favorite?
- What motivates you to put forth your greatest effort? Can you give me an example of when this happened most recently?
- Other than massage, what are you passionate about?
- What qualifications should a successful person in your career field possess?
- Elaborate on your current qualifications and those you hope to develop in the future.
- What would you like for me to tell you about this job?

Confidence is not something you can force, but thinking through potential questions, practicing, and role-playing with your peers will help you to build your confidence. One word of caution, however: avoid sounding like you are reciting memorized answers. You want to be prepared, but authentic—not rehearsed and robotic.

Lastly, recognize that some employers are not good interviewers. Without meaning to, they can make an interview difficult. If you know the main points you want to get across, find ways to communicate these, even if the interviewer isn't giving you the chance. If you have not been able to state the most important reason they should hire you, take that opportunity at the end of the interview. Before you leave, let the interviewer know that you would like to share a few final points about yourself.

Questions to Ask During Your Interview

During the interview, plan on asking effective, informative questions (Box 5.6). If you have no previous management experience, you will likely join a massage team of other therapists, so you may inquire about the structure of the massage team. You can also ask about seniority, promotional opportunities, how the hours are allocated, and what the team dynamic is like.

It is a guarantee that as an employee you will report to someone in a higher position than you. The interview is a great time to ask about the reporting structure. If your future boss is not interviewing you, ask to be introduced to him or her before you are hired. The number one reason that people leave their jobs is because of a difficult relationship with their direct boss. Taking the time to meet this person can save you future headaches, if you discover up front they do not match your style.

You can also ask questions demonstrating your knowledge of the position. For example, many employers expect employees to perform additional duties during their slow times, thus helping the department function smoothly. It is important you express your willingness to help the entire team by learning other duties. Asking the right questions during an interview will show enthusiasm and a readiness to help.

Managers want to know that their employees seek to provide excellent service. To provide excellent service, one must know the customer. Showing interest by asking questions about the client during the interview is a great first step in communicating that you care about customer satisfaction.

Just as there are great questions to ask during an interview, there are also areas to be avoided. Use caution when asking about pay, time-off, and sick policies. If you have not built credibility early in the interview, these questions may infer you are interested only in personal gain. There will be plenty of time to explore these things once you make a great impression. If what they have to offer is not appealing, then you can always decide not to work there during the next phase of the interview process.

Box 5.6 Sample Questions to Ask During an Interview

- In your opinion, which traits most help employees here be successful?
- Can you please describe the massage team you have in place?
- What is most important for a new employee to do to join the team?
- For your massage [clients, guests, or customers], what do you feel are the most important things to deliver every time?
- Are there opportunities to learn tasks within other departments so that I can assist when needed?
- What is your favorite part of working here?
- What is the average tenure of a massage therapist?
- Why do employees typically stay employed here? Why do they typically leave?
- How do you or your company define success?
- What is the company's most important core value?
- Can you describe your ideal candidate to fill this position?

Practical

For massage therapists, part of the interview process is to perform a "practical" interview, which is providing a massage for your prospective employer so that the employer may evaluate your ability. When scheduling the initial interview, you should ask whether or not a practical is part of the interview. This way, you are prepared to provide the massage. Even if you are told that a practical is not part of the initial interview, you should still be prepared in case the opportunity presents itself during the interview. This is an important point to keep in mind when deciding what to wear to the interview and when planning personal commitments after the interview. Here are a few pointers to keep in mind for a successful practical:

- Treat the practical as if it were an actual massage. If allowed, take the time to perform an intake so that you can demonstrate your communication techniques.
- Check in on the pressure early so that the recipient knows you have his comfort in mind.
- With permission, educate the interviewer about her body while you do the work. This will demonstrate your knowledge while you are performing the skill.
- The time you are allowed can vary from 15 minutes to a full-hour session, so ask the recipient what he would most like to see demonstrated.
- Not all massage rooms are created equal, so do your best with the space provided.
- Be aware that you may be asked to use equipment and supplies that are different from what you are used to. If this is the case, explain that the equipment is new to you and ask questions if needed.
- If possible, schedule a massage at the facility before your interview. This way, you will get to see the room and equipment. Plus, you can mention this during your interview to show your initiative and interest.

YOUR CAREER OPTIONS AS A MASSAGE EMPLOYEE

Today, massage therapists have more choices than ever when it comes to employers. This wide variety will allow you to find an environment that fits your personality, goals, and passions. This section covers the prospective employer options of **spas**, massage centers and franchises, wellness centers, healthcare settings, and special-interests groups. But first, let us take a look at the overall industry from a general employment perspective.

Number of Massage Therapists

According to the U.S. Bureau of Labor Statistics (BLS) *Occupational Outlook Handbook, 2010-11 Edition,* there were approximately 122,400 massage therapist jobs in 2008.[2] The AMTA reports a substantially higher number, estimating more than 280,000 massage therapists in the United States.[3,4]

Growth

The BLS expects employment of massage therapists to increase by 19% from 2008 to 2018, faster than the average for all occupations. This expected job growth is partly because people are becoming more aware of the benefits of massage. Also, massage is offered in many new places. Workplace massage is becoming a more common employee benefit, and massage services are increasingly provided in nursing homes and assisted living facilities.[2] In fact, in 2007, the Society for Human Resource Management reported that 13% of its member companies offered massage to their employees. *Working Mother* also reported that 77% of their top 100 U.S. companies offered massage at work.[5]

> The BLS expects employment of massage therapists to increase by 19% from 2008 to 2018, faster than the average for all occupations.

Compensation and Benefits

How much can you expect to earn? According to the BLS, in May 2009, the mean hourly wage for massage therapists was $19.13. The Bureau points out that, generally, massage therapists earn at least a portion of their income from gratuities, except for those who work in a medical setting, where consumers do not typically provide tips.[2] However, AMTA reports a much higher earning average at $41.50 per hour. They have also seen an increase in the average gratuity paid over the years.[3]

To help estimate earning potential, it is helpful to know that massage therapists work an average of around 20 hours a week. Therapists working in spas and fitness clubs typically work the most hours per week.[3] Many massage therapists supplement their earnings by working more than one job.

Only 16% of massage therapists receive health insurance benefits.[3] This is probably because many are independent contractors working only part-time as massage therapists or working for small businesses that cannot afford to pay for health-care coverage. However, most companies offer some sort of benefits package. Benefits can include health and life insurance, paid time off (e.g., holidays, vacations), workers' compensation coverage, disability plans, retirement savings plans, discounted services, and training.

WHERE MASSAGE THERAPISTS WORK

The most common workplace for employed massage therapists is a spa, followed by a health-care setting. In 2008, 29% of massage therapists reported they were employed at a spa or salon, 27% reported working in a health-care setting, and 8% indicated they worked in a health club.[3]

With that general overview of the industry, let us now take a closer look at the largest categories of employers and some of the fastest growing.

Spas

The largest employer of massage therapists is the spa industry, which continues to grow. According to the International Spa Association (ISPA), a spa is devoted to enhancing overall well-being through professional services that encourage the renewal of mind, body, and spirit. ISPA categorizes spas into seven primary categories, which are club, cruise, day, destination, medical, mineral springs, and resort/hotel.

To help you get a feel for the spa industry and the opportunities available for massage therapists, here are some interesting facts from the *ISPA 2007 and 2010 US Spa Industry Study:*

- Eighty-six percent of all U.S. spas offer massage, and it is, along with facials, one of the primary treatments in the spa industry.
- The top massage services offered by spas are deep-tissue/sports, Swedish, pregnancy; stone; reflexology, and couples massage (Fig. 5–7).
- The average spa employs 16 staff.
- Fifty-four percent of all U.S. spas had a vacant massage therapist position in 2007—the highest of any spa position.
- There were an estimated 24,000 open massage therapist positions in the spa industry in 2007.
- The average charge for a massage in a U.S. spa in 2010 was $85.

About 80% of all spas are day spas. The next largest categories are resort/hotel spas (9%) and medical spas (9%).[8]

Growth Potential

Spas offer a wide range of professional opportunities for massage therapists. You may have the opportunity to take on more responsibilities and roles, such as management, front desk, retail, training, and operations. In fact, most spa therapists do not spend 100% of their time providing treatments; they perform other functions, such as working the front desk or cleaning the relaxation room. This is great if you like the variety, but is not for everyone.

If you work in a resort/hotel or club spa, you can explore other related fields, such as hospitality, culinary arts, or fitness. If you work in a cruise ship spa, you get to see opportunities around the world. If you are interested in management, there are several opportunities available within most spas, depending on the size and type of facility. Most spas have a lead therapist, who may manage other spa therapists, create the schedule, hire new staff, and perform other management functions. Spas also usually have a structure consisting of a spa director and assistant spa director, who are responsible for the operations and administration for the entire facility—not just massage.

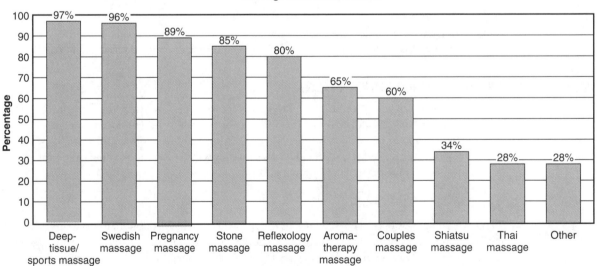

Massage Treatments Offered

Figure 5–7   The top massage services offered by spas are deep-tissue/sports (97%), Swedish (96%); pregnancy (89%), stone (85%); reflexology (80%), and aromatherapy (65%). (Source: International SPA Association 2007 Spa Industry Study.)

Compensation and Benefits

According to the ISPA 2009 US Spa Compensation Study, day and medical spas provided the lowest wages, and resort/hotels provided the highest wages.[9] Benefits offered within the industry can depend on the type of organization you work for as well as whether or not you are a full-time or part-time employee. Some common benefits include health and life insurance, professional liability coverage, retirement savings benefits, paid time off, training and education opportunities, discounted or free services and products, and use of facilities such as the pool and exercise equipment.

Massage Centers and Franchises

You may have noticed that there are a growing number of businesses whose main service is providing massage. Massage centers or franchises can now be found in many urban areas, as well as airports, throughout the United States. These businesses are usually owned by a nonmassage business person and typically employ massage therapists, front-desk workers, and someone to manage the administration and operation of the facility.

Massage centers or **clinics** can have several different business structures. The most common one is a business owned by a person or group of persons who employ or subcontract massage therapists.

According to the Associated Bodywork and Massage Professional (ABMP), "A massage clinic may have a very specific focus or it may take a broad approach to attracting clients. Some clinics set themselves apart by focusing on a select client group, such as pregnant women, athletes, or individuals with soft tissue injuries or a pathology. Other clinics take a wellness approach and offer a little of everything. A clinic may spotlight a specific modality such as reflexology, neuromuscular therapy, Eastern bodywork, or myofascial massage."[10]

Massage franchises or **chains** also focus on providing massage, but their structure is different from a locally owned massage center. National massage chains are growing throughout the United States, with the launch of new franchises as well as expansions of existing franchises. Seeing the growth of spas and the consumer acceptance of massage, these organizations have found a niche in the market—offering a branded product in numerous locations. As opposed to spas, these companies offer only massage, although some firms are testing locations that offer more traditional spa services in addition. Some massage therapists have a poor view of national massage chains, seeing them as detrimental to the profession. But as these chains continue to grow, many massage therapists see them as a place to get steady employment and potential benefits."[3]

> "As opposed to spas, [massage franchises] offer only massage, although some firms are testing locations that offer more traditional spa services in addition."
> —AMTA

Growth Potential

Locally owned massage centers are growing in popularity, but the expanding franchise niche has great future employment potential. Thanks to the availability of lower-priced massages, lots of new consumers have been introduced to massage. In addition, many centers and chains are now taking

---

5-4: Find It on the Web

For more information on spas and the various categories, visit:

- Day Spa Association (DSA): http://www.dayspaassociation.com
- Destination Spa Group (DSG): http://www.destinationspagroup.com
- International SPA Association (ISPA): http://www.experienceispa.com
- Medical Spa Association: http://www.medicalspaassociation.org
- Medical Spa Society: http://www.medicalspasociety.com

(Continued on page 165)

Peer Profile 5–1

Michele Merhib Maruniak, RMT
Founder, Elements Therapeutic Massage
Denver, CO

In 1998, after going through some tough times, I decided I needed something positive to focus on. Recognizing I wasn't as in shape as I could be, I decided to focus on my fitness level and prepare for a mini-triathlon! My personal trainer recommended a massage as part of my training regimen. I was immediately hooked, I LOVED receiving massage!

My massage therapist was in her early 50s and was ready to retire. For a year, she kept insisting that I was the right person to buy her business ... to which I kept reminding her that I was an Occupational Therapist and not trained in massage therapy. Honestly, at the same time, I was becoming disillusioned with Corporate America, HMOs, and my position as director of a Rehab Department. The thought that working with clients who were proactive about their health and wellness was intriguing.

I took a weekend introductory course to massage therapy, and by Saturday's lunch break I had decided I would be starting massage school in 2 days (on Monday). After I graduated, I revisited my massage therapist and decided to purchase her business. This included a rental space at a country club, a list of clients, a massage table, and a massage chair. I ran my own business and was happy creating my own schedule and attracting clients who needed the skills and style of massage I was offering. After a year and a half of working in this bliss, the country club sold, and I lost my first business location.

At the time, there was no such thing as a massage franchise, and many of my classmates were seeking a place to work. I chose to open a small studio in 2002 that originally was going to be a wellness center. We offered Reiki, reflexology, acupuncture, and massage therapy. Consumers were not ready for a wellness center, but they were coming in abundance for deep-tissue therapeutic massage.

I had to let go of my dream of a wellness center and focus on what consumers were demanding: a great therapeutic massage at a reasonable price and with personal customer service. At the same time, I found that therapists were looking for a place to work where they were respected and where clients were brought in for them. Many magnificent massage therapists may not be interested in marketing or running a business. Many have found, as I did, that it distracts you from being a great massage therapist. What I also brought to my first business was the belief that employees want to know the expectations of employment up front, that they crave continuing education, and that they want to have a full schedule of clients.

Within 2 years of opening my first location, we were providing more than 650 massages per month in a four-room massage studio. I opened a second location in 2005 and learned how to systemize my business with the help a business coach. Two companies approached me within 6 months of one another and were interested in taking my business model nationwide.

My business brain said, "Yes this makes sense." My emotional brain said, "But you got out of the corporate world, so are you sure you want to reenter it?" As the negotiations moved forward, I could see how I could move from being a practitioner in a massage room (sometimes up to 30-plus hours a week) to influencing how employees were treated in the massage profession, something I did not have an effect on in my previous career.

I chose to move forward with a company that mirrored my values and respected my opinions as a massage therapist and as someone who had managed massage therapists. Many of the values I consider important are the basis of Elements Therapeutic Massage's "Employer of Choice" system.

Our franchise owners buy an Elements studio because they have a core belief in massage or a personal experience with massage therapy that has drawn them to our business model. These owners are trained at our corporate support center by massage therapists. It helps our owners better understand the perspective of a massage therapist. Currently, Elements Therapeutic Massage has almost 100 studios across the United States. We are dedicated to elevating the level of massage in the industry as well as providing a great educational place to work for therapists.

advantage of the growth in demand for corporate wellness and are creating packages with local businesses. As more players enter this market and existing facilities expand, the quantity and quality of these businesses will determine their impact on future employment opportunities for massage therapists.

Compensation and Benefits

Broad compensation data are not available for this niche in the industry, but Massage Envy, a large massage franchise, says on its website that a full-time therapist can average between $32,000 and $39,000 annually.[11] We can also make some general assumptions based on what we know about business structures. For a variety of reasons, massage chains and centers are able to cut or share expenses, making the businesses themselves more profitable. In some cases, this can translate to higher earning potential for employees. However, how much the therapist is paid depends a great deal on the amount the customer is charged for the massage, quality of the business, quantity of client bookings, and many other factors. Some massage chains promote affordable or low-cost massages. With these facilities, you can expect lower wages but potentially high volume. Some facilities provide incentives and commission based on how often therapists are requested by clients, membership sales, performance reviews, and other criteria.

Most of the chains are independently owned and operated, so compensation and benefits vary, but many centers and chains will provide training, paid time off, health benefit options, and retirement savings options. Another benefit of some franchises is that massage therapists perform only massage. Unlike the spa environment, they are not expected to clean the waiting rooms, handle paperwork, or work the front desk (Box 5.7).

Box 5.7 Massage Centers/Franchises

Here are some of the main players in the massage franchise market:

- Massage Envy, a franchise concept that offers a subscription-based model, is fast becoming a large employer of massage therapists. Since 2002, Massage Envy has grown from one location in Arizona to more than 850 clinics. Massage Envy is the largest single employer of massage therapists in the United States.
- Elements Therapeutic Massage also looks to become a major franchise in the massage therapy industry. This company currently has more than 100 wellness studios. Elements Therapeutic Massage places a strong focus on the therapeutic nature of massage and is a great fit for therapists specializing in deep-tissue and other therapeutic modalities.
- XPressSpa is now located in many airports throughout the country. XpressSpa offers massage services as well as some spa services.

Other companies expanding in the market include the following:

- The Great American Backrub
- The Great Metropolitan Backrub
- Hand & Stone Massage and Facial Spa
- Massage Green
- Massage Heights[3]

Wellness Centers

Wellness centers focus on the whole person—mind, body, and spirit. They typically focus on wellness and staying healthy, but many clients come for treatment of various ailments. According to ABMP, wellness centers "emphasize the importance of paying attention to the body, mind, and spirit to promote and maintain optimum health. In this integrative medical setting, the massage therapist is one of many different types of wellness professionals. Others working at the center may include a chiropractor, physical therapist, nutritionist, naturopathic doctor, meditation leader, spiritual counselor, allopathic doctor, fitness trainer, counselor, yoga instructor, life coach, hypnotherapist, or esthetician. Wellness centers are found in many different types of locations and may be included on a college campus, in a community center, at a large corporation, as part of a hospital, in gyms, in retirement homes, or as a stand-alone facility similar to a spa."[10]

Growth Potential

Although there are limited data available on wellness centers, they have a great deal of growth potential. Consumers are increasingly interested in healthier lifestyles and complementary and alternative medicine (CAM). There are estimates that almost 4 out of 10 adults have used some type of CAM. This number is growing—specifically for the use of massage therapy as a form of wellness and treatment.

According to a report published by the National Center for Health Statistics, "Generally, persons who choose CAM approaches are seeking ways to improve their health and well-being or to relieve symptoms associated with chronic, even terminal, illnesses or the side effects of conventional treatments for them. Other reasons for choosing to use CAM include having a holistic health philosophy or a transformational experience that changes one's world view, and wanting greater control over one's own health. Many types of CAM practitioners treat not only the physical and biochemical manifestations of illness, but also the nutritional, emotional, social, and spiritual context in which the illness arises."[12]

Compensation and Benefits

Wellness center wages and benefits vary greatly by the facility and location, and national averages are not available. However, ABMP points out in its career guide, "One of the exciting things about working in a wellness center is that therapists are able to learn from other health care providers. They are exposed to new ideas for achieving health. This gives them a broader perspective when dealing with individual clients and informs their treatment choices."[10]

Health-Care Settings

Many health-care facilities employ massage therapists, including hospitals, physical therapy and rehabilitation clinics, chiropractic offices, cancer centers, and sports medicine clinics. AMTA reports that 27% of its therapists work in a health-care setting.[3]

In 2008, the American Hospital Association (AHA) released the results of their *2007 Complementary and Alternative Medicine Survey,* which reported on the hospitals that offer massage. These clients' reasons for massage included the following:

1. Pain management (66%)
2. For cancer patients (57%)
3. Pregnancy (55%)
4. Part of physical therapy (53%)
5. For mobility/movement training (45%)
6. Palliative care (41%)[3]

With the growth in both health care and massage, combined with the convergence of the two, there are substantial employment opportunities in traditional health care.

5-5: Find It on the Web

For more information on wellness centers, fitness centers, and complementary and alternative medicine, use these Web resources:

- Academic Consortium for Complementary and Alternative Health Care (ACCAH): http://www.accahc.org
- Alternative Therapy Association (ATA): http://www.alternativebalance.net
- American Association of Integrative Medicine (AAIM): http://www.aaimedicine.com
- American College of Sports Medicine (ACSM): http://www.acsm.org
- IDEA Health and Fitness Association (IDEA): http://www.ideafit.com
- Integrative Healthcare Association (IHA): http://www.iha.org/
- International Fitness Professionals Association (IFPA): http://www.ifpa-fitness.com
- International Health, Racquet and Sportsclub Association: http://www.ihrsa.org
- International Society for Complementary Medicine Research (ISCMR): http://www.iscmr.org
- Medical Wellness Association (MWA): http:www.medicalwellnessassociation.com
- National Center for Homeopathy (NCH): http://nationalcenterforhomeopathy.org

Growth Potential

The BLS reports in their *Career Guide to Industries, 2010-11 Edition on Health Care* that 10 of the 20 fastest growing occupations are health care related.[2] Also, as CAM grows, fields such as chiropractic care are also growing. These promising areas are also frequent employers of massage therapists.

According to AMTA, "health care is now a major arena that affects the demand for and acceptance of massage therapy. As massage becomes more integrated by health care providers in the United States, this will open up new opportunities for massage therapists.[3]

Compensation and Benefits

Therapists in a health-care environment typically do not earn gratuities, and their wages vary by facility and type of facility. A hospital setting is more likely to offer a wider range of benefits than a smaller, office-type setting. One of the benefits of working in a health-care environment is exposure to related health-care and wellness fields. However, AMTA points out that the growth in health care may be a primary reason that therapists leave massage therapy for related health-care careers.[3]

Special-Interests Groups

Special-interests massage opens up the field in new and exciting ways. Although special-interests massage is not yet a clearly defined employment niche within the massage industry, it is important to note that as massage therapy grows, so does the diversity of clients and potential clients. For massage therapists who have special interests, sometimes the two can be combined. ABMP highlights several in their career guide to massage therapy:

"**Geriatric Massage.** Geriatric massage supports healthy aging and may provide relief from some symptoms of age related health problems. Work with elderly clients requires the therapist to develop specialized understanding. The therapist must pay close attention to the client's medications and the ways they might interact with massage. These clients may have difficulty feeling comfortable for a full hour treatment, and the treatment time may need to be adjusted. As with all clients, the therapist must understand all existing medical conditions and any adaptive measures required.

(Continued on page 169)

Peer Profile 5–2

Ask the Expert

Lori Hutchinson
Hutchinson Consulting

Question:

What tips would you give to massage therapy students on things they can start doing now to help get them hired when they graduate?

Response:

- Take initiative to know yourself well—use some of these resources to assist you:
  - http://www.careersystemsinternational.com
  - http://www.iMapMyCareer.com
  - http://www.kiersey.com
  - http://www.caliperonline.com
  - http://www.learningfromexperience.com
  - http://www.upmo.com
  - http://www.mindtools.com
  - http://www.mydiscprofile.com
  - http://www.businessballs.com
  - http://www.authentichappiness.sas.upenn.edu
  - http://www.myskillsprofile.com
- Foster relationships with as many people in the massage/spa/fitness arenas as possible
- Attend industry networking opportunities in your area to meet potential employers and other massage therapists
- Participate in and maximize resources found within the spa community's associations (e.g., ISPA, AMTA)
- Commit to being a lifelong learner so that you always grow your knowledge
- Be positively and distinctively different in your school classroom because of your interest and behavior
- Leave your comfort zone and challenge yourself
- Select a role model to emulate and build a relationship with that individual
- Be informed—research industry news and trends
- Create a binder of accomplishments

Question:

Can you share advice on how massage therapists can find a good employment fit and the right employer?

Response:

Research, research, and more research. Identify companies that are attractive to you, then complete research through the following means to figure out if your personality matches their work culture. Companies are now more transparent about whom they are and what they offer staff members. Review the companies' websites, go visit them, Google them, talk to people who have worked for them in the past or work there now. See if you can have an informational interview with a Human Resources representative to find out answers to your questions. Speak to other massage providers about where they have worked and where they recommend (or not). Speak to your role models who may have some expert advice for you. Listen to your gut when you consider all of the information you have amassed.

Question:

What top five things must therapists do to make themselves standout above the rest?

Response:

1. Make certain your resume is perfect in every single detail. Don't complete a resume in an hour or two. Work on it over a few days, provide it to trusted friends to review and critique. Don't forget to include identification statements (company facts) about where you have worked in the past and add any accomplishments using objective (dollar signs, numbers, percentages) measurements if possible.
2. Be able to articulate your passion for being a massage therapist and why you have chosen this career. Practice your speech with trusted advisors who may provide you some excellent feedback.
3. Be flexible in your work schedule availability. Many companies need massage therapists to work on weekends and holidays, so hopefully you can be open to working on these days.
4. Demonstrate your interest in working for a specific company that you have thoroughly researched. Be able to explain in detail why the potential employer's company matches your personality and interest.
5. Be confident about why you will be a terrific massage therapist and be prepared to explain why you are able to provide an excellent massage.

Note:

Lori founded Hutchinson Consulting, and now Lori and a staff of four people, plus her husband/partner, Bill, provide spas and resorts/hotels with management recruiting services. Lori was certified in 1999 as a Senior Professional in Human Resources; she has a Bachelor's Degree in Social Work and Sociology from the University of Iowa. Lori has served as a Board Member on the ISPA Board of Directors.

5-6: Find It on the Web

For more information on medical-related massage therapy positions and facilities, use these Web resources:

- American Association of Naturopathic Physicians (AANP): http://www.naturopathic.org
- American Chiropractic Association (ACA): http://www.acatoday.org
- American Holistic Medical Association (AHMA): http://www.holisticmedicine.org
- American Hospital Association (AHA): http://www.aha.org
- American Institute of Naturopathic Medicine (AINM): http://www.ainm.org
- American Manual Medical Association (AMMA): http://www.americanmanualmedicine.com
- American Naturopathic Medical Association (ANMA): http://www.anma.org
- American Orthopaedic Society for Sports Medicine (AOSSM): http://www.sportsmed.org
- Hospital Based Massage Network (HBMN): http://www.naturaltouchmarketing.com
- International Association of Health Care Practitioners (IAHP): http://www.iahp.com
- International Chiropractors Association (ICA): http://www.chiropractic.org
- Joint Commission on Accreditation of Health Care Organizations (JCAHO): http://www.jcaho.org
- National Association of Nurse Massage Therapists (NANMT): http://www.nanmt.org
- Planetree: http://www.planetree.org

Pregnancy Massage. A therapist may specialize in prenatal and postnatal massage to work with pregnant woman and infants. Massage can provide relief from the aches and pains of a pregnant body, so long as the therapist understands how to position the client properly and deliver appropriate techniques. Most schools cover basic pregnancy massage; many offer advanced training classes in pregnancy and infant massage as continuing education.

Sports Massage. Athletes recognize that massage increases flexibility, supports the recovery process from events or hard training sessions, and improves performance. Therapists who want to move into this area will need to have a thorough understanding of muscles and their functions. They must also understand which muscles are being stressed in a particular sport; runners will likely benefit from a different approach to massage than swimmers.

Other Areas of Specialization include work with the chronically ill, physically challenged, and terminally ill, as well as mental health issues and with animals."[10]

A somewhat exotic career can develop if you decide to seek employment overseas or on a cruise ship. Working for a cruise line is often like working for a spa. You will be dealing with guests who are on vacation and most likely are seeking a pampering experience. Your hours may be long since you are always aboard the ship, but there are many perks the cruise line may offer you. If you are the adventurous type, it is worth looking into.

See Worksheet 5-5

CHAPTER SUMMARY

Becoming an employee is an excellent way to gain experience and continue your education while earning a living. In addition, employment opportunities are growing for massage therapists in a variety of exciting and diverse arenas. However, this path must be one that aligns with your goals. This is why it is imperative to your success that you fully evaluate whether becoming an employee is your best professional route.

If you determine that being employed at a company is your path, then gather further knowledge about yourself, research potential employers, and become fully prepared to build an attention-grabbing resume and ace your interviews. Once hired, you must continue to ensure your success by being flexible and working to strengthen your knowledge, abilities, and skills as well as develop professional relationships.

BIBLIOGRAPHY

1. American Massage Therapy Association. (n.d.). *Starting a Career in Massage Therapy: What You Need to Know.* Retrieved from http://www.amtamassage.org/becometherapist/starting.html.
2. U.S. Department of Labor, Bureau of Labor Statistics. (2009, December 17). *Occupational Outlook Handbook, 2010-11 Edition.* Retrieved from http://www.bls.gov/oco/ocos295.htm.
3. American Massage Therapy Association. (2009). *AMTA 2009 Massage Industry Research Report.* Evanston, IL: American Massage Therapy Association.
4. American Massage Therapy Association. (n.d.). *Demographic Study of AMTA Members.* Retrieved from http://www.amtamassage.org/news/03MemberDemographics.html.
5. Associated Bodywork and Massage Professionals. (2009, September). *Massage Therapy Fast Facts.* Retrieved from http://www.massagetherapy.com/media/metricscharacteristics.php
6. Associated Bodywork and Massage Professionals. (n.d.). *Massage Profession Metrics.* Retrieved from http://www.massagetherapy.com/media/metricscharacteristics.php.
7. International SPA Association. (2009). *Industry Stats: The US Spa Industry—Fast Facts.* Retrieved from http://www.experienceispa.com/media/facts-stats/.
8. International SPA Association. (2010). *ISPA 2010 US Spa Industry Study.* Lexington, KY: International SPA Association.

9. International SPA Association. (2009). *ISPA 2009 US Spa Compensation Study.* Lexington, KY: International SPA Association.
10. Associated Bodywork and Massage Professionals. (n.d.). *Careers.* Retrieved from http://www.massagetherapy.com/careers/..
11. Massage Envy. (n.d.). *Choosing Massage Envy.* Retrieved from http://www.massageenvycareers.com/.
12. Barnes, P., Bloom, B., & Nahin, R. (2008, December). *National Health Statistics Report: Complementary and Alternative Medicine Use Among Adults and Children: United States, 2007.* Hyattsville, MD: National Center for Health Statistics.

REVIEW QUESTIONS

1. **What is a benefit of starting your massage career as an employee versus an independent contractor or entrepreneur?**
   a. Higher income potential
   b. Building physical stamina and professional skills
   c. Setting your own schedule
   d. Determining the fees you charged for massage

2. **What is a primary reason some managers prefer employees more than independent contractors?**
   a. It is harder to create a unified team with independent contractors
   b. Employees typically come in with a higher level of ability
   c. It is easier to create consistent service with employees
   d. Both a & c

3. **Which of the following is *not* a reality of employment?**
   a. Adherence to mandated policies and procedures
   b. Paid educational and training opportunities
   c. Teamwork and relationship development
   d. Consistent job duties and opportunities

4. **Why do companies develop and enforce policies and procedures?**
   a. To reinforce the image of the company and ensure consistency
   b. For greater control of their employees
   c. As a tool to use during performance evaluations
   d. Both b & c

5. **Which of the following provides an opportunity for earning more money as an employee?**
   a. Base pay
   b. Variable pay
   c. Not reporting gratuities on your income taxes
   d. As an employee, greater earning potential doesn't exist unless you get an annual increase or promotion

6. **Which of the following is one of the most common benefits offered to therapists from their employers?**
   a. Scheduling flexibility
   b. Medical/health insurance
   c. Workers' compensation and/or disability insurance
   d. Opportunity to work in diverse environments

7. **Which of the following is a scheduling reality for employed massage therapists?**
   a. Massage therapists are not generally on-call
   b. Spas and other employers like to have a significant number of therapists available at the facility for last-minute bookings
   c. If massage appointments are not booked as expected, therapists are released from duty early or assigned other duties for their shift
   d. Massage therapists always know their schedule several weeks in advance

8. **In most facilities, particularly spas, therapists are assigned the same treatment room everyday and do not share it with others.**
   a. True
   b. False

9. **Which of the following is *not* an educational/training reality for employees?**
   a. To receive free training, you may be required to stay with the company for a certain amount of time
   b. Training is limited to technical skills
   c. You are often cross-trained in other areas
   d. Performance evaluations are conducted to provide positive feedback on performance

10. **As an employed massage therapist, which of the following is commonly expected of you between appointments?**
    a. Clean the changing or relaxation areas
    b. Perform facials if they are overbooked in that department
    c. Help with corporate bookkeeping and collecting tax information
    d. Both a & c

11. **What should an employee expect during a formal performance evaluation?**
    a. To review and plan for professional goals with your manager
    b. An annual salary increase, if performance merits
    c. Review knowledge, skills, and abilities of other therapists
    d. As an employee, you shouldn't expect evaluations to occur

12. **What is one of the greatest benefits of being an employee?**
    a. Income potential
    b. Ability to work solo
    c. Frequent performance evaluations
    d. Security

13. **Which of the following is *not* something you need to know about yourself before starting the job search?**
    a. Your personal vision and mission statement
    b. Your core values
    c. Your vision of a dream job
    d. Your knowledge, skills, and abilities

14. **Which of the following variables should you consider when evaluating potential employers?**
    a. Company age, size, and financial portfolio
    b. Company ownership, whom you'd be reporting to, and financial portfolio
    c. Company principles, age, size, and whom you'd be reporting to
    d. Company principles, strategic plan and growth projections

15. **Which of the following are vitally important in a relationship between an employee and their manager?**
    a. Developing a foundation of care and trust
    b. Clearly defined roles and expectations
    c. Similar values and goals
    d. Both a & b

16. **Which of the following is an example of a functional skill?**
    a. Dependability
    b. Punctuality
    c. Management
    d. Self-direction

17. **Which of the following is innate to an individual?**
    a. Knowledge
    b. Skill
    c. Ability
    d. Trait

18. **Which of the following should you do when drafting your resume?**
    a. Focus on actual work duties and responsibilities
    b. Have a friend read and edit your resume
    c. Place your most recent experience first
    d. Start sentences with adverbs and nouns, especially emphasizing "I"

19. **Your ability to interact with an interviewer is probably more important than how many massage techniques you know.**
    a. True
    b. False

20. **To make a great impression at an interview, _____.**
    a. Arrive exactly on time
    b. Ensure your appearance and attire show how creative and expressive you are
    c. Show your interest in the job by asking about the number of vacation and sick days you'll receive
    d. Stay aware of your nonverbal communication to ensure positive messaging

21. Which of the following is an effective and useful way to prepare for an interview?
    a. Practice potential questions and answers until they sound well rehearsed
    b. Draft and be ready to ask effective, informative questions of the interviewer
    c. Be generally familiar with your knowledge, skills, and abilities
    d. Memorize every job description you've ever had so that you can easily repeat prior responsibilities

22. It is appropriate to ask about seniority, promotional opportunities, schedules, and team dynamic during an interview.
    a. True
    b. False

23. What is attributed to the anticipated growth in massage therapy employment opportunities?
    a. The rise of animal and geriatric massage
    b. Increased consumer awareness of the benefits of massage
    c. Increase of massage in new venues
    d. Both B & C

24. In which type of facility is a massage therapist unlikely to generate a lot of income, if any, from gratuities?
    a. Wellness center
    b. Spa
    c. Health-care facility
    d. Massage franchises

25. According to research, approximately how many hours a week does a massage therapist work on average?
    a. 10
    b. 20
    c. 30
    d. 40

26. Which type of facility employs the majority of massage therapists?
    a. Spas
    b. Health-care facilities
    c. Massage franchises
    d. Special-interests groups

27. What is one of the exciting benefits of working in a wellness center?
    a. Therapists only perform massage and don't have to clean or book appointments
    b. Learning from other health-care providers in the complementary and alternative medicine field
    c. Being exposed to new ideas for achieving health
    d. Both b & c

Worksheet 5-1   Employment Realities

The below categories describe some of the realities of employment. Rank each of these items according to its level of importance to you using the following scale: 3 = very important; 2 = somewhat important; 1 = not important. When finished, consider your overall and individual answers to help determine whether the path of the employee is right for you.

_____   Having defined policies and procedures

_____   Set wage

_____   Benefits

_____   Having someone else book your appointment

_____   Schedule is fixed

_____   Uniform

_____   Treatment rooms are set up and paid for

_____   Training is offered

_____   Learning other job functions

_____   Teamwork

_____   Recurring performance evaluations

_____   Less paperwork

_____   Security

_____   Total points

The closer your score is to 39, the more happiness you will have as an employee. If your score is between 25 and 39 points, then you will probably enjoy being an employee. If you scored less than 20, review your responses to determine what may make you unhappy as an employee.

Worksheet 5–2   Self-Evaluation

Take some quiet time to reflect on the following prompts and write out what comes to mind. After you have
exhausted your thoughts in each area, put the list aside for a few days and then come back to it. Further elaborate on each area and make it a little more concrete. Once you have a list you feel adequately reflects you, then
study it and feel proud of your strengths. Discover ways to work on areas that you need to improve. Begin to
create the idea of a work environment in which you can thrive, given who you are.

As an employee, I would want to:

Exemplify these core values: _____

_____

Achieve these personal goals: _____

_____

Use my strongest skills, which are: _____

_____

Strengthen my weakest skills, which are: _____

_____

General things I am good at: _____

_____

General things I'm not good at: _____

_____

Things I love to do: _____

_____

Things I don't like to do: ————————————————————————————

——

Accomplishments I am most proud of: ————————————————————

——

Accomplishments that made a difference: —————————————————

——

Dream job description: ——————————————————————————————

——

——

——

Worksheet 5–3   Employer's Shoes

Imagine you own a business that employs massage therapists. You want to improve the well-being of your clients and wish for them to have an excellent experience they will tell their friends about. You would also like to make a profit in the process. What type of employee would you hire? Below, list some of the knowledge, abilities, skills and personal characteristics you would be looking for.

Knowledge, training, and education:

_____

_____

_____

Abilities and skills:

_____

_____

_____

Personal characteristics or traits:

_____

_____

_____

Worksheet 5–4   The Billboard Rule

Interviewers will most likely form an impression about you within the first few seconds. To help you prepare, think like a marketer who is using billboards to advertise a product. As potential customers travel the interstate, you have a few moments to attract their attention with a billboard. Smart companies choose their headline and graphic very carefully. Your image is your personal billboard. Use this space to come up with your vision of your own personal billboard, highlighting the key points you want to convey to a potential employer.

Example:

Professional Massage Therapist

I understand the importance of the guest experience and will seek to deliver a superior massage for all guests.
I maintain a level of professionalism that is respected by my peers and clients.
My appearance reflects great care and a professional appearance

Now it is your turn:

Now, when looking at the words on your personal billboard, think about how you will convey this message to prospective employers in ways other than carrying in a sign.

Worksheet 5-5   Career Pros/Cons

Think about each of the mentioned facilities in which a massage therapist can be employed, and carefully weigh the pros and cons of each. List them on the worksheet tables below.

Spas

Pros	Cons

Massage Centers/Franchises

Pros	Cons

Wellness Centers

Pros	Cons

Medical/Health-Care Facilities

Pros	Cons

Special-Interests Groups

Pros	Cons

Chapter 6

Your Path as an Independent Contractor

> *"I've always been an independent person, but that independence was in the setting of security."*
>
> —Patricia Heaton

Outline

> ## You will learn to ...
>
> - Define what a massage therapist's career looks like as an independent contractor
> - Define the differences between an employee and an independent contractor
> - Identify desirable attributes of an independent contractor
> - Define expectations, including scheduling, revenue, working conditions, office administration, tax preparation, and insurance
> - Identify types of companies that hire massage therapists as independent contractors
> - Analyze compensation and benefits for independent contractors

Key Definitions

This chapter references several key terms, which are indicated in bold. For easy reference, these terms are briefly defined here:

Behavioral control: Phrase used by the Internal Revenue Service that refers to facts showing whether there is a right to direct or control how workers do their work. Control factors are categorized by type and degree of instruction, evaluation systems, and training and are relevant when determining whether a worker is an employee or an independent contractor.

Communication skills: Skills that allow people to communicate effectively, including verbally, nonverbally, and in writing.

Empathy: Ability to identify with and understand someone else's situation, feelings, or motives.

Employee: A person hired to provide services to a company in exchange for compensation, who does not provide these services as part of an independent business.

Entrepreneur: A person who begins a business and assumes all related risks and rewards.

Financial control: Phrase used by the Internal Revenue Service that refers to the facts showing whether the business has a right to control the economic aspects of the worker's job. Financial control factors include opportunity for profit/loss, method of payment, and services available to the market. These factors are relevant when determining whether a worker is an employee or an independent contractor.

Independent contractor: A person hired to provide services, who is not hired as an employee of that person or company. The terms and specifications of work provided are outlined in a contract or agreement for short- or long-term engagement. They are sometimes called "contractors" or "freelancers."

Interpersonal skills: Skills that allow people to judge and respond appropriately to the varying needs and feelings of diverse individuals in various situations.

Professional liability insurance: This insurance provides coverage against allegations of professional negligence or failure to perform professional duties.

Relationship of the parties: Phrase used by the Internal Revenue Service that refers to the facts that show how the company and worker perceive their relationship. Factors include written contracts, extent the worker can provide services to other similar businesses, and permanency of the relationship. These factors are relevant when determining whether the worker is an employee or an independent contractor.

SMART goals: Acronym to describe goals that stands for **s**pecific, **m**easurable, **a**ttainable, **r**ealistic, and **t**imely.

Workers' compensation insurance: This insurance is paid for by an employer and covers medical and rehabilitation costs, as well as lost wages, if an employee is hurt on the job.

INDEPENDENT CONTRACTORS

When exploring the path of the independent contractor, you will discover that it is the path that lies in the middle (Fig. 6–1). In some respects, it is considered "the middle of the road" because it offers more freedom than the path of an **employee** and less risk than the entrepreneurial path. As an **independent contractor,** you are hired to do work for another, but are not considered an employee of that entity. In other words, an independent contractor is a self-employed person who works for a company on a contractual basis. These people are sometimes called "contractors" or "freelancers." The contract, or agreement, outlines the job to be performed, expectations, payment for services, termination of the contract, and length of service, which can be a short- or long-term engagement. The companies or persons you work for are "clients," not "employers." The arrangement seems fairly straightforward, but it can actually get quite complicated, especially for those contracting your services.

Becoming an independent contractor is the path most massage therapists travel. To explore this more, let us look at some of the key differences among independent contractors, employees, and entrepreneurs.

Independent Contractor Versus Employee

Massage therapists who operate as independent contractors often "feel" like an employee. They may work regularly for their clients, may develop relationships with employees and regular guests, and may even work so regularly for some clients that they come to depend financially on these arrangements. However, understanding the differences and nuances of each circumstance helps ensure that you are not taken advantage of and that you clearly understand your responsibilities and your client's (the company that contracts you) obligations.

For employers, determining the difference between an employee and independent contractor is a very gray area because there is no true test or defined difference. There are, however, several guidelines and general definitions to follow. According to the Internal Revenue Service (IRS), "The general rule is that an individual is an independent contractor if you, the person for whom the services are performed, have the right to control or direct only the result of the work and not the means and methods of accomplishing the result."[2]

When you are employed by a company, your employer has the right to direct and control the services you perform and *how* they are performed. She may not choose to tell you how to perform a massage or control how you sanitize a treatment room, but she still has the right. As an independent contractor, your clients have the right to expect certain results based on how they compensate you, but they should not tell you how to perform your job.

You may already see the gray areas. Some employees have a great amount of autonomy and independence in their jobs, but they are not independent contractors. Or, clients have some measure

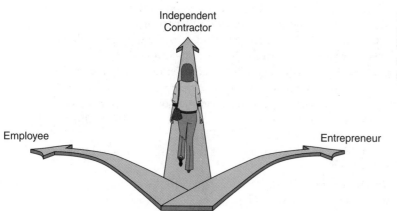

Independent Contractor

Employee

Entrepreneur

Figure 6–1 Choosing the path of an independent contractor is like selecting the "middle of the road" because it is similar to both the path of an employee and that of an entrepreneur.

of control over their contract workers, just based on the fact they are performing a job on the client's behalf and being compensated for it, but the contractors are not employees. When determining status, the key is the degree of control the employer or client has over the worker.

The IRS looks at three areas when determining the difference and level of control: **behavioral control**, **financial control**, and **relationship of the parties**. Keep in mind that just one or two of these factors alone do not indicate worker status. All of the control factors are considered and weighed collectively to determine whether a worker is an employee or a contractor (Box 6.1). This complexity is part of the reason that the determination process is so gray.[3]

Box 6.1 IRS 20-Factor Test

The IRS developed a 20-Factor Test to help guide employers and employees in determining their worker status. This test is also a good general overview of the differences between an employee and an independent contractor. However, there is no black-or-white, simple test to determine worker status according to the IRS. Depending on the occupation, some of these 20 factors will have more bearing than others. In addition, if an independent contractor does not meet one of these general guidelines, he is not necessarily an employee, and vice versa. Determining worker status involves reviewing *all* of these factors and weighing them as a whole.

Factor	Employee	Independent Contractor
Instruction	You are required to comply with direction and control regarding when, where, and how you perform the work.	You determine when, where, and how you perform the work.
Training	You are required to participate in on-the-job training, and the employer expects consistency in the service provided by all therapists.	The client may expect consistency, and you may receive orientation and general company training, but you are already highly skilled and do not receive training.
Integration	You perform work similar to others in the company, and you are an integral part of the business. The company depends a great deal on your successful performance.	Your work is different from that of other employees, and your specific work is not integral to the success of the company overall.
Services rendered personally	You provide the services yourself.	You may or may not provide the services yourself because you may have other workers who can also perform the service.
Hiring, supervising, and paying assistants	The company hires, supervises, and pays for others to help you perform the work.	You hire, supervise, and pay others to help you perform the work required under your contract, including providing supplies and other materials at your expense.
Length of relationship	Your relationship with the employer is continuous.	Your relationship with the client ends when the project or contract ends.
Set work hours	The company sets your work hours.	You set your work hours.
Full-time requirement	You are devoted full-time to the company.	You are free to work when and for whom you choose.
Location	Your employer has the right to control where you work.	You are free to determine where you work.
Order or sequence set	Your employer has the right to detail the order and sequence of how your work is performed.	You determine the order and sequence of how your work is performed.

Continued

Box 6.1 IRS 20-Factor Test—*cont'd*

Factor	Employee	Independent Contractor
Reporting	You submit oral or written reports on a regular basis.	You do not submit reports on a regular basis.
Payment	You receive your wage by the hour, week, or month.	You receive payment by the job or flat fee.
Reimbursement of expenses	Your work-related expenses are reimbursed by your employer.	You pay for your own expenses.
Equipment and supplies	The equipment and supplies you use to perform your job are purchased by your employer.	You purchase the equipment and supplies you need to perform your job.
Investment	You do not invest in the facility or equipment used to provide services.	You make a significant investment in the facility or equipment you use when providing services.
Profit or loss	You cannot make a profit, nor take a loss.	You may make a profit, or you may take a loss from the contracted work.
Number of employers	You work for only one company.	You provide services, or have the freedom to provide services, to more than one company.
Availability of services	Your services are not regularly available to the general public.	Your services are regularly available to the general public.
Termination	You may be fired, or threatened with being fired, by your employer for reasons he determines.	You may not be fired if your work is producing the expected results outlined in the contract.
Quitting	You may quit at any time, for any reason, without incurring liability.	You may terminate the contract/relationship only when the contract expires or there has been a breach in the agreement.

Behavioral Control

Employers have the right to tell employees how to perform their jobs and to control how it gets done in as much detail as they desire. They are within their legal right to tell employees:

- When to do the work
- Where to do the work
- What tools or equipment to use
- What workers to hire to assist with the work
- Where to purchase supplies or services
- What work must be performed by specified individuals
- What routines or patterns must be used
- What order or sequence to follow
- To obtain approval before taking certain actions

On the other hand, when employers hire independent contractors, they are essentially giving up their right to control those details. They can, however, provide instruction on expected results or outcomes of the work they have hired contractors to perform.

All businesses provide some level of instruction. The way the IRS views it, "the more detailed the instructions are that the worker is required to follow, the more control the business exercises over the worker, and the more likely the business retains the right to control the methods by which the worker performs the work. Absence of detail in instruction reflects less control."[3]

Control includes training, which is a primary method to describe to workers how to do certain tasks. If a business trains you about procedures or methods to use at its facility, this indicates that the company wants services performed in a particular manner. Therefore, it is an employer–employee relationship. But again, this is not a hard-and-fast rule because orientation or informational trainings about the company, general business policies, or new products and equipment are acceptable trainings for independent contractors as well.

One type of behavioral control in the massage industry that has come under great scrutiny and debate is whether contract workers can be required to wear uniforms. The traditional rationale stated that if a worker is required to wear a uniform, she is being directed what to do and thus is an employee. If she is not required to wear a uniform, she is an independent contractor. However, according to the IRS, because of safety concerns and companies wishing to allow customers to easily identify employees, this is not a clear test of employment.

Companies want to reassure clients that individuals are legitimate workers for the company. For example, imagine if a woman comes into a spa for a massage and sees everyone in the same uniform, but the person who picks her up in the relaxation room and begins the massage is wearing completely different attire. This may cause the woman to be concerned and raise questions about whether the person really works for the company.[3]

Financial Control

Financial control is about the company's control over how a worker's business is conducted. The five areas the IRS considers under financial control are as follow:

- Significant investment
- Unreimbursed expenses
- Services available to the relevant market
- Method of payment
- Opportunity for profit or loss

As massage therapists, you may or may not need to make a significant investment to work for your clients. However, you will more than likely be required to cover some expenses, such as massage equipment and supplies. Some of these may be more significant, such as purchasing massage tables, rent, advertising, licensure, professional liability insurance, and training. You may have a corporate client that reimburses you for some of these things, or one who does not require you to purchase them, but this should be spelled out in your contract so that it is clear. Any expense not spelled out in the contract will more than likely be your responsibility as an independent contractor.

Many employers may have policies that prohibit full-time employees from working a second job or from working for a competitor. Employers do not have this control over independent contractors unless a noncompete clause is agreed on by both parties in the contract. A noncompete agreement usually means the independent contractor agrees not to work for certain competitors or attempt to take clients when they leave the contract. Read these clauses carefully because they may affect the final decision. Massage therapists who work as independent contractors generally have more than one client, and there is the possibility these companies may be competitors. In other situations, there may be a company/individual competition. For example, you work for a massage center as an independent contractor but also see some of the same clients you see in the center at their home or yours during off hours. Some independent contractor situations are long-term in nature, and the contractor does not have the financial need or desire to work for other companies but still has the right and opportunity to do so.

How workers are paid is another factor in determining worker status. Flat fees, such as a fixed fee per massage, are generally considered by the IRS as evidence the worker is an independent contractor. Commissions and tips do not weigh heavily in either direction because these are common forms of compensation for both employees and contractors.

The last factor related to financial control is the worker's opportunity to make a profit or loss. Being self-employed and working as an independent contractor, you do not make a set salary or wage from one location. You have business-related costs that employees do not have, and you also have the opportunity to work more hours and at more locations than most employees. Thus, you have the opportunity to make a profit or take a loss, depending on how you manage your business and the decisions you make. Contractors are free to make decisions that will affect their profit or loss for the year. As an employee, you do not have those same freedoms. For example, as a contractor, you may choose to work 30 hours a week to increase your profit, but as an employee, you may be required to work 20 hours—no more and no less.[3]

Relationship of the Parties

The IRS reviews various relationship factors when determining employment versus independent contractor status, which include the following:

- Intent of parties/written contract
- Employee benefits
- Discharge/termination
- Permanency
- Regular business activity

Within all of these factors, "intent" is the key regarding control. The intent of the relationship is most commonly spelled out in the employer–contractor agreement or contract. This contract should state that the worker is an independent contractor of the company and define what that means as well as spell out the relationship in terms of the previously mentioned factors (Box 6.2). However, keep in mind that a contract alone does not provide sufficient evidence to the IRS to determine worker status. The IRS also looks at the other contributing factors under behavioral and financial control.[3]

See Worksheet 6-1

Box 6.2 Massage Therapy Independent Contractor Agreement

This agreement, dated _____, is by and between _____, with principal offices located at_____ and _____ ("Contractor"):

Status as Independent Contractor:
Contractor is an independent contractor and not an employee of the [enter business type]. As an independent contractor, Clinic and Contractor agree to the following:

a. Contractor has control of the means, manner, and method by which services are provided.
b. Contractor furnishes all necessary supplies and materials used in the performance of services (e.g., oils, lotions, with linens and music optional).
c. Contractor has the right to perform services for others during the term of this Agreement.
d. Contractor shall indemnify and hold Clinic harmless from any loss or liability arising from services provided under this agreement.
e. Contractor is responsible for maintaining appropriate certification, licensure, and liability insurance, including all costs thereof.

Term:
The term of this contract shall be for 1 year starting May 1, 2004, and ending April 31, 2005, after a 3-month trial period ending August 1, 2004. During the 3-month trial period, the contract may be terminated for any reason.
    This contract is for the use of massage room #2 for Wednesday, Friday, Saturday, and Sunday of each month. Other days and times can be negotiated as available.

Rent:
The contractor agrees to pay ___ at the first of each month, payable to _____ on the first of the month. A late fee of $10 per day will be assessed until the amount is paid in full.
    Included in these fees is use of massage room #2 for Wednesday, Friday, Saturday, and Sunday of each month. Other days and times can be negotiated as available. Also included are use of laundry facilities, phone with voice-mail box, phone book ad, and website page.

Box 6.2 Massage Therapy Independent Contractor Agreement—*cont'd*

Services to Be Provided by Contractor:

Contractor agrees to provide massage therapy services within the scope of licensing. Contractor agrees to dress in a style consistent with the Clinic's image and provide services in accordance with the Clinic's philosophy. Contractor shall maintain client records in a mutually agreed-on manner. Patient records are the responsibility of the contractor and will be kept by the contractor in a secure place.

The contractor is responsible for all marketing and advertising materials.

Services to Be Provided by Clinic:

Clinic shall provide the following: a safe, clean environment; a room furnished with a table, chair, stool, stereo, and storage area; receptionist area with desk and file storage area; laundry facilities and kitchen area; bottled water; and phone services with voice-mail box.

Fees, Terms of Payment and Fringe Benefits:

Contractor shall set the amount of fees for services provided to clients and is responsible for collecting all money from clients.

Local, State, and Federal Taxes:

Contractor is responsible for paying and filing all applicable local, state, and federal withholding, Social Security, and Medicare taxes.

Workers' Compensation and Unemployment Insurance:

Clinic is not responsible for payment of workers' compensation and unemployment insurance.

Insurance:

During the term of this agreement, Contractor shall maintain a malpractice insurance policy of at least $2,000,000 aggregate annual and $1,000,000 per incidence.

No Partnership:

This agreement does not create a partnership relationship. Contractor does not have the authority to enter into contracts on Clinic's behalf.

Resolving Disputes:

Any dispute or claim that arises out of or relating to this Agreement or breach thereof shall be settled promptly by mediation; however, the mediator shall have no authority to add to, modify, change, or disregard any lawful terms of this agreement. Any costs and fees of mediation shall be shared equally by the parties. If both parties are unable to arrive at a mutually satisfactory solution through mediation, the parties agree to submit the dispute/claim to a mutually agreed-on arbitrator. The decision of the arbitrator shall be final and binding, and judgment on the arbitration award may be entered in any court having jurisdiction over the subject matter of the controversy. Costs of arbitration will be allocated by the arbitrator.

Term of Agreement:

Either party may terminate this agreement, given reasonable cause, as provided below, or by giving 30 days' written notice to the other party of the intention to terminate this Agreement:

a. Material violation of the provisions of this Agreement.
b. Any action by either party exposing the other to liability for property damage or personal injury.
c. Violation of ethical standards as defined by local, state, and/or national associations and governing bodies.
d. Loss of licensure for services provided.
e. Contractor engages in any pattern or course of conduct on a continuing basis that adversely affects Contractor's ability to perform services.
f. Contractor engages in any pattern or course of conduct on a continuing basis that adversely affects Clinic's or Clinic's associates' ability to perform services.

This constitutes the entire agreement between Contractor and Clinic and supersedes any and all prior written or verbal agreements. Should any part of this agreement be deemed unenforceable, the remainder of the agreement continues in effect. This agreement is governed by the laws of Washington State.

Rider: Contractor shall have the right to use the other areas of Suite 1428 when not occupied or inconvenient to other therapists. Contractor shall also have the right to subcontract the terms of this contract to another therapist with the consent of all parties.

Continued

Box 6.2 Massage Therapy Independent Contractor Agreement—*cont'd*

Contractor and Clinic representatives certify and acknowledge that they have carefully read all of the provisions of this Agreement and understand and agree to fully and faithfully comply with such provisions.

_____

Contractor (Print Name)

_____   _____

Contractor (Signature)   Date

_____

Clinic Representative (Print Name)

_____   _____

Clinic Representative (Signature)   Date

Source: This document was found at www.thebodyworker.com/contract.doc.

Dual Status

Many massage therapists, at some point in their careers, find themselves in a dual role as both employee and independent contractor. For example, you may be a part-time employee at a local spa and also have a contract with a local website development firm to offer chair massages to their employees twice a month. There are many examples in which this exists for massage therapists, and in some cases, it even occurs within the same company. You may be employed part-time at a massage center, but you also contract with the center as an independent contractor to train new therapists. You would receive a regular wage as the employee and receive a set amount for performing the training on an as-needed basis.

Independent Contractor Versus Entrepreneur

In many ways, as an independent contractor, you are an entrepreneur. An entrepreneur is someone who owns and operates his own business, incurring any risks and rewards, including profits and losses. An independent contractor is self-employed and in that aspect an entrepreneur. However, your clients are usually other businesses who temporarily contract your services. The companies and individuals who hire contractors are paying for your services as an individual, not a company. In this text, the term **entrepreneur** describes a business owner whose clients are primarily individuals seeking massage, not businesses. Compensation is derived directly from these clients, and they pay you or your company for the services. Typically, most massage entrepreneurs are classified as small business owners, working out of their home or a facility on their property, sharing space with other therapists, or renting or leasing a small space. A massage entrepreneur may also own and operate a spa, wellness or massage center, or a massage franchise.

As an independent contractor, you may have workers, but not employees. As the name implies, independent contractors tend to work solo. As previously described, there is a difference between contractors and employees, and you may actually contract out work to other independent contractors, but they will not be your employees. If you decide to take the path of the entrepreneur, you may hire individuals to help you run your business and perform services. For entrepreneurs, these workers can be employees or contractors.

As an independent contractor, you have control over what you do, when you do it, and how you do it. You can choose to work only when there is a full moon. You may never make a living that way, but you get to decide. However, you do not have all the freedoms of an entrepreneur. As an independent contractor, you have a contract or an agreement with your client to perform agreed-on tasks under agreed-on conditions. For example, you may be contractually required to perform services on a day you are sick. As an employee, if you are sick, you may be able to take the day off and still be paid through

> As an independent contractor, you have a contract or an agreement with your client to perform agreed-on tasks under agreed-on conditions.

sick leave. As a contractor, you need to find someone else who can fill in for you and pay them for their services, unless you can make other arrangements with your client. An entrepreneur can cancel appointments, but will not receive any revenue that day. It is necessary to call in another therapist who can fill in or substitute shifts.

When you are self-employed and contract out your services, you generally do not have as many expenses, particularly start-up expenses, as an entrepreneur. To start out as an independent contractor, you can expect the expenses associated with soliciting new clients, whether they are individuals or companies; business licenses and insurance; and some equipment and supplies.

If you decide you no longer want to be an independent contractor, your exit strategy is fairly simple. You must complete your commitments, but once those are finished, you're done and can move on. Compare that to an entrepreneur who may buy in to a massage franchise opportunity that could require a commitment of hundreds of thousands of dollars, plus an incredible amount of time and personal resources. And once you own a business, an exit strategy is rarely simple and easy. You may have debt, investors, lease agreements, equipment to sell, and other liabilities. There is a significant difference in the financial commitment and the risk involved. There is also a big difference in the revenue potential. As a contractor, you typically only have yourself and your earning potential. As an entrepreneur, you may have your earning potential as a therapist as well as that of several other therapists, along with other revenue streams.

REALITIES OF BEING AN INDEPENDENT CONTRACTOR

When you select this path, your "clients" can be individuals or companies. You may have individual clients whom you treat in your home, their home, or a facility. You may also have corporate clients and go to their location to perform massage under agreed-on terms. With both of these "clients" in mind, here are some broad categories that outline key realities of being a massage therapist independent contractor.

Confusion Regarding Employee Versus Independent Contractor Status

Because the test for determining worker status is not clearly defined and somewhat difficult to grasp, many corporate clients treat their independent contractors as employees. This is an issue for the company with the IRS, but it is also an issue for you. You are not an employee, and therefore do not have the same benefits. To keep your autonomy, unless you want to become an employee, you must clearly define expectations, roles, and boundaries so that you are not taken advantage of. This is important to define and establish at the beginning of a relationship because it can be tricky to handle later on. If you have been behaving as an employee for an extended amount of time, it will be much harder for you to address this issue while still maintaining the company as a client.

Contracts

Although at times intimidating, it is important as a contractor that you have a contract with those you plan on working with. Too often contractors will verbally agree to terms and circumstances, and when things go south, they have nothing in writing to ensure equity for both parties. Oral agreements

Having a contract protects you by outlining expectations and job status.

ensure misunderstandings because there's no clear written agreement on what is to be done, how much compensation is involved, and what happens if a dispute arises. It is highly encouraged that you and your business clients have a contract or agreement that details the nature of your relationship. Having a contract protects you by outlining expectations and job status. The contract should be mutually agreed-on and signed by you and your client. It should explain roles and responsibilities of each party (Box 6.3).

Box 6.3 Items to Include in an Independent Contractor Agreement

- Job expectations and duties, specifically stating you are an independent contractor
- Payment amounts, payment schedule, and consequences if payment is not received in the agreed-on timeframe
- Milestones for payment or how and when payment is to be received
- Length of service
- Clarification on who is responsible for expenses
- Reporting requirements
- Description of how the contract is terminated and details regarding contract breaches
- Who will provide materials, equipment, and office space
- Required permits and licenses the state requires to do the work
- A statement that the independent contractor is responsible for state and federal income taxes
- A list of any benefits
- Listing of any required insurance by either party
- Circumstances under which either party can terminate the agreement
- Dispute resolution procedures

With all legal documents and contracts, there is additional required language about waivers of liability, confidentiality, conflicts of interest, and other important areas. Because this documentation is so critical to your arrangement, you should have an attorney review or draft the agreement template. The attorney can help you determine whether there are any clauses included that should be avoided. In the event you wish to change the wording in the contract provided, it is best to be honest and straightforward in your communication with the possible client. It helps to have an attorney provide you with the reasons some things need to be changed. Often a brief discussion can clarify any confusion that may exist. If the client refuses to change anything within the contract and you are not comfortable with the content, then be prepared to walk away. An example wold be a noncompete clause that prevents you from working with other companies. If you have a short-term agreement and will be unable to work for others after your contract is complete, it may not be worth the short-term benefit of this job.

Subcontracting

As an independent contractor, there may be functions you are unable, or unwilling, to perform yourself. So, you contract out work. You may have an arrangement with another massage therapist to fill in for each other on a contract basis. Or, perhaps you would like a website, but do not have the time or the ability to create one and keep it current. In that case, you may contract with a Web designer to create and update your website. There are many instances that could require you hiring a worker, so be sure you understand the IRS rules and regulations regarding subcontracting as well as any liabilities. If you decide to subcontract, you will also want to review your contract and clarify who will be covering the costs of subcontracted work.

6-1: Find It on the Web

INDEPENDENT CONTRACTOR TEMPLATES

- AllLaw.com: http://www.alllaw.com/forms/employment/independant_contractors_agr/
- Business Owner's ToolKit: http://www.toolkit.com/tools/bt.aspx?tid=indcon_m
- The BodyWorker: http://www.thebodyworker.com/businesscontracts.html
- Independent Consulting Bootcamp: http://www.independent-consulting-bootcamp.com/free-independent-contractor-agreement.html

6-2: Find It on the Web

- IRS Forms and Taxes for Independent Contractors: http://www.irs.gov/businesses/small/article/0,,id=179114,00.html
- Paying Independent Contractors: http://www.irs.gov/Businesses/Small-Businesses-&-SelfEmployed

Payments and Revenue

Before you perform services, or agree to perform services, you must work out a payment arrangement with your client. To do this, you must first determine the value of the services you provide and, second, research the market rate in your area. Once you have this information, you can set your fee. You may have different fees for different organizations, depending on needs and circumstances. However, once you've defined that fee, you must communicate it to the potential client and agree on the amount, payment schedule, and terms. You are also responsible for tracking payments and following up on past-due bills and returned checks. This is a good time to remember that once your rate is set, it is almost impossible to get a client to increase it. Set your rate appropriately to alleviate any feelings of not being compensated fairly.

For your business clients, you will make payment arrangements with them on an individual basis, unless you have established payment policies, such as all fees paid on arrival or departure. For corporate clients, you will track your hours and invoice the client accordingly, based on the hours worked, your hourly rate, and the agreed-on billing schedule. For a project, you may need to estimate the number of hours involved to determine the fee. Project fees can be difficult to determine because of the many variables. Therefore, it is a good idea to have some flexibility with project fees in your contract.

When working with corporate clients, you are typically paid by the service or by the project. Generally, you do not have a regularly scheduled "check" unless a payment plan, such as a monthly retainer, has been detailed in the contract. In this case, you may have a regular payment on a weekly or monthly basis, but it is based on you fulfilling the duties outlined in the contract. If you do not fulfill those duties, then payment is often withheld. Once a contract ends, if the relationship was favorable to both parties, then you can negotiate a new contract and new terms.

Few Paid Benefits, If Any

Independent contractors can expect to receive few, if any, paid benefits from their clients. In fact, according to the American Massage Therapy Association (AMTA), only 16% of massage therapists receive health insurance benefits.[5] This is because so many therapists work as independent contractors. Because you will not have regular, automatic paycheck deductions devoted to retirement and health benefits, you will need to set up these matters for yourself and be disciplined about financially contributing to them. It is imperative that you plan for emergencies, the future, and maintaining your health. There are a variety of ways you can reasonably address these areas of your well-being. You may benefit from seeking the advice of professional counsel in these areas to help you get started.

Training

Part of the attraction of hiring independent contractors is that they usually come already skilled and trained. Therefore, to stay on top in the industry and be sought after as an independent contractor, you need continual training in new therapies, modalities, research, and trends (Fig. 6–2). As a contractor, this training and education will be at your expense. However, if it is a legitimate business expense, then you can write it off on your taxes, which can help you at the end of the year when you figure business expenses.

6-3: Find It on the Web

There are many websites that allow you to research and compare health-care plans that can fit your needs and budget. Below are websites that will let you search plans from individual health insurance companies, a website that allows you to search multiple plans and companies at one time, and a report of the top 100 health plans in America from *US News and World Report.*

Health-care companies:

- Aetna: http://www.aetna.com
- Anthem BlueCross and BlueShield: http://www.anthem.com
- Assurant: http://www.assuranthealth.com
- CIGNA: http://www.cigna.com
- Humana: http://www.humana.com
- United Healthcare: http://www.uhc.com

Compare multiple companies and plans:

- http://www.esurance.com
- http://www.ehealthinsurance.com

Top Health Insurance Companies, from *US News and World Report:*

- http://health.usnews.com/health/health-plans

American Massage Therapy Association:

- http://www.amtamassage.org

Associated Bodywork and Massage Professionals:

- http://www.abmp.com

6-4: Find It on the Web

There are a wide variety of financial and investment firms and banks that can assist you in setting up a retirement savings plan that works for you. However, it is important that you understand the basics of retirement plans and understand the terms. Here are some helpful websites to help you do your homework:

- BankRate.com: http://www.bankrate.com/brm/news/sav/20060110a1.asp
- Internal Revenue Service: http://www.irs.gov/Retirement-Plans
- Investopedia: http://www.investopedia.com/terms/i/ira.asp
- SmartMoney: http://www.smartmoney.com/personal-finance/retirement/your-other-tax-advantaged-options-7938/

As an independent contractor, you will be subject to some training from your clients because you must be informed about their facilities, guests, and policies. You may also voluntarily attend training on behalf of your corporate clients, and any associated fees may or may not be paid by the client. Most clients prefer not to provide training to independent contractors because they are designated short-term service providers. Training expenses are usually spent on employees who will likely stay with the facility for a longer period of time, allowing the clients to achieve a return on their investment.

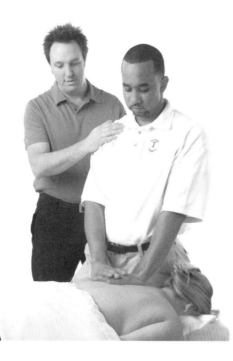

Figure 6–2   Clients expect contractors to be highly trained and skilled; therefore, you need continual training and education to stay successful.

Scheduling

Independent contractors in most industries set their own hours and work their own schedules. However, that is not always the case for massage therapists working for corporate clients. Because of the nature of the industry and scheduling of client appointments, many contractors do have set schedules.

You work when work is available, even if this is not always convenient. This is the reality of being self-employed. If you turn down opportunities because you are not available, the potential client may not call you again. Or, you may find that you have incredibly busy days or weeks, and then slower periods when you have plenty of available time.

During slow periods, take advantage of the time to promote your services to potential new clients. Being self-employed, you need to constantly promote yourself and company. It is often helpful for independent contractors to have scheduled, weekly time that is devoted to business development and administration. During this time, you can schedule networking appointments as well as handle office and administrative details.

Uniforms

As previously covered, it is a common misconception that massage therapists working as independent contractors for corporate clients do not have to wear uniforms. This is true in some scenarios, but when working for many organizations, especially spas, you are required to wear their uniform. This is primarily so that clients can recognize you easily and know their therapist is a legitimate worker for the organization. However, even if you work for an organization that does not require a uniform, or you only see individual clients, you still must take care with your appearance and attire. Ensure you have clothing that is functional for your role as well as aesthetically pleasing and presentable. As a contractor, take time and effort to look professional.

Treatment Rooms

Unless you work solely from your own facility or space, you must get used to working in a variety of treatment rooms. As a contractor, you may work in many different rooms and facilities, with different equipment and conditions, within any given week. You must learn to adapt to tables placed against walls, poor lighting and temperature control, no music or bad music, flooring that offers no physical support or comfort, and many other inconveniences. As a contractor, you can make suggestions to your client that would improve the conditions of the room for both you and the guest, but more often than not, you'll have to learn to make the best of what you've got.

You may also be provided work outside of a treatment room, such as outdoor massage or chair massage in high-traffic areas. When negotiating a contract and arrangements, be sure you know up front where you will be giving massages because this will be a critical factor for you. For example, if you are expected to give massages on the beach, you should know the tips and tricks to avoid getting sand on the client.

> When negotiating a contract and arrangements, be sure you know up front where you will be giving massages because this will be a critical factor for you.

Massage Only?

For many, one attractive component of being an independent contractor is that you determine the type of work you do. As a company contractor, you will primarily perform massage and will not be expected to do other tasks, such as check in guests or clean relaxation rooms. Although you may not perform tasks for your clients other than massage, you do perform other tasks for yourself as a business owner. You have plenty of paperwork to complete and keep track of, and you must be in constant "sales" mode, promoting your business and looking for new clients.

Working Independently

Independent contractors, as the name implies, primarily work alone. You may develop enriching relationships with clients and other peers, but you will probably not have the team camaraderie that employees have. If you work for a spa or large facility, you may develop a close rapport with the other employees, but you are not a permanent worker and often do not have the same responsibilities.

As an independent contractor, you need to be comfortable working alone and being self-motivated. You also need to create opportunities that allow you to socialize and connect with your peers. This is extremely helpful to avoid feeling isolated. You can join your state massage therapy chapter, get involved in one of the massage associations, or introduce yourself to other massage therapists in your region. This allows you to build a supportive network to ask questions, share experiences, and discuss the many joys and frustrations of being an independent contractor.

6-5: Find It on the Web

AMERICAN MASSAGE THERAPY ASSOCIATION STATE CHAPTERS

- Alabama: http://www.amta-alchapter.org
- Alaska: http://www.akamta.com
- Arizona: http://www.azamta.org
- Arkansas: http://wildwoodmassage@gmail.com (e-mail)
- California: http://www.amta-ca.org
- Colorado: http://www.amtacolorado.org
- Connecticut: http://www.amtactchapter.org
- Delaware: http://www.amta-de.org
- Florida: http://www.amtaflorida.org
- Georgia: http://www.amtaga.org
- Hawaii: http://www.amtahi.org
- Idaho: http://www.amtaid.org
- Illinois: http://www.amta-il.org
- Indiana: http://www.amtaindiana.org
- Iowa: http://www.amtaiowa.com

6-5: Find It on the Web—cont'd

- Kansas: http://www.amta-ks.org
- Kentucky: http://www.amtakentucky.org
- Louisiana: http://www.amtala.org
- Maine: http://www.maineamta.com
- Maryland: http://www.amtamd.org
- Massachusetts: http://www.massamta.org
- Michigan: http://www.amtamichigan.org
- Minnesota: http://www.amtamn.org
- Mississippi: http://www.amtamississippi.org
- Missouri: http://www.amtamo.org
- Montana: http://www.amtamt.org
- Nebraska: http://www.amtane.org
- Nevada: http://www.amta-nv.org
- New Hampshire: http://www.amta-nh.org
- New Jersey: http://www.amtanj.org
- New Mexico: http://amta-nm.org
- New York: http://www.amtany.com
- North Carolina: http://www.amtanc.org
- North Dakota: http://www.amtanorthdakota.org
- Ohio: http://www.amtaohio.org
- Oklahoma: http://www.amtaok.org
- Oregon: http://www.amta-or.org
- Pennsylvania: http://www.amtapa.org
- Rhode Island: http://www.riamta.com
- South Carolina: http://www.amta-sc.org
- South Dakota: http://www.amtasd.org/
- Tennessee: http://www.amtatn.org
- Texas: http://www.amtatexaschapter.org
- Utah: http://www.amtautah.org
- Vermont: http://www.amta-vermont.org
- Virginia: http://www.amtava.org
- Washington: http://www.amta-wa.org
- Washington, D.C.: http://www.amtadc.org
- West Virginia: http://derendoe1@aol.com (e-mail)
- Wisconsin: http://www.amtawi.org
- Wyoming: http://wyamta@vcn.com (e-mail)

Source: http://www.amtamassage.org/about/chaplist.html.

Independent State Massage Therapy Associations

Florida State Massage Therapy Association
1870 Aloma Avenue, Suite 260
Winter Park, FL 32789
(877) 376-8248
http://fsmta.org
info@fsmta.org

Independent State Massage Therapy Associations—cont'd

New York State Society of Medical Massage Therapists
P.O. Box 442
Bellmore, NY 11710-0442
(877) 697-7668
www.NYSMassage.org
info@NYSMassage.org

Oregon Massage Therapy Association

1710 Oakhurst Court
Eugene, OR 97402-8002
www.omta.net
info@bennouri.net

Tennessee Massage Therapy Association

105 Jesse Drive
Byhalia, MS 38611
(662) 890-7783
www.tmtanews.org

Texas Association of Massage Therapists

3801 Capital of Texas Highway N E240-156
Austin, TX 78746
(888) 778-9851
www.texasmassagetherapists.com
info@texasmassagetherapists.com

Formal Reviews and Opportunities for Feedback

Employees have the benefit of regularly scheduled performance evaluations as well as established systems for client feedback. This is seldom the case for contractors. Corporate clients may offer you advice and suggestions about improving your services, but typically, they are not as invested in you as they are their employees. They hired you to be a professional and perform to their expectations without guidance, feedback, or training. If you are not performing as expected, they can terminate the contract.

Individual clients do not always feel comfortable sharing how they really feel. Clients who are unhappy with a service usually never come back and do not tell you why. They simply do not make another appointment. Because of this, you must communicate your openness to feedback, and ask them for any comments or suggestions. Although comments about improving your performance can hurt emotionally, they are priceless bits of information if you are open to them. If you are not getting this regularly, then you may consider creating a way for clients to anonymously give you feedback. You can do this through e-mail surveys or by simply having a drop-box in your waiting room and asking each client to fill out an evaluation form.

Office Administration

As an independent contractor, you spend much more time on administrative and operational duties than does an employee. You may have an official "office" set up in your home, or your kitchen table may serve as your desk where you organize files. Either way, you have plenty of administrative tasks as an independent contractor. You need to keep up with your finances, which includes bookkeeping, paying bills, saving and recording receipts, invoicing and billing clients, and completing tax forms. You also have credit card statements and your business bank statements to check and track. It is important not to comingle personal funds, so it is encouraged that you keep separate records for personal and business finances. It is also recommended to have a separate bank account for your business funds. In the event you are ever sued, this becomes important so that you can protect your personal assets. You also have agreements and contracts, insurance policies and renewals, and other important documents to create and track in your business. This work can pile up quickly, so devote at least a few hours each week to administrative work, and keep all of your paperwork organized. This saves you a great deal of time and energy in the long run. If this feels daunting or you are not sure how to separate your business from your personal items, you can set up an appointment with the Small Business Association or your local SCORE office. Often, they will assist you with setting this up.

Tax Preparation

When you are an independent contractor, your clients do not withhold any taxes from your payments. Therefore, it is your responsibility to report revenue to the IRS and other relevant agencies, which includes fees paid by clients as well as any gratuities and tips you receive, even if you received these in cash. Whether you were paid by check, credit card, or cash, you must report all revenue on your taxes, or risk federal and state tax evasion charges.

You are also responsible for paying state and federal taxes as well as self-employment taxes. Self-employment taxes are a Social Security and Medicare tax for business owners, similar to the taxes that come out of an employee's paycheck. The self-employment tax rate in 2010 was 15.3%. As a business owner, you pay a higher percentage of such taxes than does an employee because employers pay some fees for their employees. These fees are now your responsibility.

You must also track business-related expenses for your own financial reporting so that you know how much you profited or lost in your business ventures. For tax purposes, you must keep copies of all receipts. Generally, you can write off business-related expenses, but you should seek tax advice on what is allowed and what is not.

There is a great deal to know and learn about company finances and tax preparation. It may be in your best interest to hire a financial or tax consultant to help you keep your financial affairs in line and compliant with all state and federal tax laws.

Many therapists have learned the hard way about paying taxes when they are due. Although it often feels like you are living paycheck to paycheck, if you do not set aside the money for your taxes, you may face some large fees when taxes are due. Ask your bookkeeper or accountant about paying your taxes on a quarterly basis to save you from a large lump sum.

Speaking of tax forms, your clients will likely ask you to complete a Form W-9, which is a request for your taxpayer identification number and certification. This provides your client with your correct name and identification number, which for most is your Social Security number. Because you are a contractor, clients who paid you more than $600 during the year must provide you with a copy of the 1099-MISC by January 31 of the year following payment.[4] You will submit the amount on your 1099-MISC form with your taxes by the April 15 deadline.

Insurance

There are several types of insurance you should consider when self-employed. These include the following:

Professional liability insurance: This insurance typically covers (1) professional liability, such as malpractice; (2) general liability, such as accidents due to negligence; (3) product liability, such as

---

6-6: Find It on the Web

For more information on the federal self-employment tax, visit the IRS website:

- http://www.irs.gov/businesses/small/article/0,,id=98846,00.html

See Worksheet 6-2

allergic reactions to essential oils; and in some cases, (4) legal expenses in the event of a lawsuit. The AMTA and Associated Bodywork & Massage Professionals are two organizations that provide professional liability insurance to massage therapists.

Workers' compensation insurance: If you have employees, many states require you to provide workers' compensation insurance for them. However, it may be an option for independent contractors as well. This rarely happens but is worth asking about. Workers' compensation insurance covers medical and rehabilitation costs as well as lost wages, if you are hurt on the job. This coverage is regulated at the state level and can be costly. Most independent contractors do not have workers' compensation insurance.

Health insurance: As previously covered, you may choose to get individual or family health insurance that covers medical, vision, and dental expenses.

Long-term disability insurance: Knowing the risk inherent in massage therapy, it may be wise to look into long-term disability insurance. This coverage can ensure income if you are unable to work for an extended period of time due to an illness or injury.

Professional Advisers

Being self-employed as an independent contractor is not as complex as being an entrepreneur with a business storefront, employees, and large investments, but it still requires a great deal of business savvy. You have many legal requirements and may need professional advice in several areas. Keep in mind that these individuals can be of great service to you, but their services, like yours, are not free. You still need to budget for their advice and assistance. Some common advisers you may want to shop around for and seek assistance from include the following:

- Attorney
- Financial and investment adviser
- Insurance agent
- Risk management adviser
- Tax preparer

If you need these services, then ask around your peer group for recommendations. It is a good idea to schedule appointments with at least two firms while you seek the one that will best meet your needs (Fig. 6–3). Some of these providers may be open to bartering their services in exchange for yours. Be careful that you are not booking all your time with trade services and also use caution in not confusing boundaries with professional providers.

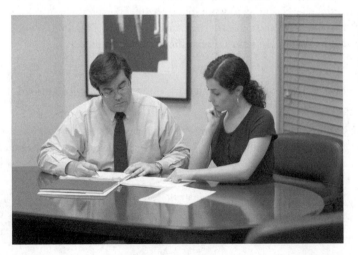

Figure 6–3 Being self-employed may require you to seek professional advice on finances, legal matters, insurance, and other technical areas.

Less Security

Being self-employed can be liberating and exhilarating. You are in charge of your fate and make the professional decisions that affect you. To a certain extent, to enjoy this freedom, you have to be willing to sacrifice security. When employed, you may rely on the security of your position. Some days, you may not perform to your greatest potential, but you still earn your wage. As long as you're not consistently performing poorly or behaving badly, you will have a job the next day.

Independent contractors have to build their client base and continue to nurture and grow it everyday in order to be successful. This involves self-directed personal and professional growth. In most cases, you will not have the security of an employer who provides you with a regular wage, withholds taxes and insurance payments, and offers training and education as well as other benefits. Often, you will be the only force that ensures you have a full day booked. Your livelihood also depends on consistently delivering a quality service. With your destiny in your hands, you have the opportunity to be wildly successful as an independent contractor, but it will take some work and commitment. Being self-employed takes courage and planning as well as diligence and commitment.

See Worksheet 6-3

WHAT IT TAKES TO BE SUCCESSFUL

Although being an independent contractor is a very popular path for massage therapists, it is not for everyone, nor is it always the right path for your entire career. There are certain traits and attributes that help make independent contractors successful.

Knowledge, Skills, and Abilities

Savvy contractors know their success depends on the quality of their work. Clients become very loyal when you exceed their expectations. With your business clients, this satisfaction can lead to more work, referrals, and higher pay. To stay on top of your game, you should have a strong knowledge of massage therapy and a willingness to learn and stay current as the industry changes. Acquiring additional training is a great way to do this.

Training gives you the opportunity to learn new skills and network with other therapists. Many students coming out of school may struggle if they do not continue to invest in their training. Clients who hire contractors expect them to be the best and to require minimal guidance or support. Independent contractors are often expected to hit the ground running and to handle situations without assistance. Know that you will make mistakes—it is normal. Remember that the most successful people are able to acknowledge the error, appreciate the lesson, and make better decisions in the future. Learning from mistakes helps fuel the continual growth and development that keeps you relevant and necessary to your clients.

> Clients who hire contractors expect them to be the best and to require minimal guidance or support.

Initiative and Confidence

Initiative and confidence are key attributes of independent contractors. You must become your own biggest fan. Initiative springs from your personality, but it can also be created by your passion and enjoyment. If you do not love what you do, then it will be hard to get yourself motivated and inspired. Initiative keeps you looking for new business and growth opportunities, spurs you to try new things, and stimulates your creativity. It gets you up out of bed each day, looking forward to the exciting work ahead of you.

Initiative is also important when problems arise. It helps you to go out and look for new business again, after you've already been turned down 10 times. When you're faced with a day in which everything imaginable goes wrong, your initiative keeps you focused on seeking solutions. With initiative, you tackle problems and do not allow them to tackle you.

Along the same lines, you also need a great deal of confidence. You have to believe you can do this. You know that you have the talent and ability that others need and want—and you must demonstrate it. Clients look for someone who is confident in their abilities, not unsure or uncertain about what they are doing. They seek assurance that they have made the right choice in you. You also need to be confident in the decisions you make, from contract decisions to the amount you charge clients. Your confidence will show in your interactions with your clients, and they in turn will have more confidence in you.

Flexibility

Flexibility is a key component to success because your work will rarely be the same. You will have a diverse group of clients and situations and will have to adapt to each of these unique opportunities. The nature of this work requires you to be flexible with people and situations as well as scheduling. Often, you are called when a client is in dire straits, meaning she has received an overflow of bookings and needs you to respond immediately. Staying flexible to her needs and responding quickly ensures that you are at the top of her list when she needs you again. Most independent contractors have to work when work is available, which is not always the most convenient timing. Responding positively is important in these situations as well. Grudgingly accepting the hours creates a negative memory for your client and reduces her chance of reaching out to you in the future.

As a self-employed person, you must learn to negotiate a variety of terms and conditions. You will negotiate client contracts, expenses, and business arrangements. When negotiating, you must be flexible. The best negotiators know they are striving to reach a win–win situation for everyone involved, which requires flexibility. However, the best negotiators also know the boundaries of what is acceptable. Their deal breakers are the rare areas in which they will not compromise because of necessity or strongly held values.

People Skills

People skills are broadly defined and can include many personality traits. No matter how you interpret the concept, you can rest assured that you will need them. A broad definition that includes all of the following traits is emotional intelligence. Emotional intelligence is ability, skill, or a self-perceived ability to identify, assess, and control the emotions of oneself, of others, and of groups.

Communication Skills

Possessing excellent verbal, nonverbal, and written **communication skills** gives you an edge. You should be able to confidently master the art of telling people who you are and why they need you. You must be an active listener to properly communicate and know when to listen and when to talk. Your nonverbal communication can say a lot about who you are and how you feel. Sharpening these skills helps you to excel (Fig. 6–4).

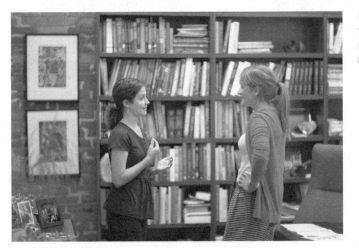

Figure 6–4 Independent contractors need excellent communication and interpersonal skills as well as empathy.

Interpersonal Skills

As a massage therapist, you need strong **interpersonal skills,** but they become even more important as an independent contractor. You must know how to respond appropriately to various needs and feelings in various situations. This is true in the relationships you build with clients and potential clients as well. Understanding and appreciating differences in emotions, then responding in a tactful, compassionate manner, can build very strong relationships. The bottom line is that successful contractors treat and honor all people with respect.

Empathy

The art of walking in someone else's shoes is essential on this path. You must be able to see other perspectives and understand other points of view. This does not mean you have to agree with them. However, you can empathize with the situation or individual and respect his position, even if you do not agree. Increasing your compassion toward others and their situation is also an important component of people skills.

   Empathy is also shown by understanding different emotions and feelings, including your own. The phrase "emotional intelligence" is becoming more popular because it defines the awareness of one's own emotions as well as others'. Sometimes, taking a mental step back is helpful. Recognizing emotions and exploring them from a neutral place allows you to better deal with and respond to them.

Fiscally Responsible

Managing money and finances is a learned skill but is not something everyone enjoys doing, even if they know how. You are self-employed as a contractor and therefore will be managing not only your personal finances but also your business finances. This includes filing taxes; keeping up with receipts, mileage, and other expenses; invoicing and billing; paying bills; monitoring credit cards and their fees; and so many other financial matters. You must make financial decisions that affect you and your business, and you need to do so in a responsible manner. At a minimum, this means not spending more than you have or can pay back within a reasonable time period. It means continually being on the lookout for revenue opportunities. You must also budget and plan appropriately, so that your expenses do not exceed your revenue, and keep reserves for slow times.

Goal-Oriented

Goals are those dangling carrots we suspend out in front of ourselves as something to strive for and challenge us. Goals are especially important when self-employed because there are generally not others around you who will challenge you to do more—it has to come from you.

> ...it is imperative that you set SMART goals, which are specific, measurable, attainable, realistic, and timely.

Because of this, it is imperative that you set **SMART goals**, which are **s**pecific, **m**easurable, **a**ttainable, **r**ealistic, and **t**imely. These goals will keep you focused on where you want to be and should include specific tactics that outline your plan of "how" you're going to reach your goal. The best goal setters also include a start date and completion date and identify others who can assist them so that they can develop an overall action plan. This keeps you focused and helps to keep you moving toward your goals.

Strong Ethics

In your work as a massage therapist, you are confronted with many situations that require you to call on your personal values to make a decision or choose a response. In your journey as an independent contractor, you may also find yourself in business situations that call on your ethics. As always, you must keep your moral compass in check and pointed in the ethical direction. This sounds easy in theory, but when presented in reality, it is sometimes a difficult choice. Your personal and professional reputation depends on the ethical decisions you make.

In some cases, your empty wallet may push you in one direction and your moral code in another. When important personal drivers and motivators compete, our boundaries can become gray and unclear. We can rationalize decisions, even when we know deep down in our hearts it was not the "right" thing to do.

Imagine you have a contract with a corporate client to train a group of therapists. The client believes its employees are in desperate need of this training and plans on you conducting at least three workshops on the subject. After the first training session, you find the employees are actually well versed and knowledgeable on the subject and do not need more training. The manager who hired you appears to be out of touch with the needs of his employees. What do you do? Do you explain your observations to the manager, knowing you may not be conducting the additional two workshops you had planned and budgeted for? Or do you assume the manager knows what he is doing, and conduct the additional training anyway? Perhaps you can overcome your fear of losing the training hours, discuss what you have noticed about their skill level, and make a confident recommendation on how you can work with the employees in another, more useful area.

Another common ethical situation is tip reporting. Your individual clients may tip you in cash. They do not report it on their taxes, so why should you? Tracing cash payments is like finding a needle in a haystack, right? Perhaps you consider reporting only a portion of your tip revenue, rather than the entire amount. Who will be the wiser? You may get away with it and not be caught for tax evasion. Regardless, it is illegal, and it becomes a legal and ethical issue—one more thing for you to worry about.

See Worksheet 6-4

MARKETING YOUR SERVICES

A critical key to success as an independent contractor is marketing yourself and your services. Whether or not you enjoy sales, you need to become good at it as an independent contractor. Unfortunately, you cannot just hang your sign outside and expect people to start booking your services. You must strategize how you plan to acquire business. The most successful therapists develop business and marketing plans that outline goals and contain tactics for filling their practices. Upcoming chapters will more fully discuss marketing.

> The most successful therapists develop business and marketing plans that outline goals and contain tactics of how to fill their practices.

WHY COMPANIES HIRE INDEPENDENT CONTRACTORS

Many managers prefer independent contractors over employees because hiring contractors can be less expensive. An employee's total compensation package includes wages, insurance, taxes, and benefits. Independent contractors often do not receive health insurance and other benefits, thereby reducing an employer's expense. Employers also do not have to withhold and pay Social Security and Medicare taxes or unemployment and workers' compensation insurance for independent contractors. In addition, they do not have to withhold and pay federal and state income tax because this is the responsibility of the independent contractor.

Because withholding and payments made to federal and state departments is different for contractors, the IRS is very interested in correctly determining who is an employee versus an independent contractor.

YOUR CAREER AS A MASSAGE THERAPIST

As previously discussed, most massage therapists are self-employed, either owning their own business or working as an independent contractor. According to the AMTA, massage therapists practice at several different sites and settings in a single day (Fig. 6–5):

- 44% travel to client locations
- 39% practice in a private office
- 22% practice in a spa or salon

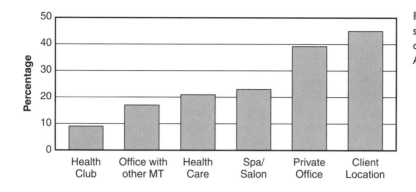

Figure 6–5 Massage therapists practice at several different sites and settings in a single day. (Source: American Massage Therapy Association.)

- 21% practice in a health-care setting
- 17% practice in an office with other massage therapists
- 9% practice in a health club

As an independent contractor, you decide where and how many hours you work. These statistics give you an idea of what other therapists are doing.

Growth

Independent contractors have growing options of venues to find work, owing to the increased demand and popularity of massage. More and more businesses, health- and wellness-related or not, are contracting out massage therapists. Companies are using therapists to reduce stress in the workplace, attract and retain new employees, and promote overall health and wellness, in an attempt to keep employee health-care costs down.

Compensation and Benefits

Generally, independent contractors can command a higher fee than employees. If you have contracted with a company to provide services, the company does not have to pay insurance, taxes, and benefits for you. They also generally expect that your level of knowledge, skill, and ability is excellent and that you require little training and no supervision, giving managers less work.

If you see clients in your home office, then you will not have to share the fee with anyone else. You also will be able to keep all tips, which can add up for exceptional therapists. It is wise to remember your business expenses come out of the total you collect. Keeping track of your income and expenses becomes extremely important and allows you to set your fees and hours so that you can make a living and save for your future.

According to the Associated Bodywork & Massage Professionals, "the amount clients pay for massage varies a great deal depending on the setting and the region of the country where they receive the massage. A common price range for massage is $40 to $90 an hour, with some lavish spas charging even more."[9] The International SPA Association identified the average price of a massage as $73 in a day spa, $83 in a club spa, and $110 in a resort/hotel spa. The fees also vary by region: spas in the North Central region of the United States have an average price of $66 for a massage, and spas in the Southwest receive an average of $87.[10] Although this fee is charged by the facility, it is not necessarily the amount the therapist receives. The spa may keep a percentage to give to other employees and to ensure it collects revenue from the massage. The fee also does not factor in gratuities, which would be extra income.

Where Massage Therapists Work

Most of the same places that hire massage therapists as employees also hire independent contractors. These include spas, massage centers/franchises, wellness centers, health-care centers, and special-interests groups. Whether or not the company hires employees or independent contractors depends on several factors, including their goals and business needs. For example, resort/hotel spas may hire independent contractors during their high season to fill in during particularly heavy booking periods. They may not have enough work to hire employees year round but need the additional manpower during certain months.

Most employed massage therapists work in a spa, followed by a health-care setting. In 2008, 29% of massage therapists reported they were employed at a spa or salon, 27% reported working in a health-care setting, and 8% indicated they worked in a health club.[5] In a 2009 AMP member survey, nearly half of members reported they spent their professional time in one location, whereas 30% worked at two locations and 11% at three locations.[8]

CHAPTER SUMMARY

The path of the independent contractor can be incredibly fulfilling and rewarding, if you are prepared for the challenges and realities of the journey. Being self-employed is something you can be proud of and may energize you to work harder than you've ever worked—and love every minute of it. However, with this freedom and exhilaration comes a tradeoff. In many ways, being self-employed is trading security for freedom. You no longer have the security of a regular paycheck or someone else handling insurance, taxes, and other affairs related to your well-being. All of these details are now your responsibility. However, you have more freedom to choose whom you contract with, what rates you charge, and how often you work.

To know if this path is the right one for you, you need to carefully evaluate yourself and the realities of being a contractor. You also need to clearly understand the law and how it relates to independent contractors and employees. This knowledge will prevent you from being taken advantage of by corporate clients and will assist you in filing all of the appropriate paperwork with the IRS. For many therapists, the hardest part is the tremendous amount of paperwork and taking care of the "business" of massage. By tending to the business of massage and the many details it involves, you are setting yourself up for success. But if the business part of massage is not appealing to you, you may prefer the path of the employee.

BIBLIOGRAPHY

1. Entrepreneur (n.d.). *Independent Contractor*. Retrieved from http://www.entrepreneur.com/encyclopedia/term/82220.html.
2. Department of the Treasury, Internal Revenue Service. (2008, May 19). *Independent Contractor*. Retrieved from http://www.irs.gov/businesses/small/article/0,,id=179115,00.html.
3. Department of the Treasury, Internal Revenue Service. (1996, October 30). *Independent Contractor or Employee? Training Materials*. [Training 3320-102(10-96) TPDS 84238I]. Retrieved from http://www.irs.gov/pub/irs-utl/emporind.pdf.
4. Department of the Treasury, Internal Revenue Service. (2009, April 21). *Forms and Associated Taxes for Independent Contractors*. Retrieved from http://www.irs.gov/businesses/small/article/0,,id=179114,00.html.
5. American Massage Therapy Association. (2009). *AMTA 2009 Massage Industry Research Report*. Evanston, IL: American Massage Therapy Association.
6. U.S. Department of Labor, Bureau of Labor Statistics. (2009, December 17). *Occupational Outlook Handbook, 2010-11 Edition*. Retrieved from http://www.bls.gov/oco/ocos295.htm.
7. American Massage Therapy Association. (n.d.). *Demographic Study of AMTA Members*. Retrieved from http://www.amtamassage.org/news/03MemberDemographics.html.
8. Associated Bodywork & Massage Professionals. (n.d.). *Massage Profession Metrics*. Retrieved from http://www.massagetherapy.com/media/metricscharacteristics.php.
9. Associated Bodywork & Massage Professionals. (n.d.). *Careers*. Retrieved from http://www.massagetherapy.com/careers/index.php.
10. International SPA Association. (2007). *ISPA 2007 Spa Industry Study*. Lexington, KY: International SPA Association.

REVIEW QUESTIONS

1. Which of the following is a self-employed person who works for a company on a contractual basis?

    a. Employee
    b. Independent contractor
    c. Entrepreneur
    d. Partner

2. What is the general rule defined by the IRS when determining whether a worker is an employee or independent contractor?

    a. If the worker wears a company's uniform, the worker is generally considered an employee.
    b. If the worker is not allowed to work for another company, the worker is generally considered an employee.
    c. If the employer controls how the worker accomplishes results or performs the job, the worker is generally considered an independent contractor.
    d. If the employer controls or directs only work results, the worker is generally considered an independent contractor.

3. Which three general areas do the IRS review to determine the level of control and difference between an employee or independent contractor?

    a. Behavioral, financial, and relationship of the parties
    b. Education/training, investment, and permanency
    c. Singular, dual, and triple Status
    d. Nature of the work, tax returns, and 1099s

4. Why does the distinction between an independent contractor and worker matter to an employer?

    a. To be in compliance with IRS regulations regarding taxes and withholding
    b. To be in compliance with the Fair Labor Standards Act
    c. It is an important ethical distinction
    d. It doesn't matter to employers, only workers

5. Why does the distinction between an independent contractor and worker matter to a worker?

    a. To safeguard the worker and the worker's rights because each status has different benefits and responsibilities
    b. It doesn't matter to workers, only employers
    c. To be in compliance with IRS regulations regarding taxes and withholding
    d. Both a & c

6. Where is the intent of a relationship between an independent contractor and client most commonly described?

    a. Job description
    b. IRS forms
    c. Agreement/contract
    d. Employee handbook

7. **As an independent contractor, your clients are usually:**
    a. Other businesses that contract your services for several years
    b. Other businesses that temporarily contract your services
    c. Individuals
    d. A 50/50 mix of businesses and individuals

8. **As an independent contractor, your client contract should outline:**
    a. Agreed-on tasks and results
    b. Agreed-on conditions
    c. Agreed-on fees
    d. All of the above

9. **Which of the following start-up expenses can you expect as an independent contractor?**
    a. Business license(s) and insurance
    b. Rent for physical space
    c. Decor and furnishings
    d. All of the above

10. **Which of the following is a reality for independent contractors?**
    a. Paid education/training opportunities
    b. Paid health and liability insurance
    c. Office administration and tax preparation
    d. Formal reviews and opportunities for feedback

11. **What are two key factors in determining the fees you charge clients?**
    a. Value of service and market rates
    b. Ability to pay and existing relationship
    c. Ease/difficulty of tasks and length of relationship
    d. Return on investment and expected bookings

12. **Once established, independent contractors do not have to devote time to business development and administration.**
    a. True
    b. False

13. **As an independent contractor, you need to be comfortable working _____ and being _____.**
    a. As a team; closely monitored
    b. Alone; self-motivated
    c. Quickly; efficient
    d. Quietly; self-reflective

14. **What are some of the common office administrative tasks you will do as an independent contractor?**
    a. Develop bylaws, a standard operating procedures manual, and book of policies
    b. Develop monthly financial reports, statements of cash flow, and financial chart of accounts
    c. Pay bills and save receipts, invoice and bill clients, complete tax returns
    d. One of the benefits of being an independent contractor is not having to do a lot of administrative work

15. Which tax is an independent contractor responsible for paying?
    a. State
    b. Federal
    c. Self-employment
    d. All of the above

16. Which of the following does professional liability insurance typically *not* cover?
    a. Malpractice
    b. Accidents due to negligence
    c. Product liability
    d. Identity or employee theft

17. As long as an independent contractor consistently performs and behaves well, the contractor will have a job the next day.
    a. True
    b. False

18. Savvy contractors know their success depends on which of the following?
    a. Quality of their work
    b. Quantity of work
    c. Bookkeeping abilities
    d. Both a & c

19. Which of the following traits/characteristics do independent contractors need to be successful?
    a. Humility
    b. Generosity
    c. Initiative
    d. Dignity

20. Which of the following best describes interpersonal skills, a trait needed by independent contractors?
    a. Verbal, nonverbal, and written communication
    b. Treating and honoring all people with respect
    c. The art of walking in someone else's shoes
    d. Emotional intelligence

21. The most successful independent contractors develop business and marketing plans that outline goals and contain tactics for filling their lives with meaning.
    a. True
    b. False

Worksheet 6-1   Pros and Cons of Being an Independent
Contractor

The IRS evaluates the degree of control and independence in three categories when determining worker status as either an independent contractor or an employee. You can use these categories and questions to help you decide whether you would prefer to be an independent contractor or an employee.

1. **Behavioral:** The company does not have the right to control what you do and how you do your job. However, it does have the right to certain expectations regarding the end results, based on the fee it pays you for your services.

Pros	Cons

2. **Financial:** The business aspects of your job are not controlled by the payer. These are things you will jointly agree on, including how and when you are paid, whether expenses are reimbursed, and who provides tools and supplies.

Pros	Cons

3. **Type of relationship:** You have a written contract or agreement that outlines expectations, payment for services, termination of the contract, any benefits received, and length of service.

Pros	Cons

Worksheet 6-2   Professional Membership Comparison

The American Massage Therapy Association and Associated Bodywork and Massage Professionals are two organizations that provide professional liability insurance to massage therapists. Use the information and work space provided below to evaluate and compare the two programs.

American Massage Therapy Association: http://www.amtamassage.org/InsCoverage.html

Annual Fees:

Specific Coverage:

Coverage Limits/Amounts:

Additional Benefits:

Associated Bodywork and Massage Professionals: http://www.abmp.com/insurance/

Annual Fees:

Specific Coverage:

Coverage Limits/Amounts:

Additional Benefits:

Worksheet 6-3   Independent Contractor Realities

The categories below describe the realities of being an independent contractor. Rank each of these items according to their level of importance to you using the following scale: 3 = very important; 2 = somewhat important; 1 = not important. When finished, consider your overall and individual answers to help determine whether the path of the independent contractor is right for you.

_____   Designing and negotiating contracts

_____   Setting fees

_____   Determining payment timing and structure

_____   Having few paid benefits

_____   Training at your own expense

_____   Having scheduling flexibility

_____   Provided treatment rooms

_____   Few other services besides massage for the client

_____   Increased administrative tasks

_____   Working independently

_____   Tax preparation

_____   Insurance responsibility

_____   Ability to hire professional advisers

_____   **Total points**

The closer your score is to 36, the more happiness you will experience as an independent contractor. If your score is between 20 and 36 points, then you will probably enjoy being an independent contractor. If you scored less than 20, review your responses to determine what may make you unhappy as an independent contractor.

Worksheet 6-4	Independent Contractor Skills and Knowledge

Using the spreadsheet below, evaluate your skills and knowledge in areas important to success as an independent contractor.

Knowledge, Skills, and Traits	High Level	Needs Improvement
Massage industry knowledge		
Anatomy knowledge		
Business knowledge		
Customer knowledge		
Massage skills		
Ability to perform effective massage		
Initiative		
Confidence		
Flexibility		
Communication skills		
Interpersonal skills		
Empathy		
Fiscally responsible		
Goal-oriented		
Strong ethics		

Chapter **7**

Your Path as an Entrepreneur

*"Whenever you see a successful business, someone once made
a courageous decision."*

—Peter Drucker

Outline

You will learn to ...

- Define what a professional's life looks like as a business owner
- Clarify the differences between an independent contractor and an entrepreneur
- Identify types and potential locations of massage-related businesses you can start

You will learn to ...—cont'd

■ Identify the desirable attributes of a business owner

■ Create a list of necessary start-up requirements

■ Build a basic business plan document

Key Definitions

This chapter references several key terms, which are indicated in bold. For easy reference, these terms are briefly defined here:

Business plan: Defines a business, identifies goals, and serves as a corporate resume.

Corporation: Type of business that is a legal entity separate from their owners. The owners of the company are its shareholders, and a board of directors oversees the major policies and decisions.

Development financing: These are long-term loans for major fixed assets, such as land or a building.

Employee: A person hired to provide services to a company in exchange for compensation, who does not provide these services as part of an independent business.

Entrepreneur: A person who begins a business and assumes all related risks and rewards.

Franchise financing: This financing is available to franchisees of recognized, nationally known franchises.

Higher purpose: A sense of contributing your passion, skills, and talents toward something bigger than yourself.

Independent contractor: A person hired to provide services who is not hired as an employee of that person or company. The terms and specifications of work provided are outlined in a contract or agreement for short- or long-term engagement. They are sometimes called "contractors" or "freelancers."

Life and disability insurance: This coverage insures your business against the death or disability of you or your business partners.

Limited liability company (LLC): Type of business that combines aspects of both the corporation and partnership ownership structures. It offers the operational flexibility of a partnership and the limited personal liabilities of a corporation.

Micro loans: These small business loans can be used for any business reason and generally range from $5,000 to $35,000.

Mission statement: Written statement that describes why a company exists and what it does.

Partnership: Type of business ownership where more than one individual own the business. A legal arrangement outlines how decisions are made, profits shared, disputes resolved, and other business details. Partners share assets and profits as well as the risks.

Professional liability insurance: This insurance provides coverage against allegations of professional negligence or failure to perform professional duties.

Property and casualty insurance: Property coverage insures the building and any property inside the building, such as equipment and furnishings. Casualty insurance covers the business itself and extends to events that may indirectly affect your business.

Continued

Key Definitions—cont'd

SBA loans: These are loans to small businesses from banks, credit unions, and other lenders, which are guaranteed by the U.S. Small Business Association.

Sole proprietorship: Type of business owned by one person. This individual generally handles all of the daily operations of running the business, owns all of the assets and profits, and assumes all the risk.

Workers' compensation insurance: This insurance is paid for by an employer and covers medical and rehabilitation costs, as well as lost wages, if an employee is hurt on the job.

ENTREPRENEURS

As you have probably noticed, massage therapy does not have a typical career ladder. You do not necessarily advance through promotions or by progressively taking on higher levels of responsibility. That is why many therapists dream of eventually starting their own practice, taking control of attracting clients and setting fees as they deem necessary. It takes effort and business and entrepreneurial skills, as well as much time, to build a practice. Once you have started a practice, income can be increased by higher productivity or raising fees; however, this is limited by the relatively intensive, one-on-one nature of massage therapy and the competitive market.

Most companies start up because someone had a passion (Fig. 7–1). The creative phase of starting a business is the act of moving from the idea phase to reality. Regardless of the product or service, someone believed she could make a difference while earning a living at the same time. She acted on this belief and developed a product or service that was attractive enough to encourage attention from others. In fact, she was so sure that her passion would be contagious that she even put a price tag on it and expected others to pay for it. Imagine that. Now, unfortunately, most businesses never make it past this point. According to the U.S. Small Business Association (SBA), more than 50% of small businesses fail in the first 5 years, with the primary reason being lack of experience. This failure rate is a great reason to plan your career progression carefully.

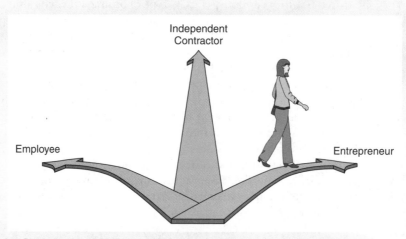

Figure 7–1   Choosing the path of an entrepreneur can be the most fulfilling choice but requires much work to succeed.

Once **entrepreneurs** make it past this first phase, they naturally progress to thinking about adding new products, services, and **employees**. In doing so, they leave the initial creative phase necessary for business creation and enter a growth strategy phase. At this phase, an entrepreneur may feel like he or she has survived the pendulum ride of fear and joy and is free to confidently explore the expansion of the business. For a massage therapist, this may look like having a full practice and exploring the possibility of renting a larger location and space for other therapists to practice and pay a percentage.

Entrepreneurship is mostly for the strong at heart and those willing to take a chance on their dreams. Owning your own massage therapy business offers freedom and flexibility as well as an opportunity to pour your heart into a personal creation that you are passionate about. It is an exciting chance to follow your dreams, but that excitement is countered with significant responsibility and stress. For many massage therapists, owning your own practice is a professional dream and ultimate goal. In fact, the American Massage Therapy Association (AMTA) reports that 96% of massage therapists are sole practitioners or **independent contractors**.[1] Many therapists start out working for someone else to increase their experience, knowledge, and skill in the profession and industry, with the ultimate goal of entrepreneurship. If you are considering starting your own practice, it is important to start planning now, even if you think your dream is several years away.

> Many therapists start out working for someone else to increase their experience, knowledge, and skill in the profession and industry, with the ultimate goal of entrepreneurship.

Typically, most massage entrepreneurs are classified as small business owners, working out of their homes or a facility on their property, sharing space with other therapists, or renting or leasing a small space. An entrepreneur may also own and operate a spa, wellness or massage center, or massage franchise, employing a small or large staff, but this is not the norm in the industry. According to the SBA, in 2008, there were 29.6 million small businesses in the United States, representing 99.7% of all businesses with employees. Showing the range of these small businesses, 52% were home-based and 2% were franchises. Census data show there were 6 million firms with employees in 2006 and 21.7 million without employees in 2007.[3]

Entrepreneur Versus Independent Contractor

As an independent contractor, you are self-employed and your clients are typically businesses. Therefore, your revenue comes from other companies. You are a contractual employee for one or more companies. You do not set their company policies or direction, nor do you have a say in their future. As an entrepreneur, you are also self-employed, but most likely your clients are individuals seeking massage, and your revenue comes directly from these individuals. As the owner, you set your company's vision, policies, and direction and have control (over those things you can control) of its future and success (Fig. 7–2). Entrepreneurs may also hire other workers, such as receptionists or other therapists, and generally promote themselves and their businesses, whereas contractors are simply promoting and marketing themselves as outsourced persons for hire.

REALITIES OF BEING AN ENTREPRENEUR

Your vision of entrepreneurship may encompass standing outside a beautifully decorated massage or wellness center, watching stressed, tense customers go in and happy, relaxed customers come out. In this entrepreneurial dream, you are not only helping and healing others, but you are also financially profitable and able to enjoy free time. Although there are various versions of this vision, the actual manifestation of the dream takes an incredible amount of hard work, significant time, unfaltering dedication, and a great deal of good luck.

See Worksheet 7-1

Most students preparing to graduate will not launch directly into entrepreneurship, but if you are considering it now, or down the road, it is important to know the realities. Also, keep in mind that the data presented here are helpful when you are developing a business plan.

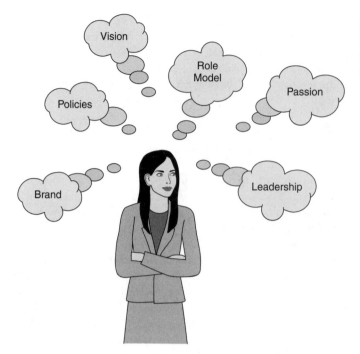

Figure 7–2   As an owner, you set the vision, policies, and direction for your company's future success.

Here are some key points about the reality of owning your own massage therapy practice.

- About 67% of massage therapists describe themselves as a sole practitioner/partner in their own business. More therapists appeared to be working as employees in spas/salons and health-care settings in 2008 than in 2005.[2]
- Massage therapists work an average of 20 hours a week. The time spent actually performing paid massages in 2008 was 15 hours per week.[2]
- Massage therapists consider a full-time practice to be, on average, 27 hours per week.[2]
- Massage therapists spend 28% of their workday on business-related tasks and 72% of their time performing massages.[2]
- About 54% of massage therapists' income is earned from jobs in professions other than massage therapy.[1]
- Of those massage therapists who earn income working in another profession, 26% practice other forms of body work, whereas 22% work in health care and 21% work in education.[1]
- Massage therapists see an average of 44 clients each month.[1]
- Of the clients therapists saw, 72%, or nearly three out of four clients, were repeat clients.[2]
- Massage therapists charged an average of $63 for a 1-hour massage.[1]
- Most physical therapy services and many chiropractic treatments are reimbursed by health insurance, whereas more than 90% of massage therapy sessions are paid out of the client's pocket.[5]

Challenges Facing Massage Therapists

The AMTA asked therapists about the challenges they face as professionals, and the top four concerns, listed in priority order, were as follows:

1. Industry perceptions, particularly being recognized and respected as health-care professionals
2. Business and economic issues, particularly a poor economy

3. Job factors, such as avoiding personal injury
4. Education issues, including finding a good school or training program[2]

WHAT IT TAKES TO BE SUCCESSFUL

There are important personal and professional components to becoming a successful entrepreneur. Most of the knowledge, skills, and traits it takes to be successful as an independent contractor also apply as an entrepreneur, such as initiative, people skills, confidence, and a strong moral compass. When determining whether you have what it takes to start your own massage therapy practice, ask yourself these important questions:

- *Am I self-motivated?* No one guides you or tells you what to do or when to work, which is attractive to many therapists. However, think about your motivation and work ethic. If no one else is pushing you, are you self-motivated enough to push yourself to put in the hours and work necessary to be successful? This includes having enough motivation to avoid distractions. When working from home, or by yourself, distractions can pull you away from the work necessary to move your business forward. You must stay focused.

- *Am I able (and willing) to do many tasks?* Entrepreneurs who own their own massage practices do much more than perform massage. According to the AMTA, massage therapists spend 28% of their workday on business-related tasks and 72% on performing massages.[2] Other common tasks include cleaning, booking appointments, accounting and bookkeeping, record-keeping, marketing, and promotion.

- *Am I willing to work a flexible schedule?* If you are used to, or desire, a predictable schedule, then entrepreneurship may disappoint you. As a business owner, you must work when the clients need you, which can be early morning to late evening. If you turn down appointments, you are turning down money.

- *Am I good at setting and achieving goals?* Setting measurable and attainable goals is important for entrepreneurs. You need to set goals and develop a plan on how you will achieve them. As with anything, you can allow flexibility as things progress, as long as you are still making progress.

- *Am I a good planner?* If you fail to plan, you plan to fail. Starting and running a massage therapy practice takes good planning from the start and throughout your business career. There are business plans, financial plans, marketing plans, communication plans, strategic plans, risk management plans, and so many others, including vacation plans. Although it may seem odd to include vacation plans in a list of business plans, it is vitally important in entrepreneurship that you take care of yourself. You are your best and most passionate employee, and many entrepreneurs get so caught up in their work and feeding their inner workaholic that many forget to plan for renewal time. So, one of the first things to write in your planner is your time off, and then you can schedule everything around that.

> Although altruistic reasons may drive your business goals, you must develop the skills required to remain financially viable.

- *Am I fiscally responsible?* Even if you have all the other skills, knowledge, and experience necessary to succeed, without this one, you will struggle. If you have strength in this area, you can manage your money and make responsible financial decisions. Although altruistic reasons may drive your business goals, you must develop the skills required to remain financially viable.

- *Am I willing to delegate tasks?* If you are not the best at managing money, or figuring out the tax codes, insurance requirements, or legalese, then you can hire professional advisers to help you. Many times, it is tough to spend money on these professional advisers because their advice is not usually inexpensive. However, if you make a wrong decision in these areas, you could lose your business or be held personally liable. As an entrepreneur, you surely want to be involved at a hands-on level in all areas of your business. Still, you must be familiar with your strengths and weaknesses and understand when delegating tasks is critical to your success (Box 7.1).

See Worksheet 7-2

Box 7.1 Points to Consider When Starting a Business

The U.S. Small Business Administration advises small business owners to consider the following points when making the decision to start their own business:

- Your vision regarding the size and nature of your business
- The level of control you wish to have
- The level of structure you are willing to deal with
- The business's vulnerability to lawsuits
- Tax implications of the different ownership structures
- Expected profit (or loss) of the business
- Whether or not you need to reinvest earnings into the business
- Your need for access to cash of the business for yourself[8]

Characteristics of Successful Entrepreneurs

A recent Entrepreneur.com article identified 25 common characteristics of successful entrepreneurs. The author recognizes the many definitions of success but found that successful business people generally shared these 25 traits:

1. Do what you enjoy.
2. Take what you do seriously.
3. Plan everything.
4. Manage money wisely.
5. Ask for the sale (in other words, ask people to buy what you are selling).
6. Remember it is all about the customer.
7. Become a shameless self-promoter (without being obnoxious).
8. Project a positive business image.
9. Get to know your customers.
10. Level the playing field with technology (such as websites, social media).
11. Build a top-notch business team.
12. Become known as an expert.
13. Create a competitive advantage.
14. Invest in yourself.
15. Be accessible.
16. Build a rock-solid reputation.
17. Sell benefits.
18. Get involved.
19. Grab attention.
20. Master the art of negotiations.
21. Design your work space for success.
22. Get and stay organized.
23. Take time off.
24. Limit the number of hats you wear (in other words, delegate when possible).
25. Follow up constantly.[4]

See Worksheet 7-3

Self-Care Is Vital for Success

A component critical to the success of massage therapist entrepreneurs is practicing what you preach. You know how important it is to take care of your mind, body, and spirit, but many people, particularly massage therapist entrepreneurs, have a tough time practicing this. As caretakers, they often work too much, do not eat right, rarely make time to exercise, and probably cannot remember the last time they got a massage, unless it was for a practical. They also seldom ask for help. Although it may seem you have no time, you have to make a conscious choice to make time to fulfill the basics of what you preach. Here are some things to keep in mind in taking care of you:

- Eat right.
- Exercise.
- Get regular massages.
- Find a stress reliever that works for you.
- Schedule time off.
- Spend quiet time meditating, journaling, or just "being."
- Ask for help when you need it (Box 7.2).

See Worksheet 7-4

- Build a strong support network.

WHAT YOU NEED TO GET STARTED AS A BUSINESS OWNER

As a business owner, you have the opportunity to make many important decisions. Although you must plan well before opening your business, remember to stay flexible—experience is the best teacher. Once you are in your business and learning realities of the business and your situation, you may need to adjust previous decisions. Be prepared by considering these areas now so that you can identify potential answers to very serious questions you may face down the road. Knowing the answers to these questions will also help you to develop your business plan.

Higher Purpose Guides the Mission

Understanding your higher purpose helps you begin to formalize the mission of your company. **Higher purpose** is a sense of contributing your passion, skills, and talents toward something bigger than yourself. Clarifying your unique higher purpose helps to answer the larger questions. Why am I here? What brings me fulfillment? How do I make a difference? If you are clear on this for yourself, you can translate it into your career. You can create a company that aligns with this sense of purpose.

To help you define your sense of purpose, you can reflect on the following statement: your purpose should reflect your reason for being—it is not a goal, it is not tied to your service or to your market, it is not tied to achieving revenue goals.

A **mission statement** describes why your company exists and what it does. It is typically focused on the present day, unlike a vision statement, which is focused on the future. A mission statement

A mission statement describes why your company exists and what it does.

is written in practical and concrete language. It describes who you are as a business but also defines the boundaries of your work and serves as a guide for future goal setting. It is a touchstone you can use when making day-to-day decisions as well as choices that affect your future.

When considering your purpose and mission, you may also want to think about your niche, or areas of specialization: is it straightforward massage, or is it therapeutic massage, pregnancy massage, or pet massage? This helps define your business and answers other questions relative to marketing

Box 7.2 Where Small Business Entrepreneurs Go for Advice

- 52% from individual mentors
- 51% from social networks
- 44% from trade associations
- 36% from business advisors
- 31% from the Internet
- 27% from Chambers of Commerce[7]

See Worksheet 7-5

and business planning. When thinking about your mission as an entrepreneur, it can be easy to get bogged down in the minutia—think in broad terms about what you hope to accomplish with your business.

Determining Your Business Structure

When you make the decision to start a business, you must also decide how to structure your business. This can have tax and legal implications for you during start-up, as well as down the road, so it is important to work with a professional adviser, such as an accountant or attorney.

There are four primary types of ownership structures:

1. Sole proprietorship
2. Partnership
3. Corporation
4. Limited liability corporation (LLC)

Sole Proprietorship

Most businesses, including massage businesses, are structured as **sole proprietorships**. The SBA describes this type of ownership as follows:

> These firms are owned by one person, usually the individual who has day-to-day responsibilities for running the business. Sole proprietors own all the assets of the business and the profits generated by it. They also assume complete responsibility for any of its liabilities or debts. In the eyes of the law and the public, you are one in the same with the business.

> *Advantages of a Sole Proprietorship*

> - Easiest and least expensive form of ownership to organize.
> - Sole proprietors are in complete control, and within the parameters of the law, may make decisions as they see fit.
> - Sole proprietors receive all income generated by the business to keep or reinvest.
> - Profits from the business flow directly to the owner's personal tax return.
> - The business is easy to dissolve, if desired.

> *Disadvantages of a Sole Proprietorship*

> - Sole proprietors have unlimited liability and are legally responsible for all debts against the business. Their business and personal assets are at risk.
> - May be at a disadvantage in raising funds and are often limited to using funds from personal savings or consumer loans.
> - May have a hard time attracting high-caliber employees or those that are motivated by the opportunity to own a part of the business.
> - Some employee benefits such as owner's medical insurance premiums are not directly deductible from business income (only partially deductible as an adjustment to income).[8]

Partnership

As the name implies, a partnership consists of two or more people sharing ownership of the business. There are three types of partnerships to consider: general partnership, limited partnership and partnership with limited liability, and joint ventures. Partnerships, as described by the SBA, are like a sole proprietorship in that the law does not distinguish between the business and its owners.

> The partners should have a legal agreement that sets forth how decisions will be made, profits will be shared, disputes will be resolved, how future partners will be admitted to the

partnership, how partners can be bought out, and what steps will be taken to dissolve the partnership when needed. Yes, it is hard to think about a breakup when the business is just getting started, but many partnerships split up at crisis times, and unless there is a defined process, there will be even greater problems. They also must decide up-front how much time and capital each will contribute, etc.

Advantages of a Partnership

- Partnerships are relatively easy to establish; however, time should be invested in developing the partnership agreement.
- With more than one owner, the ability to raise funds may be increased.
- The profits from the business flow directly through to the partners' personal tax returns.
- Prospective employees may be attracted to the business if given the incentive to become a partner.
- The business usually will benefit from partners who have complementary skills.

Disadvantages of a Partnership

- Partners are jointly and individually liable for the actions of the other partners.
- Profits must be shared with others.
- Since decisions are shared, disagreements can occur.
- Some employee benefits are not deductible from business income on tax returns.
- The partnership may have a limited life; it may end upon the withdrawal or death of a partner.[8]

Corporations

Unlike sole proprietorships and partnerships, **corporations** are separate from their owners. The SBA says:

A corporation can be taxed, it can be sued, and it can enter into contractual agreements. The owners of a corporation are its shareholders. The shareholders elect a board of directors to oversee the major policies and decisions. The corporation has a life of its own and does not dissolve when ownership changes.

Advantages of a Corporation

- Shareholders have limited liability for the corporation's debts or judgments against the corporations.
- Generally, shareholders can only be held accountable for their investment in stock of the company. (Note however, that officers can be held personally liable for their actions, such as the failure to withhold and pay employment taxes.)
- Corporations can raise additional funds through the sale of stock.
- A corporation may deduct the cost of benefits it provides to officers and employees.
- Can elect S corporation status if certain requirements are met. This election enables company to be taxed similar to a partnership.

Disadvantages of a Corporation

- The process of incorporation requires more time and money than other forms of organization.
- Corporations are monitored by federal, state and some local agencies, and as a result may have more paperwork to comply with regulations.
- Incorporating may result in higher overall taxes. Dividends paid to shareholders are not deductible from business income; thus it can be taxed twice.[8]

Limited Liability Company

A **limited liability company,** often referred to by its acronym, LLC, is a combination of features from both the corporation and partnership ownership structures. The SBA describes it as follows:

> It is designed to provide the limited liability features of a corporation and the tax efficiencies and operational flexibility of a partnership. Formation is more complex and formal than that of a general partnership. The owners are members, and the duration of the LLC is usually determined when the organization papers are filed. The time limit can be continued, if desired, by a vote of the members at the time of expiration. LLCs must not have more than two of the four characteristics that define corporations: Limited liability to the extent of assets, continuity of life, centralization of management, and free transferability of ownership interests.[8]

Acquiring Capital

Whether you are starting small by operating a massage therapy business out of your home or going big and buying into a massage therapy franchise, you need start-up money. There are four primary ways to acquire start-up money for a massage therapy business:

- Personal loans
- Loans from family and friends
- Credit cards
- Bank loans

Personal Loans

Personal loans are the best way to get started because they come with no strings attached, including interest or opinions of others also invested in the business. Let us look at this type of start-up money, using the two key words separately. First, "personal." This is your money that you invest into your company. There are differences of opinion about how much of your own money to actually invest. One viewpoint is that if you have available cash to start your business, then you must be willing to invest every penny you have in your business. You need to pull from savings, investments, and other personal sources of cash. If you are concerned about using your personal sources of cash or worried about using some of your retirement or investments, then do you really have what it takes to start a

---

7-1: Find It on the Web

FINANCIAL RESOURCES

The U.S. Small Business Administration has a wealth of information for those considering entrepreneurship. Their resources available for acquiring financial capital include:

- Developing a loan proposal
- Elements of a loan proposal
- Selecting a bank/lender
- Presenting a loan proposal
- If the loan is approved
- If the loan is not approved
- Where to turn for help
- What to do when no one will lend you money[9]

For details, visit the U.S. Small Business Administration website:
http://www.sba.gov/smallbusinessplanner/start/financestartup/SERV_LOANPROPOSAL.html

business? Do you have it well thought out and planned? Do you feel confident you will succeed? If you hesitate to invest your own money, then that is a big red flag that perhaps you have not completely thought it through. In other words, you may not truly believe you can make it, or else you would put every penny into this investment in your future. Plus, if you do not have enough faith in your business to invest in it, then neither does anyone else.

The other viewpoint on this is that starting any new business is a gamble, and there are many variables outside of your control. For example, according to SCORE, a national association focused on helping small business owners, in 2008 there were 627,200 new businesses, 595,600 business closures, and 43,546 bankruptcies. That is a lot of competition, a lot of failed business, and a lot of lost money. Because of this, it is best to not use all of your available cash to invest in the business. You must ensure that you can survive financially in the unfortunate event the business is not successful. So, you may use some of your personal funds, but you should not use all of them. If you have personal funds available, you must determine the best route for you.

The second key word is "loan." You need to treat this personal loan as a loan, even if it comes from you. Because this money is probably your emergency fund or retirement money or is earmarked for other long-term needs, you have to pay it back (Fig. 7–3). And remember, your personal money must be kept separate from your business funds. Build this into your financial plan so that you can begin to pay yourself back within the first 1 to 2 years of the business. Your accountant or bookkeeper can help you set this up.

Loans From Family and Friends

If you do not have the personal financial resources to provide yourself a loan, then you may consider reaching out to friends and family. This can be a way for those who care about you to support your vision for the future as well. Often, family and friends will loan you start-up money without asking

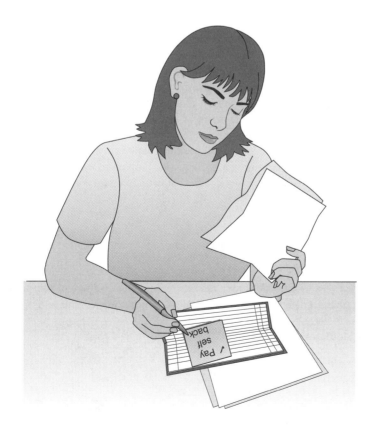

Figure 7–3   Personal loans are sometimes necessary, and a plan should be developed to pay them off.

for interest or anything in return other than their initial investment back. On the other hand, this can be a recipe for disaster if the business fails or if relationships get in the way. Managing this dual relationship may not be worth the amount they are willing to provide you. You must clearly define expectations and put them in writing. You may assume that your aunt does not want interest on the cash she loans you, but do not be caught making the wrong assumption. Clarify expectations regarding the terms or conditions of the loan, such as when the money will be paid back, interest charged, financial and operation reporting, and level of involvement from the investor.

Credit Cards

Many who do not have the financial resources for a personal loan or a loan from friends in family will turn to credit cards for small amounts of required credit. Do not be fooled by the ease of credit

> Do not be fooled by the ease of credit cards because these are still loans and sometimes have very high interest rates.

cards because these are still loans and sometimes have very high interest rates. Interest rates vary from 0% up to 37% and may change over time. According to Index Credit Cards.com, the average consumer credit card rate for the overall market was 16% in early 2010. Using this as an example, say you purchase a $250 massage table for your new business and put it on your personal credit card. Your minimum payment is $15 per month, and if you pay the minimum, it will take you 19 months to pay off the massage table at a total of $284.61. The additional $34.61 is interest payments. If you paid $50 per month, you would have it paid off in 6 months and pay $10.50 in interest. With credit cards, you always want to pay more than the minimum, so you reduce the amount of interest you pay.

It is also important to shop around for credit cards because many offer lower rates for businesses. Some offer introductory rates of 0% on purchases and balance transfers for a minimum of 6 months. Some offer even longer introductory periods, based on your credit score, of up to 1 year of 0% interest. That means your massage table costs you only $250, and the credit card company loaned you the money interest free, if you pay it off with the specified interest-free time period. However, the credit card companies are gambling that you will not pay it off early, or that you will continue to add expenses to your card. And this is where many new business owners get in trouble.

Let us look at another example. Say you have an interest-free credit card and during the first year, you put several large expenses on your credit card. You buy a massage table, lotions, linens, sound system, business cards, insurance, and uniforms. Over the first year, you do not pay any interest, and you make regular payments ranging from the minimum to a few occasional higher payments. After the 12-month introductory period, the interest rate goes into effect at 17%, and you have a remaining balance of $1,000 after 12 months. If you pay only the minimum, which is probably about $23, then it will take you 108 months (9 years) to pay off the debt, and during that time you will pay $792.87 in interest. That is almost as much as your original balance of $1,000. If you bump up your minimum monthly payment to $50 per month, it will take you 24 months to be rid of your debt, and you will pay $170.89 in interest.

7-2: Find It on the Web

DEBT CALCULATORS

Bankrate.com provides various calculators, ranging from credit card to small business types, which let you enter variables to determine interest payments, length of payments and other key indicators. Examples include the following:

Credit Card Calculators:

- Debt payoff calculator
- Loan consolidation calculator
- Credit card minimum payment calculator

> ### 7-2: Find It on the Web—cont'd
>
> - Credit card balance transfer calculator
> - Credit card debt calculator
> - Reduce credit card debt calculator
> - Find the best credit card for you
>
> **Small Business Calculators:**
>
> - Calculate your payment on any loan (includes amortization schedule)
> - Current ratio calculator
> - Quick ratio calculator
> - Debt-to-assets ratio calculator
> - Return on assets calculator
> - Gross profit margin calculator
> - Operating profit percentage calculator
>
> Visit http://www.bankrate.com/calculators.aspx to access the calculators.

Bank Loans

For small business entrepreneurs who require a bank loan to get started, there are two types of loans available to you—short-term and long-term. A short-term loan is generally for 1 year or less, meaning that you have 1 year (or less) to pay back the principal and interest. Long-term loans, as the name implies, offers a longer length of time to repay the loan and interest. They range from 1 to 7 years but can be longer for property or expensive equipment. There four primary types of loans for small businesses to consider:

- **Micro loans:** These small business loans can be used for any business reason, and generally range from $5,000 to $35,000.
- **SBA loans:** These are loans to small businesses from banks, credit unions, and other lenders, which are guaranteed by the SBA. The funds themselves are actually loaned by private lending institutions, not the SBA.
- **Franchise financing:** This financing is available to franchisees of recognized, nationally known franchises.
- **Development financing:** These are long-term loans for major fixed assets, such as land or a building.[10]

Most loan proposals include a cover letter or executive summary, which summarizes the basic intent and purpose of your loan request. The cover letter should include factual and, when possible, evidence-based information, focusing on what the banker would most want to know about you and your business (Box 7.3).

Information about you, your business background, the basics of your business, the amount you are requesting, how the money will benefit your business, and how you will repay the loan are some typical parts of the cover letter or executive summary (Box 7.4).

The SBA advises that a loan proposal and application should cover the following basics:

- **Description of business:** Include a description of the type of business and service, location, proposed future operation, competition, customers, and suppliers.
- **Management experience:** Include the owner's resume as well as the resumes of any partners or key managers.

Box 7.3 Tips for Applying for a Bank Loan

The U.S. Small Business Administration suggests the following tips when applying for a bank loan:

1. Put forth your best effort in developing the first loan proposal and application because you may not get a second chance.
2. Loan proposal formats come in many different forms, so contact your potential lender to determine which format is best.
3. Do not assume the lender is familiar with your industry or business. Be sure to include some basic background information.
4. Always include industry-specific information so that the lender can grasp how your business will be run and what industry trends may affect it.[9]

Box 7.4 The 5 Cs of Credit

When a bank loans money, it wants to ensure it gets paid back. According to the U.S. Small Business Administration, a bank must consider the 5 Cs of credit each time it makes a loan:

1. **Capacity** to repay is the most critical of the five factors.
2. **Capital** is the money you personally have invested in the business and is an indication of how much you will lose, should the business fail.
3. **Collateral** or guarantees are additional forms of security you can provide to the lender.
4. **Conditions** focus on the intended purpose of the loan.
5. **Character** is the personal impression you make on the potential lender or investor.[9]

- **Personal financial statements:** The SBA requires financial statements for all principal owners (20% or more) and guarantors. Financial statements should not be older than 90 days and must include a copy of your prior year's federal income tax return.
- **Loan repayment:** Describe how the loan will be repaid, including repayment sources and time requirements. Supporting material should include a cash–flow statement and budget.
- **Proposed business:** Provide a *pro forma* balance sheet, which combines the information in the income statement and the cash flow projection into one, easy-to-read document.
- **Projections:** Provide a projection of future operations for 1 year or until positive cash flow can be shown, in profit and loss format. Any assumptions should be explained, if different from trend or industry standards. Your projected figures should also include documentable and evidence-based explanations.
- **Collateral:** All loans should have at least two identifiable sources of repayment. Generally, the first source is cash generated from the profitable operations of the business. The second source is usually collateral pledged to secure the loan. A common type of collateral used is a home.

Other items you may need to provide to potential lenders, if they apply, are copies of the following:

- Lease or rental agreement
- Franchise agreement
- Purchase agreement
- Articles of incorporation
- Plans and specifications
- Licenses
- Letters of reference
- Letters of intent
- Contracts
- Partnership agreement
- Financial history, if purchasing an existing business[9]

CASE STUDY 7.1

Micro Loans: When Your Business Needs a Little Boost

Source: Blueher K: *The Santa Fe New Mexican.* (2008, February 3).

A few years ago, a massage therapist came to WESST Corp because she wanted to open a small office. She had a business plan and some excellent marketing ideas but not much else. She needed a small amount of money to purchase office furniture and equipment to set up her practice. What she needed was a micro loan—a small business loan to help get her business off the ground.

The massage therapist received her loan under the condition that she meet with one of our marketing consultants to help refine her ideas. She began taking classes, including a multi-week class called Marketlink that focuses on delivering a product or service to the marketplace. It wasn't long before her sales skyrocketed from a few hundred dollars a month to a couple thousand per month. Recently she returned for another loan, this time so she could move the business to a larger location and hire other therapists.

Both the original start-up loan and the subsequent loan for expansion are typical of micro loans. Helpful when the funding needs of a business are small, micro loans range from as low as $200 to as high as $50,000. Loans of this size are often difficult to find—applicants sometimes lack collateral, have suffered credit problems, or have no business experience.

WESST Corp is a private, nonprofit economic development organization. With an average loan size of approximately $15,000, WESST Corp can be very creative with collateral. The company also wants to understand the story behind any credit problems. The manner in which clients have handled past financial problems is a good indicator of character.

But don't assume that there are no strings attached. WESST Corp requires those starting a new business to write a business plan as part of the loan application. While somewhat time consuming to write, a business plan helps clients take an objective look at their business idea and forces them to understand the areas that are critical to the success of the business. Applicants also are asked to prepare a 12-month cash flow projection to help them learn how cash moves in and out of the business and how the loan will be repaid.

Once a loan is granted, WESST Corp makes sure clients have the resources they need to succeed. One-on-one counseling is provided by consultants who include WESST staff members as well as community business leaders with specific expertise. Customized solutions, targeted guidance, and support are offered.

Classes are also available, not only to those with WESST loans but also to people thinking about going into business for themselves and owners of existing businesses who want to grow their business. One of the hidden benefits of these classes is that entrepreneurs who come together to learn often end up supporting each other and making important connections.

The massage therapist is doing splendidly in her new location, and sales recently topped $6,000 per month. I wish I could say this story is representative of all of our clients, but success is truly up to the entrepreneur. It takes creativity, perseverance, and hard work to succeed. If we help a potential entrepreneur understand this, and they decide not to start a new business because they realize it will be difficult, we have also achieved.

Location, Location, Location

In deciding where to locate your business, you have many important factors to consider (Fig. 7–4). Finding space that meets your goals and business needs is critical, but not all goals and business needs are alike. For some, finding a space in a high-traffic area may be a priority, whereas others seek a space with ambiance and energy that matches their philosophy. Many massage therapist entrepreneurs make the decision to start out small, perhaps in their homes, but set a goal of leasing or renting space in the future. Or, some therapists have a natural inclination to work in a fitness centers or a chiropractor's office but may eventually realize that the environment is not compatible with long-term growth. The reality is that as an entrepreneur in the massage industry, you will most likely change locations several times. When looking at your options, below are a few of the most common business locations for massage therapists and other points to consider.

Home Studio

Many therapists start their businesses operating out of their homes. This can take various forms, from dedicated space within the home, such as a converted bedroom, attic, or basement, to shared-use space, where you live and work out of the same space, such as a living room. A home studio can also include a studio space on your property but in a building separate from the home. This dedicated space is on your property, so there is no rent, and work and home are kept very separate.

Pros

- Working from your home keeps overhead costs low.
- Commuting to work is a breeze—just walk down the hall or to the building adjacent to your home.
- If you add a building to your property, you may also increase your property value.
- Often, you can deduct a portion of your home expenses.

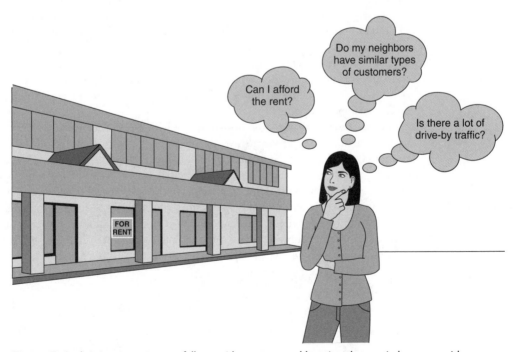

Figure 7–4   It is important to carefully consider a space and location that are in harmony with your business plan.

CONS

■ Clients may be reluctant about visiting someone's home for massage therapy, owing to concerns such as safety, privacy, and the comfort of the environment.

■ You must balance working and living in the same space, which requires you to consider issues such as separate entries, cleanliness, tidiness, odors, and pets.

■ Taking time away from work each day is incredibly important but is difficult to do when you are essentially living at work.

Rent or Lease

Renting or leasing space involves a temporary contractual arrangement to use existing space and is usually negotiated in 12-month terms for a set fee. Massage therapists often rent space from related business, such as fitness centers, chiropractic offices, or salons. In these arrangements, the rental is typically a dedicated room within the facility and with use of common areas, such as the reception area, restrooms, and changing rooms. Another option is to rent dedicated space for your business. This can be in a strip mall, office building, or other retail space and can include treatment rooms, restrooms, reception areas, and relaxation spaces that are only for the use of your clients. Definitely look into the cost of rents before making a big move. In some areas of the country, such as New York, rents are very high, and there are a lot of rules and regulations to consider.

PROS FOR SHARING SPACE WITH A RELATED BUSINESS

■ People are already coming to the location for other services so you have built-in clientele.

■ There is potential to share resources and general responsibilities, such as cleaning, laundry, and booking appointments.

■ You have a support system and sense of teamwork with others.

CONS FOR SHARING SPACE WITH A RELATED BUSINESS

■ Possible loud and intrusive noise from neighboring businesses may occur.

■ There is little room for expansion, if your business continues to grow.

■ Potential to create negative feelings and relationships, if expectations and boundaries are not clearly identified, agreed on, and upheld. For example, you may want the reception area clean and professional-looking at all times. If the facility you are renting from does not seem concerned about it, you may be the only one who picks up clutter, vacuums, dusts, and waters the plants. Over time, this can create hard feelings.

PROS FOR DEDICATED SPACE

■ You can decorate and operate the facility as you would like, without having to compromise for others.

■ There are fewer intrusions, such as noise, as well as less of the personal relationship stress that is often associated with sharing space.

■ You are able to brand the business and space as your own.

CONS FOR DEDICATED SPACE

■ Dedicated space is a more expensive option, both for start-up and ongoing expenses.

■ You are responsible for the entire business. Unless you hire employees, you are responsible for cleaning, bills, answering phones, booking appointments, and all other facility operations.

■ You have less of a support system and network, which can lead to feeling like you work on an island and have little human contact except with clients.

Cooperative

A cooperative is the term used when a small number of entrepreneur massage therapists pay for one space and then coordinate schedules. The space is shared by those in the cooperative, and so are the costs associated with the facility, such as rent, utilities, insurance, and other property expenses. Shared expenses generally also include additional support staff, such as receptionists or janitorial staff. Those in the cooperative will typically coordinate schedules, so there are hours of operation for the facility as a whole, where there is always a therapist working or available for work. In these arrangements, it is important that responsibilities, including personal, professional, and legal, be clearly outlined in writing. The financial arrangements, terms, and other key points should be put in the form of a binding contract, to protect each therapist. Typically there is one person who is in charge of ensuring that all expenses are covered in a timely manner.

> The financial arrangements, terms, and other key points [of a cooperative] should be put in the form of a binding contract to protect each therapist.

Pros

- Overhead costs are low.
- There is potential to share resources and general responsibilities, such as cleaning, laundry, and booking appointments.
- You will have a support system and sense of teamwork with other workers.
- If the relationships among partners are healthy, then the business competition may actually help your business grow, as you strive to compete with your peers.

Cons

- Although you are working in a space dedicated to massage therapy, which helps eliminate contradictory experiences such as noise, you need to select cooperative partners carefully. For example, if one partner specializes in pet massage, having barking dogs and meowing cats around the facility may not work well with human clients and partners.
- There is the potential to create negative feelings if expectations and boundaries are not clearly identified, agreed on, and upheld. For example, you may divide up duties such as answering phones and booking appointments, instead of hiring someone to do these tasks. If one of the partners consistently misses work, answers the phone unprofessionally, or does not capture appointment times accurately, then hard feelings can be created.
- If you are not as skilled as other therapists in the cooperative, or not as available to clients, then you may lose business because your clients book appointments with the other therapists.
- There are many key legal and financial responsibilities that are shared in this partnership; therefore, if a partner is unable or unwilling to fulfill obligations, then the other partners must fulfill those obligations.

Mobile Massage

Many massage therapists who own and operate a mobile massage therapy business do not need any dedicated space at all (Fig. 7–5). These therapists have a mobile massage table and go directly to the client, who is typically at home. In this case, you may have a home office but schedule appointments at clients' homes. For corporate clients, you may visit office buildings for chair massage.

Although most of the time mobile massage is very safe, there are more risks inherent with operating this type business. It is best to have a plan of action and procedure to follow if going down this route of entrepreneurship. Things to think through in advance of starting your mobile massage business include the following:

- Most of the time, you will be going to unknown locations. Plan on having a strategy for allowing others to know where you are each day. Keep a log with all contact information and times in an accessible place.
- Screen clients thoroughly. If they seem "off" during the phone interview, trust your instincts.
- Scope out the area you will be working in and have an exit strategy in mind. Place the table in a way that does not block access to exits. If things get risky, leave everything and get out.
- If upon arrival there seems to be something wrong with the client or the environment, then do not feel bad about leaving. Trusting your instincts is very important.

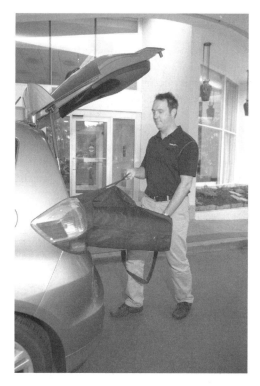

Figure 7–5   Therapists who have a mobile massage therapy business may not need any dedicated space.

Peer Profile 7–1

Tammy Gilden
Chief Energy Officer
Employee Energizer
Toronto, Canada

As a decade-plus business owner in this impactful industry I have witnessed tremendous change and potential within our industry. I bring you my successes and challenges as a way to fortify you and to pique your excitement for our unique industry of public service.

I was in management for a number of years, and needing something different, I responded to an advertisement for classes in chair massage. I had a chair massage and was definitely HOOKED! Possibilities of business burst in my head! After graduating from the Relax to the Max school of chair massage (the pilot class), I opened my business in the summer of 1998. As a pioneer, I helped build credibility for chair massage businesses at places like the Board of Trade and other networking groups, which traditionally viewed massage in a nontherapeutic (provocative) fashion.

Chair massage is an easy way to introduce someone to massage therapy because it demystifies massage. Because the client is fully clothed in an upright position, vulnerability is lessened, allowing the client to examine the value of the massage, even as they relax and enjoy it. People who have chair massage inevitably go for therapeutic treatments with massage and other massage modalities.

Mobile means setting up in any venue anywhere. Grab an ergonomically designed massage chair and go—your chair massage can make the show! Do you hear Ka-CHING? Employees spend at least 60% of their day at work. Chair massage is easy to integrate in all types of places besides the workplace—events, corporate functions, parties, beaches, airports, and elder care facilities, to name a few.

Rather than position chair massage as "wholistic" relaxation-oriented therapy, I positioned the business as corporate from the start—our name, Employee Energizer, makes our intention clear. My website has a very corporate, even technical, look. Getting the help of a media and marketing expert will help you design your own unique service offering.

How can you stay engaged in your business when you work by and for yourself? The growing can get rough, and it is definitely lonely at times. Discouragement can set in, and doubts abound, sapping your energy. Finding like-minded business-savvy massage peers is helpful, but crowding out the doubts is imperative. Crowd out doubt with affirmations; crowd out doubts by asking yourself *how* to reach your goal, not *why* you are doing this. Renew yourself as much as you can—get a massage!

Businesses need to make money to survive, so just be sure that you are making what *you* need and remember to *pay yourself first*. Saving bit by bit, putting 10% or even 5% of your income in a Certificate of Deposit, Guaranteed Income Certificate, or Registered Retirement Savings Plan (RSSP), will make the bank look at you with respect and be accommodating when you need help.

Marketing has changed so much from when I began 14 years ago! Cold calls still work, as do on-site appointments, but print advertising is losing its edge. Social media is now the queen of marketing methods. I am learning it, so you can too. Go for it!

Whether you run an on-site service, local clinic, or local storefront-based business, staffing will be a challenge. One of my challenges is how to create a relationship with the client while I myself am in the head office. I get the complaints, and the therapist/practitioner gets the compliments and forms the relationship week after week. When you have a storefront, you also need to know how to connect with the client even when your staff is giving the massages.

Contracts are an imperative—your presence is a deterrent to staff self-promotion but is no guarantee. A person without scruples and good ethics can and will find a way to self-promote. Each state government is different in how it protects your rights as a business owner as opposed to the rights of people you employ. This issue is not clear-cut like embezzlement, so the laws may be unspecific or easily construed against you, the owner. Do your best and remember that people who cheat eventually run afoul and lose what they have.

Just keep moving forward. *Now* is the time, *you* are the best one to run your business, and *you* will succeed.

- Keep a high level of professionalism. Often after services, clients will want to fix you drinks or food and talk personally. Avoid setting up an environment that could become unhealthy down the road.
- Verify with your state board regarding whether there are special considerations for this type of massage for the area you plan to work within.

Pros

- Mobile massage businesses have low overhead costs because there are no rent or facility expenses.
- You are able to separate work from home more easily because you do most of your work outside the home.
- You can realistically work from any location where you can build a client base.

Cons

- You do not control the environment and can be put into less than ideal situations, such as tight space, pets, ringing phones, and other interruptions.
- Your safety is more at risk in someone else's home.
- Drive times between appointments can eat into your available time for generating revenue.
- You must consider the additional costs in vehicle maintenance and fuel as you set your prices.

Equipment and Supplies

Determining your needed equipment and supplies is another key step. Use your own knowledge of the profession, and research what other facilities have. You can also go through massage catalogs to make sure you have a comprehensive list. Be sure to consider special requirements you may have relative to your specialty and the location of your business. Take some time to figure out the quantity of supplies you need.

Massage and treatment-specific items may include:

- Massage table
- Table linens
- Towels
- Pillows, bolsters
- Sound system
- Massage oils, lotions
- Special lighting
- Candles, scents
- Uniforms
- Rugs
- Chairs
- Tables
- Decor
- Specialty supplies (e.g., stones and heating units for stone massage)

Other equipment and supplies may include:

- Computer
- Back-up drive for business files
- Schedule and accounting software
- Printer
- Telephone line dedicated to the business
- General office supplies such as paper, paper clips, staplers, and printer ink
- Business cards and stationery
- File organizing systems such as file folders, file cabinets, labels, and binders
- Credit card processor
- Gift cards, certificates

Once you have a thorough list, begin to prioritize the items into different categories of need. Some items, such as a massage table, are critical to starting your business, and you need them when you first open. Other items, like uniforms, may be important but can be obtained after starting the business. There may even be another category of items that you do not necessarily need but really want someday, such as decor. If you have the available funds, you can purchase all of these things at once. More than likely, you may need to spread out expenses over time, once you start generating revenue.

See Worksheet 7-6

Financial Decisions and Estimates

Another aspect of becoming a successful entrepreneur is drafting a "conscious allocation of money" (i.e., budget) for your business. Doesn't that sound like fun? To complete the budget, you must make some significant financial decisions. These decisions will have a direct impact on your finances, such as the amount you charge for services. They are all also larger business questions, such as whether or not you sell retail products, if you accept insurance, where you work, and which organizations you join, if any. The budget and business plans for a start-up business go hand in hand in the business development process. It is generally helpful to work on both at the same time because it provides an opportunity to see how your ideas play out financially. In addition, working on your business plan may highlight additional revenue or expenses overlooked when creating the first budget draft.

> The budget and business plan for a start-up business go hand in hand in the business development process.

Keep in mind that budgets are estimates, but they should be based on facts obtained from researching actual prices and market conditions. Here are a few examples of the financial decisions before you:

REVENUE

- Your fees for all services
- Estimated tips and gratuities
- Additional sources of revenue, such as retail items
- Insurance payments (if applicable)

EXPENSES

- Rent
- Equipment and supplies
- Insurance
- Licensure
- Payroll (may be only yourself)
- Marketing and advertising
- Networking
- Professional memberships and conferences
- Continuing education
- Avenues of self-care (e.g., gym membership or yoga classes)

Some parts of the country allow massage therapists to affordably open and run their own business. If you live in a large metropolitan area, you may face more challenges. A therapist in New York City would pay much more in rent than one starting a practice in Chattanooga, TN. Thoroughly researching realistic costs will help you successfully plan your venture into entrepreneurship. The therapist in New York City may be able to save on rent costs by sharing space and renting by the hour.

See Worksheet 7-7

Clients

Selecting a target audience is helpful when planning your business. Of course, you can serve any client who comes to you, but your target audience is the individuals you most want to attract. There can be many reasons why you choose one group over another, which may relate to your specialty, focus, or altruistic beliefs. Business and finance may play a role so that you analyze demographic information to determine your largest, most likely, and most affluent markets. You may be interested in reviewing studies that identify certain consumers, such as the International SPA Association's consumer studies. These reports include detailed information about spa goers, who may be your target audience because they are familiar with massage.

Once you identify the people you want to target as clients, then you must determine how to reach them and develop a marketing plan with specific tactics to follow. You will explore this much more in the next two chapters.

Licensure

As a therapist, you need a professional license in almost all states to perform massage. As a business owner, you must also have a business license. Business license requirements for massage therapists vary by city, county, and state. You must identify the license you need to open your business, any associated documentation and fees, and the dates when these must be completed. In some areas, you may need to file for licenses several months before you open. You may also need to research building permits and other facility-related licenses, if you are renting a facility or operating out of your home.

Proper zoning is another area to check into. You will need to check in with your city's ordinance to find zoning rules for specific districts. You would not want to put all the work required into your new business to have the city shut it down because of zoning laws. Start your research by contacting your city or county business license office to learn the current regulations and requirements.

Insurance

There are several types of insurance you should consider when you have your own business (Box 7.5). It is best to meet with an insurance professional to go through your options and decide what type of coverage is for you. Even so, you need a basic understanding of the various types of insurance that can meet your needs. Some of the insurance types that small business owners consider include the following:

- **Professional liability insurance:** This insurance covers the business if it is sued for negligence. It typically covers (1) professional liability, such as malpractice; (2) general liability, such as accidents due to negligence; (3) product liability, such as allergic reactions to essential oils; and in some cases, (4) legal expenses in the event of a lawsuit. Two of the largest massage associations provide members with professional liability insurance—the AMTA and Associated Bodywork and Massage Professionals (ABMP).
- **Key employee insurance:** This insurance covers the life or health of a key employee, the loss of whose services would cause an employer financial loss. The policy is owned and payable to the owner/employer. Typically, the employer will pay the premium.
- **Workers' compensation insurance:** If you have employees, you are required to provide workers' compensation insurance for them. However, it is also an option you can carry for yourself. Workers' compensation insurance covers medical and rehabilitation costs, as well as

Box 7.5 Retirement Savings

"The Department of Labor has been working with a number of partners to educate small business owners about various simple retirement plan options, such as SIMPLEs (Savings Incentive Match Plans for Employees of Small Employers), SEPs (Simplified Employee Pensions), Individual Retirement Accounts, payroll deduction plans, and 401(k) plans.

The education developed by the Department and its partners include "The Small Business Advisor." This site allows businesses to review various retirement plan options available to them with a description of the features of each. Based on the responses to key questions, such as number of workers employed by the company and the decision to contribute or not to contribute to the workers' retirement, plan options are provided to the business owner."
–U.S. Department of Labor, Retirement Plans, Benefits & Savings. Visit http://www.dol.gov/ elaws/pwbaplan.htm to access the Small Business Retirement Savings Advisor.

lost wages, if you are hurt on the job. With workers' compensation, an employee is not allowed to sue the employer for on-the-job injuries; but in return, the employer must provide compensation for medical bills and damages if the employee is injured while performing work duties. This coverage is regulated at the state level.

■ **Health insurance:** Health insurance can be purchased as an individual or as a business. For business plans, a minimum number of employees is often required. If you do not meet this minimum, you can explore other options, such as individual major medical plans. This insurance can cover medical, vision, and dental expenses.

■ **Life and disability insurance:** This coverage insures your business against the death or disability of you or your business partners. The incentive for this type of insurance is to guarantee the business will continue in the event something happens to one of the partners of the business. Like health insurance, this type coverage can be beneficial when trying to attract employees.

■ **Property and casualty insurance:** Property coverage insures the building and any property inside the building, such as equipment and furnishings. Casualty insurance covers the business and extends to events that may indirectly affect your business. This insurance can be specific to events, such as natural disasters (e.g., fire, flood, and hurricanes) but may also cover incidents such as identity theft or employee theft. These plans can be purchased individually, or you can acquire an all-encompassing plan that covers all of these events and more, depending on your needs. The insured location does not have to be owned by you; you can also rent or lease it.

Health care insurance is always a topic for politicians, so staying current with bills and legislation is important to avoid costly penalties.

DEVELOPING A BUSINESS PLAN

Creating a **business plan** brings many challenges for massage therapists. It is a process that requires you to strategically analyze your business idea's probability of success. If you are seeking a loan, the potential lender will want to know that you have thought through all aspects of your idea—this helps guarantee that you will make good on your promise to repay. In the lender's opinion, if you do not take the time to think through all aspects of your business, you probably will not take the time to ensure your success.

According to the SBA, a business plan defines your business, identifies your goals, and serves as your company's resume. It is an essential part of attracting financial capital and securing business loans when starting a business, but it is also much more. Most massage therapists will not require a business loan, choosing instead to put expenses on a credit card or using personal savings to buy start-up supplies. But, the business planning process offers more for you long-term than just seeking to obtain a loan. A business plan helps you prepare for the future instead of reacting to it as it happens. A business plan has three basic purposes: communication, management, and planning. As you develop your plan as an entrepreneur, you must consider and answer a standardized series of questions and key points (Box 7.6).

> A business plan helps you prepare for the future, instead of reacting to it as it happens.

Even if you do not intend to get a business loan, you should still develop a business plan. Just thinking through the details of your business makes it seem more real and tangible. And that is where the

Box 7.6 Functions of a Business Plan

A business plan:
● Is an organizational blueprint for developing your business
● Is an organized framework that captures the relevant points of your massage practice
● Defines your business and vision of success
● Serves as an action plan to put your ideas into motion and track and evaluate your progress

real value is—in the creative process. Through this process, you address key questions, research your options, and think about your business in a way that ultimately defines your vision of business success.

The plan becomes your road map to success. You can mix creativity and strategy to map your future, and the plan can be adapted as your business grows and changes. If you struggle with timelines and goals, it provides a visible way to measure your progress.

Content of the Plan

Available business plan templates range from simple, direct one-pagers to detailed, multi-page documents with visual aids. Your needs and preferences determine the type of business plan you choose. Your first plan may start out as one page but over time may grow into something more descriptive and elaborate. Just remember that no matter what format you use, all business plans must include a description of the business as well as marketing, finances, and management information. Here is a sample business plan structure:

> Just remember that no matter what format you use, all business plans must include a description of the business as well as marketing, finances, and management information.

Executive Overview: This section briefly summarizes the key points from the entire document. It is like the *Cliffs Notes* version of your business plan. It provides a general, but solid, description of the company and includes the significant points of each section. You usually complete the executive overview after you have completed the other components.

Company Mission: Briefly state the mission and purpose of your massage practice. You may choose to mention your core values.

Company Motto: This optional portion can include a phrase you already use with your clients or feature on your literature, or you can create an expression that embodies the spirit of your practice.

Business History: In this section, you:
- Describe your therapeutic career background, certifications earned, and expertise gained
- Briefly explain the progression of your decision to open a new business location

Services: This section is where you:
- List the services you plan to offer your clients, including types of massage, therapeutic treatment such as aromatherapy, and other specialized areas
- Highlight special or unique qualities of your practice

Market Analysis: This section describes the industry and market by providing:
- An overview of the overall industry, including research-based market data
- An overview of the local market, including research-based market data

Note: You can find current massage market data on the AMTA (http://www.amtamassage.org) and ABMP (http://www.abmp.com) websites.

Target Market Strategy: In this section, you:
- Identify your target market
- Explain how you plan to reach your target audience

Competitive Market Analysis: In this section, you:
- Present an analysis of competitors, including approximate numbers and types of providers

Competitive Edge: In this section, you:
- Identify your competitive advantage
- Emphasize the unique combination of experience, knowledge, and personality you offer your clients
- Explain why your services cannot be duplicated by other practitioners

Sales Strategy: In this section, you describe how you will reach out to potential clients. You may discuss:

- Sales activities and prospects
- Promotions and specials
- Distribution channels of communication

Organization and Management Structures: Here is where you:

- Include your professional background, highlighting relevant knowledge, skills and traits.
- Include the professional profiles of other key partners or members of the management team.
- Define your primary responsibilities, as well as those of other key partners or members of the management team.

Financial Information: This section includes the financial basics, such as:

- Budget
- Income statements
- Balance sheets
- Cash flow statements
- Forecasts, including a first-year monthly projection and a multi-year projection

Appendix: This is a place for support material, which can include legal documents such as domain name ownership and professional licenses. You can also include any brochures, logos, or marketing pieces here.

SAMPLE MASSAGE BUSINESS PLAN

Executive Overview

Total Relief Massage is a Sole Proprietorship owned by Michelle Smith, Licensed Massage Therapist (LMT). Ms. Smith has been an LMT in the State of California since January 2002, running her business from a home-based location. In the years since obtaining her certification, Ms. Smith has continued her education, completing classes in reflexology, hot stone massage, deep-tissue massage, and sports massage. She has advanced training in deep-tissue and sports massage and plans to specialize in these areas. Ms. Smith evaluates her clients with respect to their individual needs and preferences and offers the combination of expertise that best serves each individual.

After many months of searching for the perfect location, Ms. Smith is expanding her business and allowing it room to grow by moving from a home environment to a centrally accessible, business-centered area. She has located a place for rent at 348 Executive Avenue in the downtown area.

In pursuit of our objectives, Total Relief Massage is seeking loan financing for $10,000. This loan will be paid from the business's cash flow and collateralized by the company assets, backed by the solid reputation, experiences, and personal guarantees of Ms. Smith. Currently, there is enough profit being generated by her current clients to cover the estimated monthly payment.

Our Mission

Total Relief Massage provides pain and stress relief to our clients an effort to improve their overall health and well-being.

Business History

Michelle Smith, LMT, owner of Total Relief Massage, has been licensed by the State of California since January 2002. While working as a Massage Therapist at a Los Angeles spa, she built her massage expertise and mastered the techniques that allowed her to establish a loyal clientele once she moved her business primarily to her home office. Ms. Smith also offered in-home service and built a reputation as a deep-tissue and sports massage expert.

In 2006, Ms. Smith joined the American Health Specialties Network, which increased her credibility as a health-care provider and allowed her to easily help more clients who carry alternative health-care coverage. As her practice has grown steadily, Ms. Smith is planning to relocate to a business-oriented location to increase her availability to the day workers who seek massage for stress and pain relief purposes. Incidentally, her chosen location is near a hospital and will expose her business to potential clients who are recovering from injuries and illness.

SAMPLE MASSAGE BUSINESS PLAN —cont'd

Our Services

Total Relief Massage provides a range of therapeutic massage services, including reflexology, relaxation, deep-tissue, and sports massage.

Market Analysis

The following are facts regarding the current positive state of massage industry growth and supports Ms. Smith's decision to have her location near a hospital:

1. Data compiled by American Massage Therapy Association (AMTA) estimates that in 2009, massage therapy was a $16 to $20 billion industry.
2. The 2008 and 2009 AMTA Consumer Surveys showed that between July 2008 and July 2009, roughly 48 million adult Americans (22%) had a massage at least once.
3. The 2009 AMTA Industry Survey indicated that more than two thirds of massage therapists (76%) indicate they receive referrals from health-care professionals.
4. The number of hospitals offering complementary and alternative medicine grew from 7.7% in 1998 to 37.3% in 2007. Of those hospitals that offer complementary and alternative medicine therapies, massage therapy was offered by 70.7% as indicated by a National Survey conducted by the Health Forum/American Hospital Association in 2007.

Ms. Smith proposes to move her home-based business to a high-traffic location in a business area, taking advantage of the day workers who are employed in the surrounding businesses. Ms. Smith's business will be ideally positioned for lunch and after-work appointments because her location will be convenient for many corporate workers.

Also, the planned site is in close proximity to Standard Memorial Hospital and will draw the attention of patients traveling to and from the hospital. People who are injured and recovering represent a lucrative market for massage therapy. Ms. Smith has already contacted many of the physicians and medical offices surrounding the hospital and provided them with an information packet and referral cards.

Target Market Strategy

Total Relief Massage tends to receive clients from two general categories—stress and pain reduction and injury management. In its new location, the company is poised to serve clients w ho seek stress reduction because of its proximity to industrial business parks and is ideally situated to serve the needs of those seeking pain relief because of its proximity to a major hospital and the surrounding medical offices. With Ms. Smith's existing, loyal clients, most of whom will find the new location convenient, and the inflow of new clients from these neighboring areas, her practice is ensured to thrive and grow.

Competitive Market Analysis

Within a 10-mile radius of Total Relief Massage's proposed, new location, there are approximately 20 individual massage providers working out of their homes or private offices, in addition to LMTs working in spas, fitness centers, chiropractic offices, and other settings.

Because of the intensely personal nature of massage services, it is reasonable to conclude that Ms. Smith offers unique services that cannot be duplicated by any other massage provider. She brings her own combination of healing touch, sensitivity, and therapeutic expertise to her clients, benefiting their health in ways that cannot be replicated elsewhere.

Competitive Edge

Total Relief Massage carries its competitive edge in its singular focus on stress and pain relief, thus attracting a specific clientele much more likely to become loyal. Her networking abilities also offer her a competitive edge because she will aggressively build relationships with the hospital and medical offices in the area.

The new location will be uniquely positioned to serve the needs of stressed and overworked corporate employees who work in nearby buildings and complexes. She will be providing materials and offering on-site demonstrations arranged by the human resources department of several companies. Finally, its main street location may make the business more accessible to existing clients, who previously had to travel to Ms. Smith's residential neighborhood to obtain treatment.

Sales Strategy

Total Relief Massage understands that providing the best possible massage services is in itself a sales strategy. By conforming treatment to meet the specific needs of each client, Ms. Smith will incorporate her creative passion for therapy to provide a massage experience that would be difficult to find elsewhere. In her current practice, she has implemented a client return program that has resulted in a 30% return rate for new clients.

Ms. Smith has a three part sales strategy that will ensure her practice stays full:

1. Using marketing materials focused specifically on pain relief, she plans to ensure that every medical office within a 5-mile radius receives her information and referral packets. She will accomplish this through direct mail, face-to-face contact, and local event attendance. With her current materials, she has already experienced some client referrals, approximately 6 clients, and expects with her new materials to gain even more.

Continued

SAMPLE MASSAGE BUSINESS PLAN —cont'd

2. To ensure she is also known within the corporate community, she will create marketing materials focused on stress relief and tension. As with the medical offices, she will contact all corporate offices within a 5-mile radius with these materials.

3. Understanding the importance of on-site visibility, Ms. Smith has identified signage for her office making it more visible. Part of this loan will help pay for this high-profile signage. Ms. Smith intends to place these signs outside her highly visible new office, so that they can be easily viewed by commuters going to work and people traveling to and from the hospital.

Organizational Structure

Michelle Smith, owner and sole proprietor of Total Relief Massage, has been an LMT in the state of California since January 2002. She graduated from the LA School of Massage in late 2001 and achieved her diploma with 650 hours of massage training. In the years since obtaining her schooling and certification, Ms. Smith has continued her education, completing classes in reflexology, hot stone massage, deep-tissue massage, and sports massage. Ms. Smith also is also a member in good standing of the American Health Specialties Network and a member of the American Massage Therapy Association.

Before entering massage school, Ms. Smith was the office Manager for a health clinic for 4 years. She acquired all the necessary skills to ensure she has the ability to run her own business.

Ms. Smith is solely responsible for the day-to-day operations of the business, including providing treatment, scheduling, billing, procuring supplies, and maintaining the facility. Once her business expands and she is able, she plans to hire a part-time office worker, freeing her up to do more massage, and she will investigate sharing her office with other massage therapists on a rental basis, earning her additional income.

Financial Documents

See attached proposed budget, sales forecast, cash flow statements, and balance sheets. (These are unique to each business. Refer to Chapter 2 for suggestions regarding what to include in your financial section.)

7-3: Find It on the Web

- Sample Business Plans: http://www.bplans.com/samples/sba.cfm
- Interactive Business Plan Development: http://www.canadabusiness.ca/ibp/eng/index.cfm
- Small Business Administration, online tutorial of how to develop a business plan: http://app1.sba.gov/training/sbabp/index.htm
- Small Business Administration, information, and resources on developing a business plan: http://www.sba.gov/smallbusinessplanner/plan/writeabusinessplan/index.html

See Worksheet 7-8

CHAPTER SUMMARY

Most companies begin because someone had a passion for something. Regardless of the product or service, someone believed he could make a difference while earning a living at the same time. Entrepreneurship is a popular avenue for therapists in their professional careers, usually after they have had some experience in the workplace. In fact, 67% of massage therapists identify themselves as sole practitioners or partners in their own businesses. The reality is that many of these therapists also work a second job to make financial ends meet.

There are important personal and professional components to becoming a successful entrepreneur. Most of the knowledge, skills, and traits it takes to be a successful independent contractor also apply to an entrepreneur, such as people skills, confidence, strong moral compass, and initiative. When determining whether you have what it takes to start your own massage therapy practice, ask yourself these important questions: Are you self-motivated? Are you good at (and willing to do) many tasks? Are you willing to work a flexible schedule? Are you good at setting and achieving goals? Are you a good planner? Are you fiscally responsible? Are you willing to delegate tasks?

To get started as an entrepreneur, you need to know and understand a lot about yourself as well as your vision for your business. You must begin sketching out the type and structure of your business, where it will be located, whom you want to serve, and your financial landscape. All this information is identified in a business plan, which serves as a blueprint in the process of developing your own business. And remember—if you believe you can do it, you can.

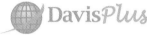 **For additional resources visit Davis*Plus* at http://davisplus.fadavis.com** (keyword, koerner).

BIBLIOGRAPHY

1. American Massage Therapy Association. (n.d.). *2010 Massage Therapy Industry Fact Sheet*. Retrieved from http://www.amtamassage.org/news/MTIndustryFactSheet2010.html.
2. American Massage Therapy Association. (2009). *AMTA 2009 Massage Industry Research Report*. Evanston, IL: American Massage Therapy Association.
3. Small Business Administration, Office of Advocacy. (2009, September). *Frequently Asked Questions*. Retrieved from http://www.sba.gov/advo/stats/sbfaq.pdf.
4. Entrepreneur (2009, Mar. 13). *25 Common Characteristics of Successful Entrepreneurs*. Retrieved from http://www.entrepreneur.com/homebasedbiz/article200730.html.
5. Associated Bodywork and Massage Professionals. (2009, September). *Massage Therapy Fast Facts*. Retrieved from http://www.massagetherapy.com/media/metricscharacteristics.php.
6. U.S. Census Bureau. (2009, June 25). *Census Bureau Reports Increase of Nearly 1 Million Nonemployer Businesses*. Retrieved from http://www.census.gov/newsroom/releases/archives/employment occupations/cb09-96.html.
7. SCORE. (n.d.). *Small Biz Stats & Trends*. Retrieved from http://www.score.org/small_biz_stats.html.
8. U.S. Small Business Administration. (n.d.). *Choose a Structure*. Retrieved from http://www.sba.gov/smallbusinessplanner/start/chooseastructure/START_FORMS_OWNERSHIP.html.
9. U.S. Small Business Administration. (n.d.). *Finance Start-Up*. Retrieved from http://www.sba.gov/smallbusinessplanner/start/financestartup/SERV_LOANAPP.html.
10. Business Finance.com. (n.d.). *Small Business Loans*. Retrieved from http://www.businessfinance.com/small-business-loans.htm.
11. U.S. Small Business Administration. (n.d.). *Small Business Readiness Assessment Tool*. Retrieved from http://www.sba.gov/sbtn/sbat/index.cfm?Tool=4.

REVIEW QUESTIONS

1. **How are most massage entrepreneurs classified?**
   a. Small business owners
   b. Medium-sized business owners
   c. Large corporate shareholders
   d. Limited liability company board members

2. **More than 50% of an average massage therapists' income is earned from:**
   a. Performing paid massage
   b. Performing Swedish or deep-tissue massage
   c. Jobs in other professions
   d. Gratuities

3. How is time approximately distributed between the average massage therapists' workday?

    a. 6% doing business-related tasks/94% performing massage

    b. 28% doing business-related tasks/72% performing massage

    c. 50% doing business-related tasks/50% performing massage

    d. 91% doing business-related tasks/9% performing massage

4. Which of the following was *not* one of the top four concerns of massage therapists, according to a 2009 AMTA study?

    a. Industry perceptions

    b. Business and economic issues

    c. Widespread growth of new, unproven techniques

    d. Job factors

5. If you are used to, or desire, a predictable schedule, then entrepreneurship may disappoint you.

    a. True

    b. False

6. Which of the following is *not* an important factor in becoming a successful entrepreneur?

    a. Self-motivation

    b. Ability and willingness to do many tasks

    c. Self-care

    d. A well-crafted exit strategy

7. Which of the following is *not* a characteristic of successful entrepreneurs?

    a. They ask for the sale and are shameless self-promoters

    b. They have a positive business image and become known as an expert

    c. They invest in themselves and take time off

    d. They remember it is all about them and take what they do lightly

8. Which of the following do you need to get started as a business owner?

    a. Compile a complete list of items you want to eventually get for your business

    b. Find a business location that is in harmony with your goals and needs

    c. Financial capital

    d. Both b & c

9. Creating a company that aligns with your personal mission or higher purpose can give you a deep sense of:

    a. Self

    b. Purpose

    c. Your clients

    d. Financial freedom

10. How are most massage businesses structured?
    a. Sole proprietorships
    b. Partnerships
    c. Corporations
    d. Limited liability companies

11. Which of the following is *not* one of the four primary ways to acquire start-up money for a massage therapy business?
    a. Kiva
    b. Personal loans, or loans from family/friends
    c. Credit cards
    d. Bank loans

12. The greatest benefit of personal loans is that the money doesn't really need to be paid back.
    a. True
    b. False

13. When starting your business through capital loaned from family and friends, you should:
    a. Clearly define expectations and put them in writing
    b. Always ask for a line of credit, instead of a set amount
    c. Guarantee it with the Small Business Administration
    d. Both a & b

14. Which of the following is a type of small business loan used for any business reason, generally ranging from $5,000 to $35,000?
    a. SBA loan
    b. Macro loan
    c. Micro loan
    d. Loan from friends or family

15. Which of the following contains a description of your business, management experience, personal finance statements, and business projections?
    a. Bank loan proposal and application
    b. Personal loan proposal and application
    c. Credit card application
    d. Purchase agreements and contracts

16. Which of the following is a disadvantage of operating a massage business from a home studio?
    a. Employee concerns about privacy, safety, and comfort
    b. Client concerns about privacy, safety, and comfort
    c. Possible loud and intrusive noises from neighboring properties
    d. Low overhead costs

17. **What types of businesses do therapists most commonly rent space from?**
    a. Occupational therapists, personal trainers, and spas
    b. Childcare centers, nursing homes, and hospitals
    c. Chiropractors, fitness centers, and salons
    d. All of the above

18. **What is an advantage of a cooperative?**
    a. Costs are shared between therapists
    b. General responsibilities are shared between therapists
    c. Support system and sense of teamwork with others
    d. All of the above

19. **An advantage of renting or leasing dedicated space is your ability to brand the business and space as your own.**
    a. True
    b. False

20. **Which of the following is a disadvantage of a mobile massage business?**
    a. You don't control the environment and can be put in less than ideal situations
    b. Work and home are more easily separated
    c. Little room for expansion if your business continues to grow
    d. Both a & c

21. **Which of the following is *not* a common expense for entrepreneurs?**
    a. Insurance
    b. Equipment and supplies
    c. Marketing and advertising
    d. Food and beverage

22. **In addition to financial estimates, what does a budget help you to do as a new entrepreneur?**
    a. Attract and retain new clients
    b. Complete your tax returns
    c. Answer larger business questions, such as whether to sell retail products or accept insurance
    d. A budget only helps you determine the financial requirements of your business

23. **In addition to being a tool to acquire a business loan, what other purposes does a business plan serve?**
    a. Fiscal accountability, personal responsibility, and client expectations
    b. Determining income, expenses, and earning potential
    c. Business structure, location options, and insurance requirements
    d. Communication, management, and planning

24. **A business plan defines your vision of success and how you intend to get there.**
    a. True
    b. False

25. **All business plans must:**
    a. Be one page in length
    b. Be detailed, multi-page documents with visual aids
    c. Define what your life looks like as a business owner
    d. Include a description of the business, including marketing, financial, and management information

Worksheet 7-1   What Owning a Business Means to You

Find some quiet time to reflect and journal on what owning a business means to you. Here are some key questions to consider:

- Why do you want to own your own business?

- What does your business look like?

- What is special about your business?

- Who will you serve?

- Who will you solicit for help?

- Who will support you through this process?

- How will it feel when you put out your "Now Open" sign?

- How will you feel after 30 days?

- How will you feel after the first year?

- How do you define success?

- What do you think your obstacles will be?

- How will you handle obstacles?

Worksheet 7–2 Entrepreneur Self-Analysis

Complete the following self-analysis of key traits you need as an entrepreneur by listing examples of strengths and opportunities.

Self-Motivation

Strengths	Opportunities to Improve

Performing Multiple Tasks

Strengths	Opportunities to Improve

Working Flexible Hours

Strengths	Opportunities to Improve

Setting and Achieving Goals

Strengths	Opportunities to Improve

Planning

Strengths	Opportunities to Improve

Fiscal Responsibility

Strengths	Opportunities to Improve

Delegation

Strengths	Opportunities to Improve

Worksheet 7-3   Entrepreneurial Readiness Assessment

The U.S. Small Business Administration designed an assessment tool to help entrepreneurs better understand their readiness to start a small business. This assessment encourages potential business owners to consider many important elements during the planning process, including skills, characteristics, and experience.

Consider the questions below and complete them with a "yes," "no," or "mushy middle."

GENERAL

- Do you feel ready to start your own business?

- Do the people in your life think you are ready?

- Have you ever worked in a similar business?

- Would family and friends support you in your business?

- Have you ever taken a course or studied how to start and manage a small business?

- Have you discussed your business plan with a business coach or counselor?

- Are there any business owners in your family?

PERSONAL CHARACTERISTICS

- Are you a self-starter?

- Would other people say you are a leader?

- Are you ready to invest your personal financial resources to get your business started?

- Do you believe in yourself and your abilities enough to ride out the tough times?

- Do you enjoy being in charge of your own decisions?

- Are you prepared to make sacrifices, if necessary, in the standard of living you are accustomed to until your business is up and running?

- Do people come to you for advice and help with decisions?

- Are you willing to regularly put in the hours needed to make your business work?

- Do others see you as a team player?

SKILLS, EXPERIENCE AND TRAINING

- Do you have a business plan yet?

- Do you understand what makes up a business plan?

- Which form of legal ownership (sole proprietor, partnership, or corporation) is best for your business?

- Do you understand the importance of business planning and how it can affect your business's success?

- Do you know whether you require a special license or permit and how to obtain it?

- Do you know how to research your customer base?

- Do you know how to determine whether your business is breaking even?

- Do you know how to determine the start-up costs for your business?

- Are you aware of the loan programs offered by banks in your area and the SBA?

- Do you know how a business loan can affect your credit score?

- Are you familiar with using balance sheets and income or cash-flow statements?

- Do you know why small businesses are considered riskier loan prospects?

- Will your business fill an existing market need?

- Do you know who your potential clients are?

- Do you understand how to deal with taxes as they relate to your business?

- Have you prepared a marketing strategy for your business?

- Do you know how to research and learn about your business competitors?

- Do you understand marketing trends in your business industry?

- Are you comfortable with using computers and technology to help advance your business?

- Have you thought through a payroll process?

- Have you come up with a strategy for customer service?

- Do you know how to go about getting an EIN (Employer Identification Number)?

- Do you know whether your business needs intellectual property protection?

- Do you know where find out about regulations and compliance requirements relating to your business?

There is an online version of this available at http://www.sba.gov/sbtn/sbat/index.cfm?Tool=4, where you can take the assessment and receive an automatic statement of "Suggested Next Steps" based on your score.[11]

Worksheet 7-4   Your Support Network

Identify the friends, family, and organizations that could make up your entrepreneur support network by acting as resources, providing information, or personally helping you to stay positive. This can also include people you do not know, such as authors, speakers, or leaders who motivate you, as well as books, movies, songs, articles, and other sources of media. For the following categories, think about whom you would reach out to for assistance.

Requirement	Identified Support
Business plan development	
Financial management	
Setting goals	
Acquiring a loan	
Bookkeeping	
Legal concerns	
Morale booster	
Peer advice	
Professional organizations	
Marketing	
Purchasing advice	
Employee management	
Continuing education	
Mentor	
Other	
Other	
Other	

Worksheet 7–5   Drafting a Mission Statement

A simple way to get started drafting a mission statement is to answer the following six questions:

1. How would you describe yourself?

2. What is your special place or role?

3. Who do you serve? Directly? Indirectly?

4. What do you do?

5. Why do you do it?

6. What does your end product look/feel like?

Worksheet 7-6   Equipment and Supply Checklist

Take a good look at massage supplier websites and catalogs to familiarize yourself with available equipment and supplies. Then, make a thorough list of what you need to start your business. Some of the supplies and equipment you need depend on the location you anticipate working from (e.g., shared retail space, dedicated space, home). Once you have completed the list, then prioritize the items into the categories of phase I, II, or III and indicate an average price and quantity you need for each item:

Phase I: must have to open business; phase II: must have eventually; phase III: not required but desired

Item	Phase I	Phase II	Phase III
1. _____	_____	_____	_____
*Price per Item:*_____	*Quantity:*_____	*Total Price:* _____	
2. _____	_____	_____	_____
*Price per Item:*_____	*Quantity:*_____	*Total Price:* _____	
3. _____	_____	_____	_____
*Price per Item:*_____	*Quantity:*_____	*Total Price:* _____	
4. _____	_____	_____	_____
*Price per Item:*_____	*Quantity:*_____	*Total Price:* _____	
5. _____	_____	_____	_____
*Price per Item:*_____	*Quantity:*_____	*Total Price:* _____	
6. _____	_____	_____	_____
*Price per Item:*_____	*Quantity:*_____	*Total Price:* _____	

Continued

Item	Phase I	Phase II	Phase III
7. _____	_____	_____	_____
*Price per Item:*_____	*Quantity:*_____	*Total Price:* _____	
8. _____	_____	_____	_____
*Price per Item:*_____	*Quantity:*_____	*Total Price:* _____	
9. _____	_____	_____	_____
*Price per Item:*_____	*Quantity:*_____	*Total Price:* _____	
10. _____	_____	_____	_____
*Price per Item:*_____	*Quantity:*_____	*Total Price:* _____	

Worksheet 7-7   Estimating Your Start-Up Costs

The following two forms will help you as you begin to estimate your start-up costs. The first form provides an overview of the basic items every therapist should consider purchasing.

Basic Start-Up Costs

Item	Low	Medium	High	Your Estimate
Portable table ($300–$1000)	$ 300.00	$ 500.00	$1,000.00	
Stool ($50–$100)	$ 50.00	$ 75.00	$ 100.00	
(3 Sets) Table linens ($60–$180)	$ 60.00	$ 110.00	$ 180.00	
Bolster ($20–$40)	$ 20.00	$ 30.00	$ 40.00	
(3 mo.) Lotions ($100–$200))	$ 100.00	$ 150.00	$ 200.00	
(3) CDs ($10–$20 each)	$ 30.00	$ 50.00	$ 60.00	
CD player ($30–$100)	$ 30.00	$ 50.00	$ 100.00	
Booking calendar/software ($25)	$ 25.00	$ 50.00	$ 100.00	
General office supplies ($100–$150)	$ 100.00	$ 125.00	$ 150.00	
Accounting ledger/software ($25–$100)	$ 25.00	$ 60.00	$ 100.00	
Application and state licensing fee ($100–$300)	$ 100.00	$ 200.00	$ 300.00	
First-year CE requirements, vary by state ($0–$500)	$ —	$ 250.00	$ 500.00	
Total				

Undertaking an entrepreneurial venture, such as starting your own business, involves many obvious and some hidden costs. Filling out the following worksheet of common business start-up costs can help you estimate what your costs might be. This list may not apply to every venture, so think through what your ideal business looks like and be sure to include any estimates not listed below.

Rent	$_____
Improvements/build-out	$_____
Salaries/wages	$_____
Payroll expenses	$_____
Equipment leases/purchases (copiers, fax machines, telephone system, computer)	$_____
Furniture	$_____
Supplies	$_____
Inventory	$_____
Advertising	$_____
Utilities	$_____
Licenses/permits	$_____
Insurance	$_____
Accountant's fees	$_____
Attorney's fees	$_____
Other expenses	$_____
Other expenses	$_____
Other expenses	$_____
Other expenses	$_____

Worksheet 7–8   **Business Plan Worksheet: Bullet Format**

Identify key points relative to each section in bullet form below and draft your initial thoughts.

I. **Executive Overview:**

Describe your company. Who are you? Why are you seeking a business loan? What do you envision for your massage business?

-

-

-

-

-

II. **Company Mission:**

What do you want your business to contribute to the world? What do you strive to provide to your clients? List some of your core values.

-

-

-

-

-

III. **Company Motto:**

This is a simple but memorable statement or phrase that embodies your practice.

-

-

IV. **Business History:**

What is your therapeutic background? What training and education have you pursued? How did you arrive where you are today?

-
-
-
-
-

V. **Services:**

What core services do you plan to offer your clients? Include any areas of specialization or add-on services.

-
-
-
-
-

VI. **Market Analysis:**

Mention significant overall industry points, growth, and variables.

-
-
-

State significant local market points: How will your local market support your business?

-
-
-

VII. **Target Market Strategy:**
   Who are the clients you aim to draw? What are their typical characteristics? Where will you find them?

   -
   -
   -
   -
   -

VIII. **Competitive Marketing Analysis:**
   Briefly describe your competition.

   -
   -
   -
   -
   -

IX. **Competitive Edge:**
   What makes you stand out? What can you provide that other practitioners cannot duplicate? (Use the work from Chapter 8.)

   -
   -
   -
   -
   -

X. **Sales Strategy:**

How will you reach out to potential clients and encourage existing clients to return? Include promotions, advertising, and marketing plans.

-

-

-

-

-

XI. **Organizational Structure:**

Your professional background: List your training and anything else that contributes to your chances for business success. Will you work alone or have a hierarchy?

-

-

-

-

-

Professional profiles on other key partners: If applicable, list people you plan to include in your business.

-

-

-

Your primary responsibilities: What roles will you hold?

-

-

-

Key responsibilities of partners, if applicable:

-

-

-

XII. **Sales Strategy**

What is your strategy to attract and retain clients? Mention specific avenues you plan to use to attract clients.

-

-

-

Communication: How will customers find out about you?

-

-

-

Do you plan to participate in special events or offer specials?

-

-

-

XIII. **Financial Information**

To be attached. (Use the work from Chapter 2.)

- Budget

- Income statements

- Balance sheets

- Cash-flow statements

- Forecasts

XIV. **Appendix**

Attach applicable items.

CAREER SKILLS FOR SUCCESS IN MASSAGE THERAPY

Chapter 8

Preparing for Marketing Success

"Before everything else, getting ready is the secret to success."

–Henry Ford

Outline

You will learn to...

- Define the areas of massage that most attract you
- Identify the clients you wish to work with
- Understand common client fears
- Define what makes you different from the rest
- Successfully locate the training you need
- Build a design for your materials that reflects you and your business

Key Definitions

This chapter references several key terms, which are indicated in bold. For easy reference, these terms are briefly defined here:

Benefits: Statements that translate how specific features, or strengths, benefit your clients.
Differentiation: The ability to separate yourself from your competitors.
Features: Statements of specific strengths about your service.
Marketing: An activity used to attract clients, share a message, or develop a brand or image that shows value.
Target Audience: A specified group of people you want to receive your marketing message.

MARKETING PREPARATION

There are two phases to your marketing success; the first is marketing preparation. This encompasses all the things to be accomplished and thought through before you begin broadcasting your unique business idea. Second, you must select the avenues you will use to communicate your product and services, such as print advertisements, fliers, or event sponsorship. Client expectations are being set long before they attempt to make an appointment with you. These expectations are formed from personal beliefs and past experiences but are also influenced by the marketing items you put out into the world. Whatever they view that represents your service will begin to set their expectations for what they will receive when they arrive for their massage. Always remember this as you begin to create the materials and messages that will represent you. For example, it is easy to grab a piece of paper and make a sign to hang in your window—but is that how you truly want to represent yourself?

This chapter will assist you in thinking through your strategy while you are still in the creative phase of business development so that once you are ready to launch, you will have a better chance of success. The goal is to prevent you from becoming one of the many therapists who leave the industry because of business naivety.

By now, you should have a good idea of who you are and why you chose massage therapy as your career. You have identified some of your strengths and opportunity areas. This work is important because as you begin to build your business and marketing strategy, you can always return to your core values. These will help you as you decide what type of business you want to have, what services you will offer, and who you want to work with. It is exciting to be in this phase!

When you are in the creative phase of a business, the sky is the limit. Anything you can imagine is possible. In your imagination, you are running a mobile massage business, you have become known in your community as an expert in prenatal massage, or you work at a local chiropractor's office and have a steady stream of appreciative clients. At this phase, you envision that your practice is full, your clients are wonderful, and you happily go to the bank every week and deposit enough money to pay your bills, with some extra to spend on enjoying your life. This phase is so exciting. This, however, is the phase most people get stuck in. Having your dreams become reality takes attributes that deter many—attributes such as courage, a willingness to take risk, an openness to invest, and most important, an ability to take action.

The formula for success is the combination of truly understanding your innermost desires, setting an intention to fulfill those desires, and then taking action to achieve these dreams.

Desire + Intention + Action = Long-term success and happiness.

> Desire + Intention + Action =
> Long-term success and
> happiness.

Setting up your marketing strategy is one of the action steps required for success.

Narrowing Your Focus

Here is some good news. A national survey conducted in July 2010 found that the complementary and alternative medicine (CAM) industry is a $34 billion dollar industry, with about 35% of these dollars being spent on services such as yoga, chiropractic, and massage.[1] As the demand for CAM services continues to increase, so does the money being spent on massage. With this growth, you have a great opportunity for success. As a strategic marketer, you know you cannot possibly create something that will be attractive to every single one of those massage clients. Therefore, it becomes vital to narrow your **target audience** and become specific about the kind of clients you wish to work with. Knowing this helps you to focus your time, energy, and money. A first consideration is whether you want to work with individual clients or have businesses as your clients. For example, if you chose to focus on individuals who see you in your home, you would take a different approach than if you wanted to have business clients such as spas and massage centers.

As the massage industry continues to grow and flourish, so do the types of massage. In fact, the Association for Bodywork and Massage Professionals (ABMP) states there are as many as 250 types of massage and bodywork. However, Swedish and deep-tissue massage are, by far, the top two types, making up nearly two thirds of all massage sessions conducted by ABMP members.[2] This is supported by the International SPA Association (ISPA) 2007 Spa Industry Study, which found that 97% of all spas offer deep-tissue/sports massage and 96% offer Swedish massage.[3] The ISPA also reported that Swedish massage is the most popular spa treatment among U.S. spa-goers, with 63% having received a Swedish massage in 2005.[4]

To ensure a successful start, it is important for all new graduates to have a high skill set in delivering a basic Swedish massage, followed by acquiring skills in deep-tissue work. This basic knowledge will ensure that you are able to get a job and sustain yourself while you gain experience and determine what type of work you are drawn to most. As time passes, you will gain new skills and the confidence to begin exploring other modalities within massage therapy. As you take continuing education classes, you will be exposed to many new ways to work with your clients. This is a great way to begin exploring and paying attention to what type of work attracts you.

Too often, people in business try to be everything to everyone. They view the whole world as their potential marketplace. This broad view usually stems from fear of not having enough business, of missing out on a customer, or of not pleasing everyone. The most successful enterprises understand the value of becoming very narrow in their products or services so that they can become experts at fewer things. Take the Irvine, California fast-food restaurant In-N-Out Burger as an example. The menu of this burger chain is the shortest in the fast-food burger category, consisting of hamburger, cheeseburger, the double, fries, milk shakes, and soda. While other hamburger places are waging price wars and competing by menu expansion, In-N-Out Burger stays steady—and profitable—by keeping its menu small and unchanged. This company's success shows that you don't have to be fancy, you don't have to be all things to all people, but you do have to be consistent to be successful.[5] It would be hard for In-N-Out Burger not to be an expert when its selection is so small, and this ensures that its customers have the same high-quality food and service every time.

For a massage therapist, applying this concept means choosing an area to become an expert in and focusing most of your energy on elevating that choice (Fig. 8–1). Too often, therapists succumb to the fear of losing potential clients, and this may show when they try to represent themselves as experts in numerous modalities. Many think this will attract more clients, when it actually may confuse potential clients and cause them to wonder how a therapist who does so many different things could possibly be good at any of them. If you visit massage therapy websites, you will see some therapists who do a great job of defining their area of focus with a site that is on-point and specific. You will also find therapists who list every kind of training they have ever taken, related or not.

It is important to narrow your focus and specialize. Become known in your area as the expert in something, and you will begin to notice more referrals and "on-target" clients coming your way.

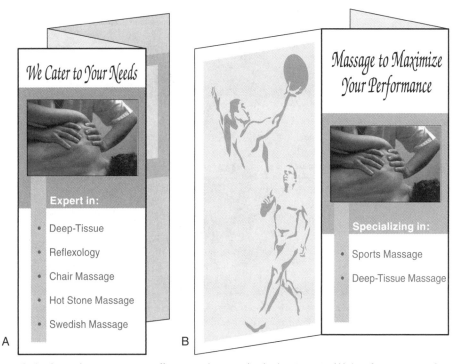

Figure 8–1   It can be tempting to offer everything you've had training in (A), but focusing on what you are really good at will pay off in the long run (B).

> Become known in your area as the expert in something, and you will begin to notice more referrals and "on-target" clients coming your way.

See Worksheet 8-1

This does not mean you will no longer do basic massage. You will most likely continue to attract clients who are looking for a massage outside of your specialty— and that is great news. You will accommodate their needs and potentially introduce them to your level of expertise in other areas. As time progresses, you will notice your client ratio begins to shift as you fill your practice with more clients seeking you out for your specialty. You can become more selective about whom you work with. For example, if you have little interest in relaxation massages, you can take on fewer sessions as you build the expert side of your practice.

Client Selection

Here is a novel concept—you have the ability to purposefully select your clients before they show up. This is not only beneficial but also highly recommended. When you narrow your focus based on your passion and think through whom you wish to attract, you can save yourself from future backtracking and redoing materials that you created before you had focus. You will avoid the problem of having to work with clients you would prefer not to. Redoing your materials is time-consuming and can be expensive. By skillfully choosing your clients, you will be able to focus all your energy on creating an experience that will attract and keep your chosen group.

Before choosing your clients, it is important to understand what kind of massage you love doing. Once you have narrowed that focus, you can determine whether there are enough clients within this category to support you (Fig. 8–2). For example, if you decide that you love to work specifically with women older than 70 years with scoliosis, you might recognize that there are not nearly enough of these clients in your small town to build a thriving practice. In this case, you might have to broaden your focus to ensure that there are enough clients near you to keep your practice full. You might expand your potential client base to people who experience chronic back pain,

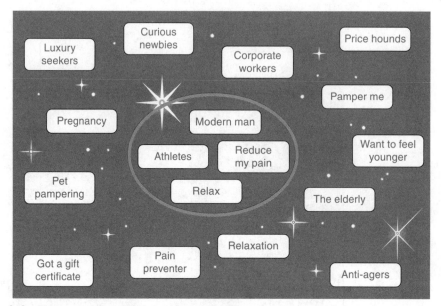

Figure 8–2   There are millions of potential massage clients in the universe. Recognizing that you cannot build a business aimed at satisfying them all is a smart move. Choose those clients you are most passionate about working with and differentiate your business from the rest.

See Worksheet 8-2

while specializing in geriatric work. You then become known in your area as a back-relief expert with a special program for older people. It is still specific and viable, but not so narrow that you eliminate your chance for success.

The worksheets in this chapter will begin the process of helping you narrow your focus. Choose what you love to do, and then begin exploring the clients this work will attract. It is fine to change your mind as your practice develops. Reality and experience have much to teach us. Early on, you may find working with athletes very fulfilling, but as time goes on, you may find yourself drained physically. This reality can lead you to other areas of specialty. Or, you may take a continuing education course and fall in love with the new modality you learn. You can then begin to change direction and rethink what this practice will look like, whom it will attract, and where you will find these potential clients.

Know Thy Client

Before you can build great client interactions, you must understand the needs and desires of those you hope to work with. Savvy companies understand the value of continually investing in methods that delve into what truly satisfies guests and encourages them to return. In fact, the most successful businesses invest the time and financial resources to fully understand their customers. This consumer knowledge keeps their products and services relevant for the real world. The most successful spas, for example, go beyond the generic understanding that many spa guests seek stress relief. They also try to understand the nuances of their guests' perceptions. For example, a company planning to invest in opulent design may find that their core customers would instead prefer a knowledgeable and highly skilled staff over a new, high-tech, salt-infused relaxation room. In this case, the company's money would be better spent on in-depth employee training than on cosmetic building development. Gaining this understanding early can save the company money and help focus resources on experiences that meet and exceed the customer needs.

Entrepreneurs who start out thinking they have a great idea, without taking time to understand their potential clients, more often than not have a business that eventually fails. Just because you think something is really great, doesn't mean anyone else thinks so and would be willing to spend money on it. The real magic happens when you match your passion with something that enough people want and are willing to pay for, and you have an in-depth understanding of who they are.

In a perfect world, you would graduate from massage school with a complete understanding of who massage clients are—what they are looking for; what they look like; where they live; what they do; and, most important, how to find them. In this perfect world, a complete research book would give you such great information on massage clients that you could artfully create a business strategy they couldn't resist. This type of data, however, usually exists only for corporations that have hundreds of thousands of dollars to invest in full-blown consumer segmentation research. As of this writing, there is no such level of research on massage customers.

> "The aim of marketing is to know and understand the customer so well the product or service fits him and sells itself."
> —Peter Drucker

Fortunately, there is information that can be extremely helpful in increasing your understanding of the massage consumer. The American Massage Therapy Association (AMTA), ISPA, and ABMP have conducted consumer research that can help you understand your future clients better.

Who Gets Massage

It has been reported that 42% of all adult Americans have had a professional massage at some point in their life.[2] To break this down further:

- About 22% of adult Americans (48 million) had a massage at least once between July 2008 and July 2009. An average of 34% of adult Americans received a massage in the previous 5 years.[6]
- In July 2008 and July 2009, 40% of women and 29% of men reported having a massage in the past 5 years.[6]
- Baby boomers aged 55 to 64 years have doubled their use of massage during the past 10 years.[7]
- Baby boomers aged 65 years and older have nearly tripled their use of massage during the past 10 years.[7]
- Americans who have completed college are four times (28%) more likely to get a massage than those who did not complete high school (7%).[7]
- Of the adults who received a massage in 2009, those with a combined household income of $50,000 or more were three times more likely (24%) to receive a massage than those from households making $25,000 a year or less (7%).[7]

According to the ABMP, there are three principal reasons why these adults seek massage—relaxation and restoration (34%), relief from pain or muscle soreness (31%), or receiving it as a gift (27%).[2]

The AMTA looked at reasons for going to a massage therapist slightly differently, but their results are similar:

Thirty-two percent of adult Americans who had a massage between July 2008 and July 2009 received it for medical or health reasons.

Nineteen percent of adult Americans say they've used massage therapy at least one time for pain relief.

Of the people who had at least one massage in the last five years, 31 percent report they did so for health considerations such as pain management, injury rehabilitation, migraine control, or overall wellness.

Eight-six (86) percent agree that massage can be effective in reducing pain.

Eighty-five (85) percent agree that massage can be beneficial to health and wellness.

In July 2009, 32 percent of adult Americans said they had at least one massage in the last five years to reduce stress or relax—up from 22 percent reported in 2007.

Forty-nine percent of consumers said they have considered a massage to manage stress in the last year, as compared to 38 percent in 2008.[6]

Both the ABMP and AMTA report that spas are where the majority of clients receive a massage, followed by a therapist's office.[2,7] During the past decade, ISPA has done extensive research on the spa-goer and has developed a detailed profile, which also provides insight on the massage client:

> The typical spa-goer is female (69 percent), non-minority (85 percent), in her early to mid 40s. She has been going to spas for over a year, but not as long as 9 years (60 percent) and her first spa visit was to a day spa (49 percent). Although she usually visits a day spa when she goes to a spa (77 percent), this average spa-goer also uses resort or hotel spas on occasion (64 percent). On that first visit, she had a body massage (68 percent) or facial (13 percent). Over time, she's added other services … [including] deep tissue massage (48 percent). Her main reasons for going to spas are to alleviate stress (77 percent) and soothe sore joints and muscles (38 percent), but sometimes a trip to the spa is just to maker her feel better about herself. While she does go to spas with close female friends, most of the time she goes alone (69 percent) and her usual spa visits only last 1-2 hours (65 percent). This spa-goer tends to be married (60 percent), has a college degree (81%) and above average ($50K+) household income (85 percent).[4]

Putting the Research to Use

So, how do you make use of these data? Let's put on our marketing hat for a while and parse the information down to what is most important. The following statements can be validated and may help you decide which customer groups have the largest populations.

- Women receive massage more often than men, so where would you most likely find women who are open to massage?
- As people get older, their use of massage increases dramatically, so where would you find groups of people who are 55 years and older?
- Recipients of massage are more likely to have an annual household income above $50,000, so where would these people live, frequent, and work?
- One third of those seeking massage are motivated by pain relief, so where might you find people who are in pain?

By answering these questions, you can begin to decide how to reach these likely clients with your advertising message. Another important point is that you do not always have to go where the masses are going. Although the largest volume of clients falls within certain areas, some of the most successful businesses succeed because they carve out a specific niche. For example, research shows that the incidence of men seeking massage is increasing, but they are more hesitant to discuss it, or fear that it may reflect negatively on their masculinity if too closely associated to pampering. A great niche to explore, if it matches your interest, is to create a therapeutic environment that caters more to men than women. Everything would be different, including your advertising, messaging, waiting room, and the way you communicate with your clients. Create an atmosphere that reinforces the type of therapeutic work you are doing, rather than spa pampering. Your messaging might focus on improving sport performance, offering pain relief, and providing specific conditioning work. Make it okay for your clients to refer you to their male friends.

Understanding Client Fears

When you understand what your potential clients are afraid of, you can build in support processes that will alleviate these barriers to a great experience. Think about some transactions that have potential to cause alarm. In the automotive repair industry, for example, customers often approach their service providers with apprehension. Because most people seeking automotive service are not knowledgeable about these matters, they might be afraid they will be sold items they do not need. They might fear that the employees working on their vehicles are not trained properly, or that they might be kept waiting for hours while the work is completed. Smart automotive companies that recognize their customers' fears will put in processes to help alleviate these concerns. For example, they may print a list of what the manufacturer recommends for servicing so that they are backed by the manufacturer. They may promote the level of training or certification their employees must undergo, and they can train their staff to accurately assess wait times based on current volume and level of work. These subtle techniques can go a long way in ensuring that their customers are comfortable with their choice to do business.

Most people fear the unknown. Therefore, new clients have anxiety about their massage experience, from the time they set up the appointment to the time they pay for their service. They may have some knowledge of various massage experiences from their social networks, and this may comfort them—or may create more anxiety. For example, they may hear an awkward or uncomfortable story from a friend, or even a friend of a friend, about something they had never even considered. In fact, many consumers tend to fear activities that their network of friends and family have not tried. Consumers are more likely to try a spa treatment, like massage, if they know someone close to them has tried it and can get some feedback on the experience and outcome.

This is particularly true for women, who like to share their experiences with their networks. However, this is not the case with most men. Although men would also feel more comfortable going to a spa if they knew their friends did, most men tend to be uncomfortable talking with other men about spas and spa treatments. More men are openly admitting that they like to indulge in spa treatments; however, most are uncomfortable about disclosing this, unless their reason for going is to treat pain. This reasoning helps reduce the stigma associated with men going to get "pampered" and lessens their chance of being teased by the men in their social networks about going to a spa or indulging in a "feminine" activity.[8]

The actual massage experience incorporates many steps, including the greeting, the service, transitions, different therapists, and locations. Such unpredictability can cause anxiety even among seasoned massage clients. No massage is ever the same, nor is there consistency among centers and therapists about tipping, voicing complaints, amenities, room temperature, procedures, relaxation rooms, and other aspects. Seasoned clients may have a defined idea of what they want, but if they visit a new center, they may be introduced to a new process or procedure, which can create anxiety. These differences can be slight, such as what to do with used robes or towels in the changing areas; or they can be more significant, such as visiting a center that incorporates massage of the gluteal muscles when they have never had this experience. Therefore, the term "new" can apply to not only new clients but also to seasoned massage clients who are visiting a new center or trying a new treatment or therapist.

The ISPA Consumer Trends Report revealed that spa-goers, particularly "newbies," have anxieties about the various stages of the spa experience and want some guidance on what is going to happen—before it happens. Here are several key points consumers want to know before the visit:

- How much clothing they need to remove for their treatment to be effective
- How long the treatment itself will last
- How treatment may affect their skin
- Their right to customize and adjust the temperature of the room and pressure level of the massage
- How the treatment may affect their body when they return home
- How long they can use the lounge, sauna, hot tub, or other facilities before and after the treatment
- Which facilities and spaces are open to both genders
- How and when they will be accompanied at various points in the visit[8]

The ISPA Consumer Trends Report identified three common fears among spa-goers:

1. *Arriving at the appointment early enough.* Many new spa-goers will schedule a 1-hour appointment and block off their calendars only for the 1 hour, plus driving time. This does not give them time to complete paperwork, use the facilities, get changed, or relax and unwind before their treatment. They do not realize this until they arrive, which creates anxiety upon arrival. If they were informed when they made the appointment that they should arrive a "bit early to change and unwind," this too can create a concern about how early they should arrive and what activities and services are available.

2. *Nudity and clothing removal.* Just stating, "Remove your clothing," is too vague for new spa-goers, and they are unsure about what articles of clothing they need to remove. Some may feel comfortable with all of their clothing removed, but others may prefer to keep on their undergarments, bathing suit, or other clothing. The anxiety lies in what clothing they should remove to keep them comfortable without interfering with their treatment. There are also fears around draping procedures, locked doors, and even changing rooms because of their fear of being seen without clothing. If the changing room is in a public area, such as a locker room, many clients will be fearful of changing clothes in the open and would prefer a more private area.

3. *Pain during massage.* This common fear centers on receiving a massage with too much pressure or in an area that is tender or sore. Spa-goers often do not want to criticize the therapist or are afraid speaking up will ruin the mood or the rest of the treatment. These stories of pain or awkwardness often make their way around many social circles, leaving a lasting impression and fear for many spa-goers, who do not realize that they can and should speak up about any pain or discomfort.

Two other fears identified in this ISPA report were uncomfortable temperature and skin reactions, which are concerns primarily for spa-goers receiving wraps, scrubs, or facials, but also for massage clients. For example, clients may worry about the room temperature becoming too warm or too cold or about stones used in hot stone treatments being too hot. Clients may also have some concern about their skin's reaction to massage oils and lotions.[8]

Three other common causes of concern and fear are important to mention specifically:

1. *Tipping.* Tipping policies and procedures are not always posted or communicated to guests. Clients are unsure how much to tip; how to not tip if the service was not acceptable; and how to pay. For example, in some instances, a tip may automatically be added to the total, and this can make some clients uncomfortable. They may not have felt that amount was warranted for the service they received and don't know how to change it. Or, they may not know whether to pay the therapist directly or add it to the bill.

2. *Transitions and wait times.* After a massage, therapists often tell their clients to stay as long as they need, and then leave the room to give them some privacy. The clients are smart enough to know the room is probably being used by someone else after them, or the therapist has another appointment, but the therapist has just told them to stay as long as they need. Exactly how long is too long? Can they take a nap, which they would really like to do, or should they hurry so that the therapist doesn't think poorly of them for delaying the next appointment? This uncertainty is not conducive to relaxation and can cause fresh anxiety at the end of the treatment. Another transitional time concerning to clients is changing clothes before and after treatment. They are usually left alone for privacy, and an attendant may or may not be around to help. Clients are not always sure about where to change; where to put used towels; whether to wear their towel in the sauna or not; and which areas are for men, women, or both. Many clients are fearful of "doing the wrong thing" and aren't sure of what is expected of them during transitional times. Clients are also uncertain about what to do while they are waiting for the therapist. This can cause anxiety about the therapist finding them indulging in an activity that may or may not be free or appropriate for their treatment or, again, doing something "wrong."

3. *Voicing complaints.* Some facilities encourage comments and clearly state what to do in the event a client has a complaint. However, most facilities do not provide such instructions, leaving it up to the client to figure out. For a variety of reasons, many consumers hesitate to state during their visit what went wrong, what they didn't like, or what didn't meet with their needs or expectations. They simply will not return. This does not give the therapist or owner any chance to right a wrong or to smooth ruffled feathers.

The bottom line to easing concerns and fears of clients is to communicate openly and be as specific as possible. Some tips to accomplish this include providing material to clients about common questions and concerns; finding out if they are new to the spa or treatment; asking questions and remembering their answers; and carefully considering your statements to ensure they are clear and precise.

See Worksheet 8-3

Here are some inexpensive ways you can gather information about your clients:

- Acquire industry-level research such as that provided by the AMTA, ABMP, and ISPA.
- Send surveys to guests in your database, paying special attention to loyal customers and those who came only once. Ask them questions that pertain to what they are seeking, what frustrates them, and anything else relevant to the massage experience you are trying to create.
- Interview frontline staff or pay attention to your clients' behaviors for key insights.
- Host customer focus groups by having a social hour at your facility. You can use this group environment to talk about massage therapy and ask questions of your clients. You might consider having door prizes or rewards for those who attend.

Differentiation

Imagine this for a moment—a potential massage client is interested in getting a massage. He has about 300,000 licensed massage therapists he could call and book an appointment with. Where would this client start, and how would he know how to find the one matching his needs? **Differentiation** is the ability to separate yourself from the 299,999 other massage therapists in practice.

Being different for the sake of being different will not always work. You have to differentiate yourself in a manner that is extremely important to your potential clients. For example, singing a customized chant to every massage client will definitely set you apart from all the competition, but most likely is not something that will keep clients coming back for more. Setting yourself apart just because you want to stand out is not enough, and actually is not worth the effort or extra costs that are sometimes involved. After you think thoroughly about the types of clients you will be working with, you should incorporate things that they will find appealing.

When you think about differentiating yourself from everyone else, revisit your selection for favorite modalities and types of clients you want to work with. Spend time thinking about who they are and what experiences you could create that would be unique and meaningful for them. For example, if you primarily attract clients looking for a spa-type setting or experience, you might consider adding in some of the following items: a spa-sounding name for your massage business; fruit-infused water in your waiting area; spa magazines; scented, warm washcloths for after the massage; and sounds of nature in the waiting area. All these items are inexpensive but would differentiate you from the massage therapist down the road.

See Worksheet 8-4

Crafting a Message That Speaks to the Chosen Client

After you narrow your focus and identify the clients you are most interested in working with, you can begin to think through how you will speak to them with your materials so that they want to come see you. Your choice of words, tone, and inflection will affect how potential clients view your business. Let's say you have advanced training in prenatal massage; what benefits would clients receive from working with you? Would it be of interest to them that you are nationally certified or a member of the Better Business Bureau? Might it be helpful to emphasize to future mothers the safety of your massage environment?

Knowing your **features** and translating them into **benefits** is a great sales technique and helps you determine your marketing message. Instead of just listing your accomplishments, translate them into specific benefits for your clients—explain how and why your accomplishments benefit others. It is fine to list some of your credentials because this builds credibility, but find space to hone in on the benefits the client will receive. For example, instead of just listing that you have taken training in Thai massage, state that adding Thai massage to a wellness regimen can result in more flexibility and greater range of movement. This shifts the clients' perspective to what they will receive, which is much more appealing than just your training accomplishments.

Using this information, you can define short and long marketing messages as well as features and benefits.

See Worksheet 8-5

Training Support

Another important aspect in preparing for **marketing** success is getting the training you need to deliver on the promises of your marketing materials. Finding the right educational resources that will allow you to confidently represent yourself as an expert is key. There are many options for you to explore. It is best to begin familiarizing yourself with the available options and see what sounds the most interesting. Continuing education is an investment in your future, so it is best to have an idea of the type of training you are attracted to so that you can find the providers who meet your needs. Often, busy lives intervene, and therapists find themselves facing their license renewal. They may quickly scan their area and take whatever is being offered at the time. Although you might accidentally discover some great training, it is leaving too much to chance. Planning your education is a strategic step toward ensuring long-term success as you purposefully acquire the skills necessary to set yourself up as an expert.

> Planning your education is a strategic step toward ensuring long-term success as you purposefully acquire the skills necessary to set yourself up as an expert.

After you decide which modalities seem the most appealing, you can begin to look into available training. There are many experts in the field, and having the opportunity to spend time learning with them can be very fulfilling. Finding these training opportunities is usually not difficult. There are numerous ways to discover the educational opportunities that are accessible for you.

Where to Find Training

Most states have an AMTA chapter that offers learning events. You might receive fliers providing you with event details. These events not only provide you with education but also offer you a chance to connect with your massage community. These events are usually well attended and affordable.

The massage industry has several trade publications that can provide you with important training information. Many continuing education providers and schools advertise their programs in them. Another great way to track down educational opportunities is to search online. There are specific sites that advertise massage classes, and random searches will reveal some hidden gems. If trying a random search, enter the key words that interest you, along with the words "massage continuing education," and see what comes up. To help narrow this search, you can enter your state or the state's initials.

Word-of-mouth also goes a long way in helping you find the right teachers. Ask your peers or massage school teachers who they recommend in your chosen modality. They can also be great

---

8-1: Find It on the Web

Begin your exploration by reading about the different types of massage.
The ABMP has a full listing of massage modalities at http://www.massagetherapy.com/glossary/.
massagetherapy.com also has a listing located at http://www.massagetherapy.com/glossary/.

resources and let you know about training they took that didn't work out well, potentially saving you time and money. Training is such a valuable investment that it is worth thinking through before you spend your money.

As you take a good, deep look at what motivates and interests you the most, every focused decision you make brings you closer to realizing your dreams. In the next section, you will find ways to share your passion with the world.

MAKING A GREAT FIRST IMPRESSION WITH YOUR MATERIALS

As you know, you have only one chance to make a great first impression. Just as personal appearance can influence success in a job interview, your business materials can influence whether you book a corporate event or secure a personal client. These items of influence will speak about you even if you are hundreds of miles away. So, everything matters during the development of the items that represent who you are and what you do. What you hand to your clients will most likely set an impression that will be hard to forget.

When creating materials, another important consideration is to ensure that everything in it is an accurate representation of what clients will receive when they show up (Fig. 8–3). Pictures and words should always communicate what really happens during the service. For example, massage therapists would not have long nails. Most hot stone therapists do not leave their clients alone with stones on

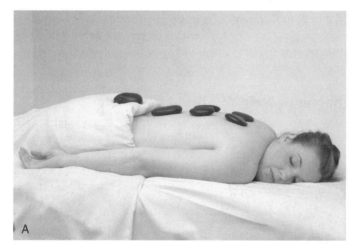

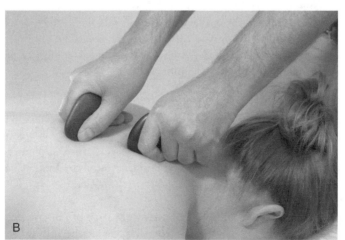

Figure 8–3 Choose your photos carefully. They will represent the level of work you do. Using a picture showing a client abandoned with stones on the back does not capture the benefit of hot stone therapy (A), but showing the stones being actively used during a massage will communicate the therapeutic benefits of hot stone massage (B).

their backs, which many pictures portray. This kind of picture can undervalue the therapeutic benefits a client will receive from their session. Choose pictures and then assess them for overall impression—do they convey relaxation, therapy, or pain relief? Choose graphics that match what you will be offering.

Business Name and Logo

Another decision to make before marketing your business is whether or not you will have a branded logo to represent who you are as a business. There will be some cost involved in the design of your logo, but the professional representation it provides you might be invaluable. Legally, there are some restrictions about using names, so contact your attorney if you plan to establish a formal business name and logo. Your attorney can guide you on the availability of your name and the trade marking process.

Here are some things to consider when making this decision. If you plan to operate only as an employee or an individual entrepreneur who works primarily with clients, it may not be necessary to create a logo that represents your business or practice. Most of your materials will simply feature your name, contact information, and information on your specialty. If you think you might ever have someone who works with you under a company name, then a business name and logo become very important. For example, what if your practice becomes very successful and you are approached by another therapist who wants to create a joint venture or come to work for you? It is much easier to do this if there is a brand established outside your name. You both become therapists working under the umbrella of that business name and logo. If you plan to work with businesses, then having a business name and logo can boost your professionalism higher than other therapists who may be trying to work with the same corporations. This is not something you have to figure out as soon as you graduate, but it warrants some thought as your business grows.

See Worksheet 8-6

Finding Someone to Help You Build Materials

Before creating your materials, you have to think about how you will build them. There's a chance that you have the creative skills to do it yourself, and if not, finding someone to help you build your look is not as hard today as it was in the past. There are a variety of ways to get the help you need if you do not have the skills or software programs to build your own. Because these items represent your professionalism, do not settle for something that looks homemade or has errors.

Software Programs

There are several inexpensive programs that have templates for you to work with. These programs are recommended only if you have the computer skills and somewhat of an artistic flair. Most of these programs contain templates for business cards, postcards, fliers, brochures, and other business stationery. Having a professional design your materials is preferable, but creating your own is better than not having these items at all, and it is a viable starting point. As your income increases, moving to more professional-looking materials is recommended.

Virtual Designers

A more current way to build your printed items is to hire a designer online. There are numerous providers looking to work from their home, and because of their unlimited access to a worldwide audience, these providers are often affordable. Sometimes you can even find creative designers in other countries who will do the work for a fraction of the cost in the United States.

Pre-Created Materials

Another option for you to consider is to choose from the array of pre-created materials available. There are companies who have designed blank templates that are specifically for massage therapists.

8-2: Find It on the Web

The websites http://www.elance.com and http://www.guru.com are great sites to search for your virtual designer. Both sites will allow you to create your job and then contemplate bids. You can review the credentials and costs of the providers to make a choice that fits your need.

They already contain pictures and words that apply to your message. These range from generic pieces focused on the benefits of massage to pieces focused on a specific modality such as hot stone massage. Within the template, you are allowed to customize and add in your contact information. These might be a good option to start with as well. You can find suppliers by searching the Web for "massage marketing materials" or "massage marketing supplies."

Working with a Local Person

It is sometimes best to work with a local person to help you design your marketing pieces. There is value in connecting face-to-face with someone and explaining what you hope to accomplish with your materials. This avenue might be more expensive than others, but the level of work is often higher. If you can find a recent graphic artist graduate who is in need of establishing a portfolio, you can access the artist's energy and skill at a better price. Most local graphic designers can be found in the phone book, on the Web, or through word-of-mouth referrals from peers.

Business Materials

The initial lack of clients and cash flow often causes new massage therapists to put off professionally creating their business and marketing materials. Unfortunately, many choose to design their own or decide to hire an amateur, friend, or relative to create their new look. Although in some instances this might work out great, the odds are you will not be satisfied with the final product.

There are many reasons that you would want to create a professional portfolio of business materials:

- They make you look more stable. Even if you have been in business only a short while, professional materials infer that you have been in business for some time, giving clients more confidence in your abilities.
- They encourage the perception that you are a bigger business. Everyone wants to do business with entities that seem to be growing and doing well. Having homemade materials might infer that you are small and possibly not well run.
- They help you look polished. Your materials help show that you care about your business and what you are doing. They are also a great opportunity to list your values and mission statement, further encouraging the perception of a well-put-together business.
- They help you appear organized. When all your materials coordinate and look similar, it communicates a sense of organization in your thinking. This is a trait many clients seek in a professional therapist and also begins the branding process so that your look will be associated with your work over time.
- They help you stand out from the competition. When you have organized and professional marketing materials, you stand out from all the other ads and literature in the marketplace. Many therapists need this edge to succeed!

Business Cards

If you are responsible for recruiting clients to your practice, then it is imperative that you have a business card. This is the first step to cementing your professionalism as a practitioner. Regardless of whether you use a local designer or buy a premade template, remember that a business card is often the first impression of your level of professionalism. Because people might keep your card, it also has long-term potential to remind them of their first impression of you.

The following basic information should always be contained within a business card:

- Your name and credentials
- Logo and business name if applicable
- Location information (to your level of comfort)
- One method of contact—probably phone or e-mail

Secondary information can include:

- Areas of specialization (features and benefits)
- Regular specials

If you have a business name and logo, then the business card should match their style and essence. You want all your materials to be similar in look and feel.

<aside>See Worksheet 8-7</aside>

Try to avoid putting too much information on your business card. Its purpose is to help with your introduction and serve as a reference for future contact. If you have to include more than basic information, you might explore using the back of the card or even using a fold-over card.

Stationery

In addition to business cards, you might want to create stationery. This can include letterhead, notepads, envelopes, address labels, receipt pads, and sticky notes. These items enhance the professionalism of your business and help brand your name and look. You can usually find a small business package of these items at office stores or from online print companies.

Brochures

Beyond the basics of a business card and stationery, you should consider having a brochure created. If you are not prepared to launch a website, having a brochure is a great way to communicate about your business with words and graphics. The purpose of a brochure is to educate the client about the subject of the brochure and encourage the client to contact you.

A well-done brochure should provide all the information a client needs to make the decision to contact you, including how to either book an appointment or contact you for more information. Do not expect that the brochure will make the sale for you. Its primary purpose is to provide enough information and benefits to allow someone to contact you for more details.

The first step in creating a brochure is to write the copy. You should write from the client's point of view. It's not what you want to say—it's what the potential customer needs to know.

Brochure Tips

Here are some tips to get you started with your brochure:

- Write out the copy and then go through it again with the intent to eliminate some of the excess words and unnecessary information. In other words, go lightly with the text.
- Think of pictures that will effectively communicate what the client will experience. Find images that match what you are doing and can replace sentences.
- As you move to the design phase, ensure that the design matches the look and feel of any other materials you have already created, including fonts, type, colors, and logo.
- Stay focused on what your services do for clients, not on all the features of your training. An example of the difference in marketing a blender might be;
    - Feature focus—12-speed blender with a 5-horsepower motor
    - Benefit focus—makes ultrasmooth smoothies in half the time of other blenders

    The benefits sentence helps the potential customer envision what it would be like to own one.

- Try not to be too formal in your writing. Pretend you are talking to your favorite client and explaining the benefits.
- To stimulate your thinking, make a point of gathering up brochures from local businesses to get ideas that appeal to you.

Brochures can be used at conventions, for business calls, to give to people requesting more information, and for current clients to pass on to others. Like your business card, people often keep it, and it will communicate who you are and what your business is like even months after you have given it to someone (Fig. 8–4).

Intake Forms

Although most do not consider intake forms to be marketing materials, they do in fact provide an impression of your business, and therefore you should think about how they appear from a marketing perspective (Fig. 8–5). If you have decided to have a business name and logo, then the intake forms

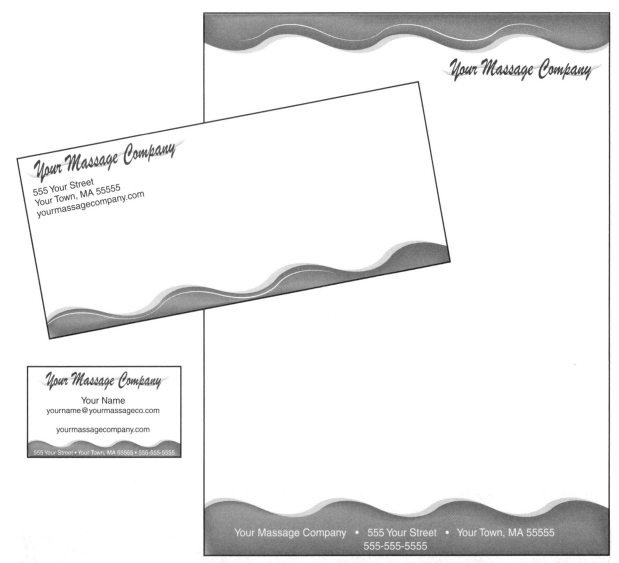

Figure 8–4   Professional business materials make you look more stable, organized, and polished.

Your Massage Company

yourmassagecompany.com

Three-Session Treatment Plan

Client Name: _____   Date: _____

Strengths and Resources: _____

_____

Presenting Complaints: _____

_____

Short- & Long-Term Goals: _____

_____

Therapeutic Objectives: _____

_____

Session 1: Preparing the Way

_____

_____

Session 2: Exposing the Complaint

_____

_____

Session 3: Integration

_____

_____

Suggested Ongoing Maintenance:

_____

_____

Client Signature: _____   Therapist Signature:_____

Note: Document is intended for use in conjunction with a thorough health history form.

Your Massage Company • 555 Your Street • Your Town, MA 55555   555-555-5555

Figure 8–5   Intake forms are a great place to continue your branding. Uniformity and consistent branding of your business make your unique look recognizable by your clients. (This form was created by imassage, inc.)

become a great way to continue branding these, creating a consistent look and feel to all your materials. You can capture the essence of your business within the framing of the document. These forms, along with any other materials you make, will create an effortless connection among your documents, and your own unique look will become recognizable by your clients.

As another consideration, all internal forms being provided to clients must always be crisp, clear, and free of typos. Too often, businesses do not view these forms as important, and they appear misaligned and blurry and contain misspellings. Being in the health-care profession, you do not ever want to imply that you do not pay attention to details. This is one way to avoid creating unnecessary concern in clients.

Printing Your Materials

Like the options you have for finding a designer to help create a look for your business, there are many accessible and affordable options for printing your materials.

There are numerous local printers to consider. You can find a small, family-owned printer or use a large national office company. The benefit to working with a local company is you have the ability to proof your materials in person and deal with a person face-to-face. This allows you the opportunity to fully explain your needs. One recommendation, if working with local printers, is to get several price quotes and samples of their previous work. There can be a lot of variance in printing costs depending on whom you work with.

There are also many online printers who advertise great rates and fast turn-around. It is worth checking into these companies to compare pricing to local printers. Simply go to a search engine and type in "online printing." You will have a plethora of options to explore. It is again worth mentioning that you do not always have to reinvent the wheel—preprinted templates are a viable option. The same companies that provide the templates will also send you the quantities you order, alleviating special printing needs. These templates may be a great place to start, but as your business matures, you should consider creating your own design and look to communicate your own unique message.

Peer Profile 8–1

Tamika J. Harris, CA-CMT, NCTMB, YI
Southern California

Marketing Preparation

A common question I get asked by massage therapists is, "Do I have to do marketing?" The answer for everyone is, Yes! Fortunately, this wonderful profession has become very diverse in allowing therapists the choice to be an employee, independent contractor, or business owner. Within each role, a key to generating business is making sure potential clients know who you are, where to find you, and—the very essential—what you can do for them.

As a new massage therapist, or even a veteran therapist getting involved with a fresh outlook, the excitement of the creative aspect of marketing can sometimes lead to poor decisions. For this reason, take some time out to do planning and implementation. Begin with a simple but effective tool: brainstorming. This is a process beginning with thinking. Prior to engaging into any tangible item, be certain about your personal concept, mission, and target market. Who you are as a therapist in the realms of marketing is not the same as your resume presented to a company. This is your statement and reflection of your inner being. Know the services you offer and create a common thread so that your services have a personal, recognizable stamp. For example, if the majority of your services and focus is built around prenatal and infant massage, but you happen to offer sports massage on occasion, develop your self-concept around prenatal and infant massage to prevent consumer confusion. Then, take a moment to write a mission statement about four or five lines long. Having a mission statement will help your marketing to be reflective of your overall business ethics and character. A portion of a mission statement may be, "Through massage, the goal is to provide clients an outlet to find personal peace while receiving compassionate service." However, if all your marketing material contains highlighting with big, bold letters, with oranges and reds in the background, this wouldn't convey a message of "personal peace," even if the marketing choice were an eye grabber.

After your self-concept is established, create a to-do list or a checklist. Just as in going to the grocery store to make purchases for the home, a list can ensure that crucial details are not forgotten. Many affiliate the word "marketing" with "advertisement," but marketing involves much more than putting out and ad for informative reasons. Marketing must create a response, desire, and need for potential clients to contact you. It also reflects the way you present yourself professionally in person and includes everything with your name or your business's name on it, such as the following:

- Business cards, brochures, and postcards
- Signage, website, and e-mails
- Gift certificates, coupons, and discount cards
- Press releases and mailing labels

As a new massage therapist, do not ignore the fact that marketing is essential but can be costly. Therefore, you should choose effective but manageable tools at first (business cards, brochures, and the least expensive, word-of-mouth). Put on your to-do list the marketing tools you plan to use, when you want to have them completed, and the method you plan on using to distribute them. This will keep you on task and help you to create a game plan for implementing the benefits of marketing to build your client base. If you are putting out an announcement or ad, create a heading beyond one that says "Massage Therapy." Headings, especially on coupons, press releases, or blogs, should be client focused to ensure that potential clients know that your business can solve their problem (i.e., stress, headaches, fibromyalgia). Use a comparative method before publishing marketing material. For example, hold up your postcard next to one belonging to a local competitor—which is more convincing? If it's not yours, then revise it. Potential clients can seek any massage therapist, so why should they choose you? Reward your clients after providing a set number of referrals, and don't ever ignore the great outcomes a simple thank-you card can achieve. But don't count on print materials to do all the work. Your personality, social abilities, customer service, and courage to network will accomplish a very important task: building retention and creating new clients. Join your local chamber of commerce, get involved in community events and programs, and stay in contact with a professional association; tell everyone you are a massage therapist. Your personal passion and joy for what you do will be reflective to those around you, and before you know it, your appointment book will begin to fill up.

CHAPTER SUMMARY

The time invested in preparing for marketing can save you from losing money, losing time, and losing self-esteem. Your materials play a strong role in this, helping you define yourself and your business in the eyes of the world. When you present potential clients with your best first impression, you set a positive tone and clear expectations for future interactions. By preparing for your career with thoughtful contemplation of your marketing strategy, you will launch stronger and more confidently into your next phase of success—marketing.

BIBLIOGRAPHY

1. Associated Press. (2009, July). *$34 Billion Spent Yearly on Alternative Medicine.* Retrieved from http://www.msnbc.msn.com/id/32219873/ns/health-alternative_medicine/.
2. Associated Bodywork and Massage Professionals. (n.d.). *Massage Profession Metrics.* Retrieved from http://www.massagetherapy.com/media/metricscharacteristics.php.
3. International SPA Association. (2007). *ISPA 2007 Spa Industry Study.* Lexington, KY: International SPA Association.
4. International SPA Association. (2006). *ISPA 2006 Spa-Goer Study.* Lexington, KY: International SPA Association.
5. Green, F. (2003, July). *In-N-Out Burger Carves Niche in the Fast Food Market.* Retrieved from http://www.qsrweb.com; http://www.qsrweb.com/article/111666/In-N-Out-Burger-carves-niche-in-the-fast-food-market; http://www.qsrweb.com/article.php?id=493&na=1.
6. American Massage Therapy Association. (2010, February 12). *2010 Massage Therapy Industry Fact Sheet.* Retrieved from http://www.amtamassage.org/articles/2/PressRelease/detail/2146.
7. American Massage Therapy Association. (2009). *AMTA 2009 Massage Industry Research Report.* Evanston, IL: American Massage Therapy Association.
8. International SPA Association. (2004). *ISPA 2004 Consumer Trends Report: Variations and Trends on the Consumer Spa Experience.* Lexington, KY: International SPA Association.

REVIEW QUESTIONS

1. **Which of the following are the two phases to your marketing success:**
   a. Marketing preparation and selecting marketing avenues
   b. Narrowing your focus and client selection
   c. Defining features and defining benefits
   d. Understanding research and analyzing data

2. **How are client expectations set or influenced?**
   a. By personal beliefs and experiences
   b. By marketing items
   c. By policies and procedures
   d. Both a & b

3. **When it comes to marketing:**
   a. Use a buckshot approach and try to hit everyone
   b. Use a blanket approach to cover your immediate geographical area
   c. Narrow your target and be very specific about the kind of clients you want
   d. Both a & b

4. **Why do some successful companies decide to narrow their product and service offerings?**
   a. To be all things to all people
   b. To become experts at fewer things
   c. They are limited in what they know
   d. They're fearful of losing business

5. **It is highly recommended that you select your clients before they show up.**
   a. True
   b. False

6. **What allows you to focus your energy on creating an experience that encourages loyalty?**
    a. Skillfully choosing your clients
    b. Redoing your marketing materials
    c. Desire + Intention + Action
    d. A strong brand

7. **Why is it necessary to know what kind of massage you love performing before choosing your target audience?**
    a. To better select whom would be your best clients
    b. To narrow your focus
    c. To ensure you don't eliminate your chance for success by being too narrow
    d. All of the above

8. **Why do many successful massage businesses invest their time and resources to fully understand their customer?**
    a. To understand their competitive advantage and differentiation
    b. To know which retail products to stock
    c. To ensure they love the same type of massage as you do
    d. To keep their products/services relevant and understand their clients' perceptions

9. **According to the Associated Bodywork and Massage Professionals, how many adult Americans have had a massage at some point in their lives?**
    a. Nearly one fourth
    b. Nearly half
    c. Nearly three fourths
    d. There is no research to determine this figure

10. **What demographic doubled and tripled its use of massage between 1999 and 2009?**
    a. Caucasian women
    b. Hispanic men
    c. Individuals aged 55 years and older
    d. Teens

11. **It has been reported that 85% to 86% of adult Americans agree that massage can be effective/beneficial to:**
    a. Keeping a youthful energy
    b. Reducing pain
    c. Health and wellness
    d. Both B & C

12. **According to research, most men are uncomfortable admitting they indulge in spa treatments unless it is to:**
    a. Brag to their friends
    b. Treat pain
    c. Relax
    d. Receive a couple's massage

13. **Which of the following tips help(s) ease client concerns and fears:**
    a. Provide frequently asked questions (FAQs)
    b. Client testimonials
    c. Asking questions and remember their answers
    d. Both a & c

14. **Interviewing frontline staff and paying attention to client behavior is an example of which of the following?**
    a. An inexpensive way to gather information about your clients
    b. Determining your differentiation
    c. Developing loyal clients
    d. Guerilla marketing

15. **Which of the following is *not* an example of effective differentiation?**
    a. Serving fruit-infused water in your waiting area
    b. Singing a customized chant to every client
    c. Scented, warm washcloths for after the massage
    d. All of the above

16. **Which of the following creates a message that skillfully speaks to your client?**
    a. Listing your credentials
    b. Knowing your features
    c. Narrowing your focus
    d. Translating your accomplishments into specific benefits for your client

17. **Your marketing materials should:**
    a. Be carefully crafted to list everything you do and know
    b. Be carefully crafted to create a great first impression
    c. Accurately represent what clients will receive
    d. Both b & c

18. **Who should invest in a company logo?**
    a. All massage therapists need a company logo to differentiate themselves
    b. Massage therapists who plan to work primarily with individuals
    c. Massage therapists who plan to work with other businesses or employ another person
    d. No massage therapist really needs a company logo

19. **Which messages do professional business materials send?**
    a. They help you to appear polished and organized
    b. They help you to differentiate yourself from other therapists
    c. They encourage the perception that you are a bigger business
    d. All of the above

20. **What is often the first impression of your level of professionalism?**
    a. Business card
    b. Stationery
    c. Brochure
    d. Intake form

Worksheet 8-1   Choose Your Favorite Modalities

Circle five of the following popular modalities that interest you the most. If something is not listed, write it in the empty boxes. Then review your choices, and ask yourself if you had to choose only three areas to specialize in long-term, what would they be?

Lomi Lomi	Lymphatic drainage	Aromatherapy
Deep tissue	Canine	Equine
Rolfing	Sports	Chair
Prenatal	Therapeutic	Stone therapy
Cranial sacral	Relaxation	Shiatsu
Reflexology	Thai/stretching	Geriatric
Mayan abdominal	Reiki	Esalen
Swedish	Other:	Other:
Other:	Other:	Other:

Of those circled, choose your top three favorite modalities

Choice 1:

Choice 2:

Choice 3:

Worksheet 8–2   Identifying Potential Clients

Reviewing your favorite modalities from Worksheet 8–1, draft some sentences that describe the clients your favorite modalities would attract. Write about these clients, describing traits and physical characteristics such as age, gender, inclinations, and physical conditions. In the next section, add notes on where you might find these clients. Where do they live, work, play, and hang out? What associations, civic activities, and events are they involved with?

Example:

Modality 1: Canine massage

Client description: People who own dogs, people who take care of dogs, people who work at pet stores, families with pets, breeders. They could be male or female, more likely to live in subdivisions—higher income areas are even better—and members of dog associations

Where would you find these clients?

Pet stores, parks, grooming shops, veterinarians, the pet section of book stores, participating in dog events, dog shows, pet-friendly walking trails, and social networking sites about dogs

Based on your favorite modalities, complete the following worksheet.

Modality 1:

Client description:

Where would you find these clients?

Modality 2:

Client description:

Where would you find these clients?

Modality 3:

Client description:

Where would you find these clients?

Worksheet 8–3   Easing Client Fears

How can I reduce my clients' anxiety about nudity?

How can I prevent my clients from worrying about tipping and when to pay?

How can I encourage my clients to speak up if their treatment is painful or inappropriate, and let me know if they have specific requests?

How can I help ease my clients' anxiety at transitional times, such as arriving, changing clothes, waiting for treatment, and departing?

Worksheet 8–4   Differentiating Your Practice From the Competition

Reviewing your favorite modalities from Worksheet 8–1 and your client descriptions from Worksheet 8–3, draft some ideas you have about what you could consider adding to your massage experience that would differentiate you from the competition.

Modality 1:

Differentiators:

From your above list, what is the least expensive but would have the most positive impact on the client?

Why would these matter to your chosen client?

Modality 2:

Differentiators:

From your above list, what is the least expensive but would have the most positive impact on the client?

Why would these matter to your chosen client?

Modality 3:

Differentiators:

From your above list, what is the least expensive but would have the most positive impact on the client?

Why would these matter to your chosen client?

Worksheet 8-5   Features and Benefits

Use the following worksheet to define your personal and professional "features," which include your knowledge, skills, abilities, personal traits, and accomplishments. Then, next to each "feature," define how that translates into a "benefit" for potential clients. The benefits become the speaking points you will use in your materials to encourage client bookings. As much as possible, validate these statements with facts and research, ensuring that you are not promising more than you can deliver.

Feature: Skill, Training, Personal Trait	Describe the Benefits
Swedish Massage	Improves circulation, induces greater relaxation, removes toxins

Now, take the benefits you have listed and draft sentences that you could put in a brochure.

Example: A great addition to your wellness plan is Swedish massage, which promotes relaxation and improves circulation, leaving you feeling refreshed and ready for your next task.

Benefit statements:

Worksheet 8-6 Naming Your Business

It is fun and creative to think of a business name. Imagine that you are opening your own massage business. Write down some names that you would consider for it. After you write the names you like, go to the Web and type in the name you have chosen and see if you can track down any other businesses with this name. This is where your attorney will come in very handy. She can keep you out of trouble by researching the legal availability of the name.

Business Name	Are There Others With This Name?

Now you can be creative and start drawing a potential logo. What images come to your mind that would represent your business? What colors do you like the best? Are there any words that have significant meaning for you? Take a few moments and draw an example logo that would represent your business. If you need ideas, you can type in "massage logo" on the Internet and then click the "images" feature. There are some very creative therapists who have built great logos for their business.

Worksheet 8-7   Creating Your Business Card

Now, you can draft some ideas about what you would like your business card to look like. Use your ideas about your logo and business name to keep a consistent look for your materials. If you need ideas, you can type "massage business card" into an Internet search engine and then click the "images" feature.

Things I definitely want on my business card:

Other ideas for my business card:

Chapter 9

Filling Your Practice With Clients You Want to Work With

"Next to doing the right thing, the most important thing is to let people know you are doing the right thing."

— JOHN D. ROCKEFELLER

Outline

You will learn to...

■ Identify and learn about your market competitors

■ Set a fair price for your services

■ Find the best ways to target your audience

■ Analyze the forms of advertising available to you

■ Write your own press releases

■ Use your social network to connect with new clients

■ Choose the ideal social media outlets for you

Key Definitions

This chapter references several key terms, which are indicated in bold. For easy reference, these terms are briefly defined here:

Advertising: Method of communication that will end up in the presence of a targeted client.

Article query: An inquiry from a writer to an editor regarding the interest in publishing an article in their publication. The inquiry is usually a one-page letter that outlines the proposed article.

Audience profile: The demographics of the audience exposed to an advertisement.

Blog: Software that allows someone to post content on the Web, which is often free or inexpensive to set up.

Client referral program: A program that rewards loyal clients for recommendations made to friends and family.

Connectors: Individuals who have an exceptional ability to communicate with many other people and who do so frequently.

Cost-per-point (CPP): The basis for evaluating cost-effectiveness, which is the cost to reach 1% of the target customer population.

Direct mail: A marketing effort that uses a mail provider to deliver a printed piece to your scheduled audience, which can include brochures, catalogs, postcards, newsletters, and sales letters.

Frequency: The number of times an advertisement will be heard, read, or watched.

Marketing: Process and activities that attract potential clients.

Nontraditional media: Basically any outline besides the traditional mediums of television, newspaper and radio. It can include cell phones, web sites and blogs.

Promotions: A broad term describing any avenue to make a product or service known to potential customers. Some forms of promotion include advertising, onsite promotions, sponsorships, public speaking, and word-of-mouth.

Public relations: Activities a business undertakes to educate the public about its products, services, values, and mission. They are not usually paid advertisements, but points of interest or noteworthy stories.

Reach: The number of people who will hear, read, or watch an advertised message.

Social network: An online community filled with friends, family, coworkers, and new acquaintances drawn to similar topics and themes.

Traditional media: Television, radio, and newspapers make up the traditional media outlets.

MARKETING AT ITS FINEST

This chapter will be most relevant for those of you ready to launch into the world of entrepreneurship. Even if you are not quite ready to do that, it helps to understand basic marketing concepts. **Marketing** is the process and activities you will be involved in that will attract your potential clients to your massage products and services. Good marketing involves research, promotion, sales, and product and service distribution. In the marketing preparation chapter, we explored the earliest stages of marketing, which include defining your unique service, deciding which clients you want to work with, and figuring out how to communicate with them in an appealing way. This chapter will discuss further aspects of marketing, such as setting your pricing structure, and will explore the avenues available to you for putting your message out into the marketplace. There are many choices available to promote yourself, so it becomes even more important to send your message through the right marketing channels. It can become very expensive to place ads in venues not accessed by your potential clients.

Keeping an Eye on the Competition

Within your market, you most likely will have competition. It is a good idea to become familiar with what is offered in the community where you plan to practice. By familiarizing yourself with the competition, you learn who is practicing massage, how they position themselves in the community, where they are located, and how much they charge. If you plan to work as an employee at first, this is also a great way to figure out who the prospective good employers are.

Here is some sound advice when it comes to competition. It is good to stay aware of what they are up to, but do not spend too much time envying them, copying them, or criticizing them. You have the ability to create and manifest the dream massage job you desire. It is important to keep your attention focused on what you are doing—not on what everyone else is doing. You need all your mental and emotional energy to stay in tune with what you are building. So, do not waste time worrying about the competition. Rest confidently in the knowledge that you will create what you need to be successful. Many small businesses spend too much time focused on what their competitors are doing, and they lose sight of what they should be doing. As a start-up business, keep your focus on your brilliance.

See Worksheet 9-1

Setting Your Price

The best strategy for pricing is to charge the most you can without deterring the clients you want. This sounds simple, but it can be challenging to figure out the right amount. If you are a new graduate and have been giving away your services to friends and family, it may take a leap of faith to believe in your talent and begin assessing a fair price for what you offer. If you lack confidence in your abilities, it might be difficult to confidently set a price that will generate enough income to keep you going. So, how do you know where to price yourself? There are a few things you can explore to find the right price point for your services.

First, research how massage is priced in the area where you plan to practice. Start paying attention to advertisements. Make some calls, send some e-mail inquiries, and talk to other therapists to gather your pricing data. Nationally, the average amount charged for a massage is about $60, but this varies geographically and by type of setting. If you live in a large metropolitan area, specialize in a specific modality, or are extremely confident you can fill your practice, you will be able to charge more than this.

See Worksheet 9-2

A second thought to consider while setting your price is not to let fear make the decision for you. The fear of setting your price too high, or overpricing, is usually a result of thinking your price will scare potential clients away. It is tempting to think that if you set your price lower than others, you will have a fuller practice. This is not always the case; in fact, the truth is that cheap prices attract cheap customers. Price-sensitive customers are less likely to be loyal, are more vulnerable to being

> ...the truth is that cheap prices attract cheap customers. Price-sensitive customers are less likely to be loyal, are more vulnerable to being swayed by a competitor's advertisement, and are harder to keep satisfied.

swayed by a competitor's advertisement, and are harder to keep satisfied. In short, it takes a lot of work to keep the "cheapies" happy. Another good thing to remember is that lowering your price is a lot easier than increasing your price once you have already set it.

Finally, when setting your price, consider the type of clients you are hoping to attract. What value will they find in your service and how much are they willing to pay for this? For example, if you decide to operate a primarily portable massage practice, you will have to charge enough to compensate for travel time between clients, fuel, and portable supplies. These clients are willing to pay more for this kind of service because not only are they receiving massage but they are also saving the time of commuting to your office, they are relaxed in their own environment, and it is convenient. It would be unwise to set a low pricing structure and aim toward a price-sensitive client base. You will run yourself ragged and end up with no money to show for it. A better plan would be to specifically target highly populated, wealthy areas and offices and to keep your appointments contained within a certain area, allowing the most visits in the least amount of time while charging the highest amount (Fig. 9–1).

In previous chapters, you learned about the importance of specialization. Other key benefits of specialization from a marketing perspective are that you can communicate more easily what your business is and you can charge more. When you set yourself apart as a knowledgeable expert, you will attract clients more willing to pay you for your specialization. They in turn will be more loyal, be willing to pay more, and have higher satisfaction levels.

A final note on pricing to consider is that if you begin to develop a practice that includes many clients who will be using their insurance to pay for massage, you may be restricted in the amount you charge. Insurance companies will not accept premium prices for massage services, and often clients are resistant to paying the difference. This is something to keep in mind as you begin to choose the demographic of clients to work with.

> See Worksheet 9-3

Avenues of Marketing

Most of you will not have unlimited budgets that allow you to explore different marketing options without fear of running out of money. You will most likely err on the side of caution and try to minimize how much you spend promoting your business, while hoping for maximal results.

Marketing communication falls into different categories. These include advertising, promotion, and public relations. Social and Internet marketing have also begun to strongly affect some businesses and will be discussed in this chapter as a separate channel of marketing. As you learn a bit about

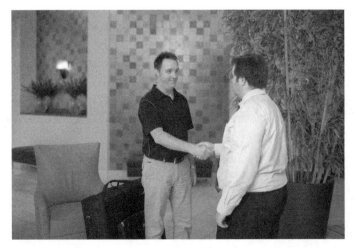

Figure 9–1   A portable massage practice will have to charge enough to compensate for travel time, fuel, and portable supplies. These clients are willing to pay more for the convenience and additional benefits of staying home.

each category of potential marketing choices, remember that the smaller, locally focused, grassroots efforts are likely to pay you the best dividends. When it comes to choosing the avenues that work best for your business, there is a formula to keep in mind. You have two areas of resource to pull from: your financial resources, or the amount of money you spend marketing your business, and your energetic resources, which represent the amount of time and energy you are willing to invest to fill your practice. Most likely, you will need to pull from both areas, knowing that one or the other will not work alone.

Using Advertising to Fill Your Practice

Advertising is the method you choose to place a communication that will end up in the presence of a client you are trying to attract. Examples of advertisements are radio and television ads. The advertiser pays the channel (radio and television stations) for the time it takes to air their message. Advertisements can be spoken, video, or print.

Even more important than finding the right channel to place your message is ensuring you have the right message. As you begin the process of building your ads, recognize that the content may be extremely interesting to you but is likely less than riveting to most people who read it. Honestly, people are bombarded with advertisements everywhere they go, and they tend to glance past the ads that look and sound like every other ad. Much money has been wasted by companies placing ineffective ads.

A potential client may have to see your ad several times before feeling motivated to call. Those who are willing to keep placing their ads in the most effective channels will reap long-term benefits.

Discounting

Offering discounts can become like a drug. You see quick results as clients come in to get the special price. Eventually, you have to offer your services at full price in order to make a profit. Working at discounted or lower prices means you will work much harder to break even; this will take a physical toll on you. If you do decide to offer a discount, have a really good reason so that the value of your service is not undermined. For example, you can correlate the discount to a holiday or special event. Also, consider using time or product upgrades as incentives, instead of lowering your price (Fig. 9–2).

Acquiring Advertising Proposals

Once you begin to reach out and solicit information on your advertising options, you will be bombarded with proposals from many different sources. It can become overwhelming. Advertising representatives will most likely send you enticing packages and media kits. Seasoned salespeople may try to convince you to spend your advertising budget on their advertising campaign. As you review all your options, keep in mind that you are seeking to reach the people most likely to desire your services. You are looking to spend less money than you will gain by attracting them, garnering you a nice return on your investment.

Box 9.1 Creating Focus in Your Advertisement

Consider the following factors before choosing your avenue of advertising:

1. Build ads that speak directly to your chosen customer. Explain the benefits of having a service performed by you.
2. Focus on what you are excellent at doing, not how you plan to do it.
3. Be persuasive and concise. Do not let the fear of missing something result in a long, unfocused ad.
4. Speak directly to your audience's need by using clear, direct communication and pictures.
5. Consider creating some urgency so that even procrastinators have a reason to contact you quickly.

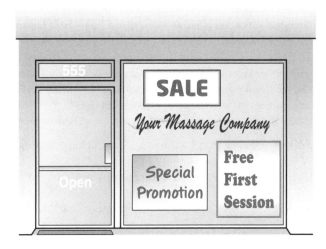

Figure 9-2   Be cautious about offering discounts. You may see quick results, but you will work much harder to break even. It's often better to use time or product upgrades as incentives instead of lowering your prices.

As you begin to consider your options, keep in mind these four things to consider when evaluating proposals: audience profile, reach, frequency, and cost-per-point (CPP). **Audience profile** means the demographics of the audience exposed to your ad. If you decide to specialize in canine massage, a local, dog-oriented weekly newspaper may be a much better idea than running your ad in a career woman magazine. Although many career women have pets, the dog newspaper is geared specifically for a pet-interested audience. Ask the salesperson to provide data about their viewers, listeners, or readers. **Reach** is the number of people who will hear, read, or watch your message. **Frequency** is the number of times they will hear, read, or watch your ad. **Cost-per-point (CPP)** is the basis for evaluating cost-effectiveness. CPP is what it costs to reach 1% of your target customer population. This is a good way to compare quotes from different outlets. Some of them will use a different name for CPP, but it is important to understand how much you are paying per exposure to your ad. Your goal is to compare all the different proposals and find the option to reach the most qualified audience the maximal number of times at the lowest cost. Make sure to buy enough frequency to guarantee that your message is heard by the correct audience more than once.

Until you reach a point of financial success, you probably will not use traditional forms of advertising. The cost of a single campaign would more than likely tap out your entire marketing budget. However, it is possible to team up with others or trade services for some exposure in these avenues.

Traditional Media

What is known as **traditional media** is advertising placement in television, radio, and newspapers. For many years, these were the standard categories companies used to create good presence within their chosen marketplace. With the onset of the Internet and instant access, these channels have begun to dwindle in relevancy for some advertisers, but they still remain strong as vehicles to reach the masses. As a new massage therapist, the cost of this type of advertising will most likely be out of your reach, but it is still good to be familiar with what is available and how to use it most effectively. Someday, you may share advertising costs with others, increasing your chances of using a form of traditional media.

Television

Advertising on television can include broadcast on the major networks—NBC, CBS, ABC, and FOX—or you can choose to advertise with your local cable company. Advertising on cable television allows you to target more customized viewers and often is more affordable. Of all the media, television is the most expensive. You will have to pay for the 30 or 60 seconds your commercial will run, in addition to creating your commercials.

The price you pay for television advertising is determined by viewership and the time slot when the commercial runs. Having commercials run overnight may be affordable but most likely will have very limited viewership. If you try to place your ad in a popular evening show, you may end up being able to afford only one commercial. The best way to determine your ad placement in television is by knowing exactly who your potential customers are and exactly what shows they are most likely to watch. If you are targeting young mothers or pregnant women, for example, then you most likely would want your ads to run during women's daytime programming.

Some of the advantages of advertising your small business on television include the following:

- TV reaches a much larger audience than local newspapers and radio stations.
- People watching TV are usually attentive.
- Your message comes across with sight, sound, and motion, which can give your service credibility.
- It gives you an opportunity to create a personality for your business, which can be effective if done well.

Some of the disadvantages to advertising your small business on television include the following:

- Television advertising is very expensive.
- Once your commercials are created, it is hard to make changes.
- It is harder to target your select audience with general broadcast television.

Radio

Another traditional outlet for your advertising is radio. Even with the other alternatives available, listening patterns appear to be stable, indicating that radio remains a popular choice. Radio reaches more than 239 million people 12 years and older over the course of a typical week, according to the RADAR 106 National Radio Listening Report, which was released on September 20, 2010. In a nutshell, that is a lot of people listening to their favorite tunes and talk shows.

A radio sales representative should be able to share with you the types of stations available and the demographics of their listeners to create a package that is personalized for your business. Be sure to ask about sponsorships, such as weather and sports, because these are often more affordable than regular radio spots.

Some of the advantages of advertising your small business on the radio include the following:

- Radio advertising is much more affordable than television.
- You can use your voice to build a relationship with listeners, making them think they "know" you.
- Ads can be created relatively quickly and can start running almost immediately.

Some of the disadvantages to advertising your small business on the radio include the following:

- Just because radios are on, does not mean people are listening.
- It is hard to track effectiveness because there is no coupon or ad to bring in.

If you decide to go with radio advertising, there are a few things that will help you be successful. When you create your 30- or 60-second story, engage your listeners by covering your service's key benefits in an efficient but entertaining way. Finish up with a call to action by offering a special, and provide your phone number and website. Write the ad the way you would talk to someone about the benefits of massage.

Newspaper

Newspapers are the oldest form of media. Although newspaper circulations are expected to decline with the onslaught of the Internet, they continue to be one of the largest avenues for advertising, as measured by volume of advertising dollars. Small, local businesses especially find newspapers an effective way to advertise. Every community has its own newspaper. There are more than 1,600 paid-circulation daily newspapers in the United States and several thousand other local papers as well.

Newspaper advertising can be very confusing because they use terms like "column inch," "points," and "picas." Ask the sales representative to show you example sizes in actual papers so that you can decide on the type of ad you would like to place. Explain to your salesperson about the clients you are seeking and the services you offer, and ask for guidance in choosing the appropriate section of the newspaper. Once you choose the section where you would like to run your ad, ask to see the proof before it prints. This will help alleviate any costly errors (Fig. 9–3).

Some of the advantages of advertising your small business in the newspaper include the following:

- Newspapers permit you to reach a large number of people within a specified area.
- Your newspaper ad can be saved and viewed later by readers.
- Newspapers publish frequently, so you can place an ad and have it running within a few days.
- Various ad sizes are available. If you don't have a large budget, you can still run a series of small ads.

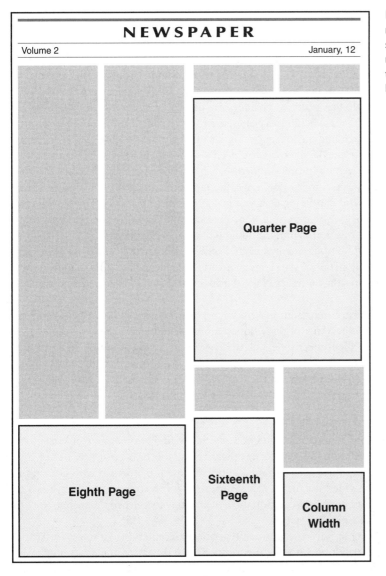

Figure 9–3 Buying newspaper advertisements can be confusing, so ask the sales representative to show you example sizes in actual newspapers and ask for his or her guidance on the right section for you in which to advertise based on your specific target audience.

Some of the disadvantages to advertising your small business in the newspaper include the following:

- There is a lot of competition within the newspaper, making it very important to have an ad in the right place with the right message.
- Most newspapers have a short life span, so running ads frequently is key.
- Not everyone who receives the paper will see your ad.
- These ads lack movement and sound and generally will run in black and white.

If you decide to use newspaper to advertise your massage business, there are ways to stand out from the clutter. You want visual appeal that draws attention, so your headline and photo are very important. If you could have only a headline, what would be the most effective thing to say? The eye actually likes white space, so try to not put in too many words. People will avoid reading the small print, and you should avoid black backgrounds on small ads. Try to make only one point with your ad; resist the urge to include all kinds of specials and focal points. Remember to speak directly to your target audience so that they see and understand your message.

Nontraditional Advertising

Advertising is a rapidly changing industry, with ads appearing on websites, cell phones, blogs, and other nontraditional media. A good definition of **nontraditional media** is basically anything besides the traditional media of television, newspaper, and radio. As you commute around your city, you see many examples of nontraditional advertising, often in forms that catch you by surprise. You may have noticed over the past decade that many companies have become very creative in how they use advertising space. You may see banners behind airplanes, barns with painted roofs, taxi-cab toppers, urinal boards, and even people standing on corners swinging a sign around. Nothing seems off limits to place your business information. Marketers realize it takes more than a television campaign to capture the interest of our highly mobile, preoccupied society. Marketers are also looking for ways to promote their products and services for less money. Although not mainstream, this kind of advertising is often more affordable and can be especially valuable to small businesses. For a beginning massage therapist, nontraditional ways of getting your message out might be the perfect choice, especially if you research all your options before deciding what works best for you.

The wide selection of nontraditional media can be exciting. You may be on the receiving end of many ideas as enthusiastic salespeople try to convince you that advertising your business on top of a taxi cab is the best decision you can make. Take the time for due diligence and find the best place to put your message.

If you are considering forms of nontraditional media, be sure the salesperson can clearly speak to you about their audience profile. Many of these outlets are small and locally owned, so they may not have the budget to analyze their effectiveness or audience. Start paying attention to the media and ads present where your chosen audience is. If you decide you want to work with career professionals, you might explore the businesses around their offices to see what forms of advertising they are being exposed to when they prepare for work, take their lunch breaks, and commute home.

Niche Print Pieces

Stop by your local grocery store or restaurant, and you will likely find any number of small, local magazines and newspapers. This nontraditional form of advertising can be a great way to get your feet wet with advertising. Usually, these forms of media are franchised to a person who lives in the area. Most of the content is provided for them, and part of their job is to get some local news to keep it relevant for the local audience. Most importantly, their job is to get people, such as you, to advertise so that they can make a profit.

If you find yourself wanting to advertise in these types of publications, make sure you have as many facts as possible about distribution amounts and locations. Ask them not just about how many papers or magazines they take to different locations but also how many they retrieve back when the new edition comes out. If they are unable to answer this question, it is worth asking a couple of the distribution points whether they have to throw a lot of them away. You may find yourself drawn to the ones you typically read, but resist the temptation to put your advertising in just your favorites. You want to place your ads in the ones most likely to be read by your potential clients.

Most communities have specialty papers targeted to specific readers such as seniors, pet owners, working moms, and people seeking a healthy lifestyle. Spend time collecting all these publications and assess their relevance to your potential clients. Also, pay attention to who is advertising in them already. Are they businesses that would be appealing to your chosen client base?

See Worksheet 9-4

Direct Mail

Direct mail is a marketing effort that uses a mail provider to deliver a printed piece to your selected audience. It can include brochures, catalogs, postcards, newsletters, and sales letters. Direct marketing to potential and existing clients can be an effective strategy for a small business. For a new massage therapist, this is probably a strategy that will come later in your practice. Once you begin to build a network of contacts, then you can begin to send them information encouraging revisits. Acquiring a qualified mailing list may be too costly for you at first, but once your practice is growing, you can seek to expand by looking into this option.

A better option might be to inquire into shared direct mail in your area. These pieces arrive in your mailbox as magazines or envelopes with other businesses included. Valpak® is an example of this type of advertising. Before you begin planning your direct marketing campaign, start examining the ones you come across. You probably receive many in your mailbox already. Begin saving the ones that capture your attention. Pay attention to how they use color, size, headers, shapes, and graphics to communicate their messages. Create a pile of the ones you really like, and place in another pile the ones that annoy you. Look for any shared direct marketing offers such as Valpak® as well. These will usually contain contact information so that you can find out costs and other pertinent details.

Although most forms of direct mail use a printed piece and a mail service, you do have the option of directly contacting potential and current clients through e-mail and e-blasts. You create your professional piece using a digital template and then send the message to a database you have on your computer. There are many inexpensive companies that provide professional templates for you to create some attractive ads to send to your clients. For your database, you can manually enter names, have a sign-up form on your website, or try to add your information to like-minded organizations that distribute to large databases. Two popular e-mail marketing companies are Constant Contact and Vertical Response. You can search for and find these on the Web.

Tapping Into Existing Lists

There are many customers searching the Web to find massage therapists, so it is important to make sure your name is listed in areas they are likely to go. For example, both the American Massage Therapy Association (AMTA) and Associated Bodywork and Massage Professionals (ABMP) offer a listing service for members that consumers can access to find a massage therapist in their area. Visit your state board's website and see if they have an area where massage practitioners can list their contact information. The National Certification Board for Therapeutic Massage and Bodywork also offers a listing service for nationally certified massage therapists.

One example of a national service to explore can be found at http://www.massagetherapists. healthprofs.com. Type in your zip code and see what comes up. Another way to track down some listing sites is to go to your search engine and type in "find massage therapist (enter your town and state)." Ask your peers where they have listed their information to help get you started.

Creative Signage and Ad Placement

An often-affordable way to use nontraditional advertising is by placing ads or signage in unique locations that build awareness for your business. You will want to check the zoning laws in your area before you order any signage to prevent the loss of your investment. Outdoor signage comes in all shapes and sizes. Some standard uses of signs include banners; A-frame signs near entries; window posters; and small, pegged directional signs. Some nonstandard uses of signage include air-filled mobile signs, lighted digital signs, and temporary signs that promote a special offer. To get a bigger picture of what is available, you can always stop in at a local sign company and ask them to show you all the options available for creative signage.

Once you are clear about the kind of signage you can have around your place of business, think creatively about how to make some professional, attractive signs to build awareness for your business. There are some rules to follow for any signage that is placed outside for people on the move to read. Your headline must capture the essence of your entire message. You have to assume that people will only glance at your sign, so make the headline do all the talking. Use large fonts. If you use a picture, choose it carefully. Often, a picture will catch the viewers' attention first, and if they like it, they might read your headline. Avoid putting too much information on outdoor signage because it will only make your graphics and fonts smaller, ensuring that no one reads the sign. Ask to proofread your sign before it prints so that you can view it for accuracy and effectiveness (Fig. 9–4).

The professionalism of your signage sends messages about the professionalism of your business. It can be expensive to replace old and tattered signs, but if they look worn, then they need to be replaced or removed. You should never chance the possibility of a forgotten sign sending negative messages about your business and deterring potential clients from stopping in (Fig. 9–5).

You can also get creative with your signage placement. Some businesses use their cars as forms of advertisement. This can be done through custom paint, clings, and magnets. There are companies that specialize in putting your advertisements in unique locations around town, such as on park benches, walls, and even pizza boxes. It is probably best to stick with some mainstream ideas at first, but some of the best advertising has been done in wacky ways. Start noticing all the ways companies advertise their businesses in your town.

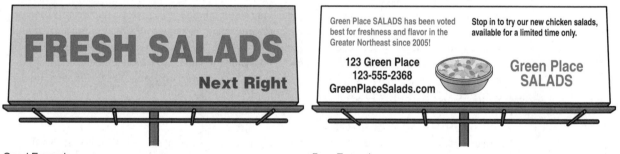

Good Example   Poor Example

Figure 9–4   People on the move only have a moment to glance at your banner or sign, so make the headline effective; use large fonts; don't include too much text; and use minimal, but powerful, graphics and/or pictures.

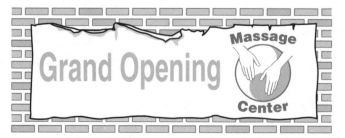

Figure 9–5   Although it can be expensive to replace old and tattered signs, never chance the possibility of a forgotten sign sending a negative message about your business and deterring potential clients.

USING PROMOTION TO FILL YOUR PRACTICE

Promotion is a broad term for using any avenue to make your product or service known to potential customers. Advertising is one form of promotion. There are numerous ways to promote your business that do not fall within traditional and nontraditional advertising avenues. On-site promotions happen at your place of business and are often centered on an activity designed to increase the number of products or services you sell. An example of an on-site promotion might be a local car dealer who decides to have a picnic on the lot. He brings in some costumed characters and inflatable rides and places festive decorations on the lot to draw in people. His real intention is to encourage people to visit, take a test drive, and purchase cars. He uses the promotional aspects of a party to do the work of drawing people in, instead of running a basic sales ad in the newspaper. He can choose to advertise his promotion but is still placing the focus on the event and special deals over his normal message.

For a massage business, you might decide to run a gift certificate promotion before Mother's Day. You advertise that all gift certificates will be 25% off during a certain time frame. You create some excitement around this offer by hanging signage inside and outside your place of business, e-mailing all your current clients, and running a small ad in a local magazine. Although you hope to bring people in to purchase the gift certificate, you are also hoping to increase your bookings after the ad. You use the gift certificate promotion to increase purchasing excitement and awareness and also make a goal of filling your schedule for the next couple of weeks. To measure success, you will keep track of gift certificates sold and the number of bookings that come in as a result of your promotion. If this is less than the amount you paid to run the promotion, it may be time to go back to the drawing board and come up with another idea.

Promotion at Events

Most cities have a variety of events going on at any given time. Often, you can become involved with these events through sponsorships and participation. As a massage therapist, it will be important to choose only events that your potential clients are most likely to attend. If we use the canine massage therapist as an example, you can look into events aimed at pet owners. Most pet stores, training programs, and grooming facilities will have information about upcoming pet events for you to check out. Often, there are events centered on charities, pet adoption, and pet play time. You can become very creative in finding ways to make your services known to potential clients who attend these events. Many of these event coordinators may be willing to offer you promotional advertising in exchange for the donation of massages as door prizes.

In another example, a massage therapist who wants to work with athletes can promote at events that cater to athletes and people who are physically fit. You can look into local races for charities, gym events, and fitness fairs. Plan to visit local shops that cater to athletes, such as running, biking, swimming, and active wear shops. They often have a bulletin board full of upcoming athletic events and may even let you post your information if you ask them.

See Worksheet 9-6

Once you discover a few promising events, you will have to become assertive in seeking information. You can call, ask for the event coordinator, and tell them you would like to become involved in the event. Be open to their ideas, and do not hesitate to share your own. Many times, they need volunteers and are willing to accommodate some personal promotion in exchange for free labor or complimentary products and services.

Once you decide to become involved, there are many ways to share your information with participants. You can put your information in bags, have a table, put your name on tee shirts, become part of the event program, and even hang signs. Be creative and think of ways that allow every participant to see your information.

Another way to use events to your advantage is to host your own. You can choose to arrange a grand opening event, educational seminars, meet-and-greets, and receptions. The key to success for these events is to make sure the word gets out through a combination of press releases, e-mails, direct mail, social media, shared advertising with neighbors, and other advertising. Small events can disappoint the planner if there is insufficient build-up.

Group and Club Memberships

Becoming a member of local groups can be rewarding for your business as well. It is even better if the group is filled with your potential clients. Your local chamber of commerce should have a listing of all the active groups in your area, as well as keeping a calendar of community events and meetings. Plan on stopping in to get as much information as you can about your groups of interest. You can also ask your clients, boss, and coworkers what organizations they are involved in. Once you attend a couple of meetings, you can ask the members for information about similar groups in your area.

When you find a group that interests you, you can find ways to promote your specialization within the group structure. As an example, lets' assume that you are a therapist who decides to specialize in infant and toddler massage. Your first goal is to explore and discover the groups that would most likely attract parents of young children. Start with the event promotion work we discussed and visit all the stores in town that are likely to cater to pregnant couples and to new moms and dads. Once in the store, make note of the local events that are advertised there. These local events are usually sponsored by an organization catering to your selected group. Often, staff members at these locations are familiar with local groups and how to contact them. It is important to have a good idea of the groups you are looking for so that you can ask efficient, to-the-point questions.

Visit your local chamber of commerce and tell them about your business. Let them know that you would like to have information on any local groups or events that cater to young families. You can also search on the Web for local groups that support your client base. In this example, you can search for "pregnancy groups *your city, your state*" or "new moms groups *your city, your state*." Experiment with different searches until you find what you need.

Joining and becoming involved with groups can be very rewarding when you find those most relevant to the clients you are trying to attract. Be aware, however, that group membership can pull from your energetic resources; try not to give too much of your time away.

Public Speaking

Introverts are probably shrinking in their seats after reading the header of this section. Never fear—public speaking can take place in small, informal groups, such as the groups you join and become active with! Many small groups are looking for speakers to come in and educate their members. This can be a financially inexpensive way to create a loyal following. As we continue to use the infant massage example, you may consider approaching several groups and offering to lecture and demonstrate at their next meeting. You can start by providing an educational session on the benefits of infant massage and end with a demonstration on what a real session would be like. You may need to line up the baby client in advance; possibly ask a current client or someone you know. Plan in advance how you will

---

9-1: Find It on the Web

Another way to find groups of interest is to search the Web. Here are some sites to get you started.

- **Meetup.com** allows you to enter your topic of interest and search by geographical area.
- **Active.com** provides a great resource of upcoming meetings and activities in your area. On the home page, you can enter your state as the key word and choose the type of activities you would like to see.
- **Meettheneighbors.org** offers people in work areas and subdivisions a chance to get to know each other. This site is probably most beneficial for those in large areas.

gain business from your efforts. Take plenty of business cards and educational handouts with your contact information. You could even create a form for attendees to enter their contact information. It is important to provide an easy way for them to take your contact information with them.

Sampling

Offering samples of your work can also go a long way toward filling your practice. A word of caution, however: do not give away the farm, especially to the wrong people. If your business relies heavily on walk-in clients, it may be a good idea to get a massage chair and set up outside during slow times. It is important to have a strong call to action for those who take you up on a free 10-minute back massage. You can offer each person a printed piece with your hours of operation and an incentive or discount for an immediate booking. Your handout can include educational information about the type of massage you do.

You can also use sampling to fill your practice by visiting businesses or attending group meetings that are filled with your potential clients.

Word-of-Mouth

Word-of-mouth business often happens by accident, but smart massage marketing can make it happen on purpose. Many therapists admit that they have built their entire practice on word-of-mouth efforts. This effective method can take a long time to fill a practice, however. To make this easier you could create a **client referral program**, which is a program that rewards loyal clients for recommending you to their friends and family. You can create printed pieces with basic information on your specialization for them to distribute to their connections. At the very least, ensure that all your clients have several of your cards so that they can pass them out to those they think can benefit from your services.

Connectors

Another inexpensive way to get the word out about your business is to link yourself with **connectors**. Take Mary, for example. She is a busybody who loves to go out. She volunteers; she has a job in sales and an active social life. More than likely, you will find her on several social networking sites. Mary is a connector, and your goal is to find people like her and make them raving fans of your work. Connectors are not always in your tight circle of friends and family, but they may be acquaintances who run in completely different circles. Start asking people you know if they know people like Mary. Once you solidify relationships with connectors, you are literally one person away from hundreds of potential clients.

One therapist said he sought out connectors he knew and offered them a free massage. He was upfront with them and acknowledged their ability to communicate with many others. He let them know he wanted them to experience his work and talk about it with their connections. This simple tactic translated to eight regular clients. Another therapist found a connector in a small community. She decided to travel one day each week and do massage in the connector's hometown. The connector even helped the therapist set up the appointments because she liked having the therapist come to her hometown and work with her friends.

Another way to find linked-in people is to increase your networking by attending local events, business meetings, community classes, and social gatherings. You are bound to run into great people who will help you grow your business.

See Worksheet 9-7

USING PUBLIC RELATIONS TO FILL YOUR PRACTICE

Public relations are the activities a business undertakes to educate the public about its products, services, values, and mission. Usually, public relations are not paid advertisements, but points of interest or newsworthy stories.

Most entrepreneurs dream of seeing their business positively featured in the local newspaper or on television or being asked to speak as a subject matter expert at a big event. However, with thousands of small businesses competing for this precious air time, it is not always easy. Even so, with a little planning and strategy, you can set yourself up as a valuable resource and make the headlines of your local media outlets.

Here are some pointers to get you started on the right track:

1. *Separate yourself from the sea of press-hungry businesses.* Recognize that when you send in a press release, there are likely to be hundreds of others also waiting on the desk of the person who decides what to focus on. You have to present your idea in a way that is very clear and unique. Pick out three interesting or inspiring points in your journey and weave these into a compelling story. Make it easy for the reader to follow along and understand the essence of your message.

2. *Have your 30-second pitch ready to go.* If you get lucky and are contacted by an interested party, you need to have your pitch nailed down. Practice how you would share your story in 30 seconds, capturing the most important elements of the release.

3. *Create a topic that is unique.* Most reporters are not going to get too excited when another ribbon-cutting release crosses their desk. They may find it interesting that your massage studio has services dedicated to helping seniors improve mobility so that they can stay independent longer. In relation to that, they may discover that you have created and coordinated a volunteer massage program that works with the local senior center. Adding client testimonials would be a bonus, but make sure you get a signed form stating that you can use each client's information.

4. *Give your topic local flavor.* If you can, tie in your local community with the topic you choose. Most likely you will not be seeking national coverage, so build subjects that will be attractive to your local media. Try to quote or highlight local members of the community or clients you have worked with. Reporters especially like a great personal story that pulls at people's emotions.

5. *Make it easy to contact you.* Clearly identify who people should contact and how to do this. Make sure to include your name, phone, address, and e-mail so that you are easily reachable.

6. *Choose your contacts wisely.* For most news outlets, you want to send your releases to only one contact. Often, reporters are vying for the next great story, and you do not want conflicting versions of your release. Plan on contacting your local news shows and newspaper print offices to find out who receives press releases. A large outlet may have different people for different categories. Once you identify your recipients, ask how they prefer to receive releases.

7. *Use the holidays to promote your business.* Often during the holidays, reporters are looking for new and interesting topics. They will not be interested in any holiday-focused discounts you are running, but they may be very interested in how their viewers can reduce stress during busy shopping seasons.

8. *Get featured in the new business section.* Most local newspapers and business magazines allow notices of new jobs and businesses. Take advantage of this and send them a quick release about the creation of your new business, your profile, and a headshot.

9. *Create an exciting event.* You may be able to get together with your business neighbors and brainstorm on an idea that will not only generate a lot of traffic but also gain the interest of the media. Introduce yourself to your neighbors and start discussion ideas for a group event. These can work especially well around the holidays; for example, you might create a "safe" trick-or-treat event, or work in conjunction with a charity.

10. *Believe in yourself.* You must truly believe in what you and your business stand for. Interviewers will be able to tell immediately if you are not passionate about what you are promoting. Sharing your ideas with friends and family can help build your confidence for when it is time to talk to a media person. Go even further and show up at local events to share your information with others. Your excitement can be contagious, and eventually you will run across someone who wants to help promote you and your business.

> You must truly believe in what you and your business stand for. Interviewers will be able to tell immediately if you are not passionate about what you are promoting.

(Continued on page 319)

Peer Profile 9-1

Debra Locker,
President
Locker Public Relations

Press Releases 101
Ask the Expert
So, you want to write a press release? Good for you for taking this proactive step in promoting your massage therapy business. Press releases are a tried and true tactic in public relations. They are beneficial to the media, can land coverage for you, and, perhaps best of all, you don't have to be a PR pro to write a release!

Timely and newsworthy pitches and releases will position your company as a trusted contact in the eyes of the media. Releases should be generated throughout the year and can focus on holidays, specific events or promotions, new offerings, new personnel, innovative treatments, updated products, and programming.

Telling Your Story
There are two main things to consider before writing a release—your story and its validity as news. Let us discuss both of those, starting with your story. Defining your story is a critical first step to PR. A good story takes a lot of time to develop, and it constantly changes and evolves. A story always has a beginning, middle, and end. To begin writing, think about why you created your company or practice, your mission and vision, and what your company or product is meant to do.

For example, let us say you are the lead massage therapist for a chain of day spas in Ohio. These questions will help you create a story that sets you apart from other therapists:

- Are you offering therapies, products, or services that can be found only in the spas where you work?
- What are your success stories? Collect testimonials from loyal customers.
- Are you giving back to the community—do you participate in charitable events, auctions, and other nonprofit activities?
- Educational programming is a great news peg. Classes and seminars offered by you or your team offer can position you as experts in your field.
- What do you do better than any other therapist? What does your spa do better than any other spa?

To craft your story, you want to use key messages. The key messages should be simple and memorable statements. They support your story and build your reputation. You can think of key messages as points you ultimately want to read as sound bites in an article.

You now have the basis of your story—congratulations! No one else has your history, your experiences, or your story. You own it, so use it! Your story is what makes you PR-able.

News Pegs
As mentioned earlier, you also need a solid news peg or angle in order to produce a valuable press release. What makes you or your company PR-able? When your clients leave your practice or spa, what do you want them to remember most?

To help you figure out what is PR-able, here are some tried and true news pegs:

- *Offering commentary, Q&A, or articles for your areas of expertise.* Perhaps you create a release with your tips and research, containing the top 10 reasons why massage is beneficial, or seven ways to give yourself a stress-relieving break at home.

- *Money—sales, donations, record-breaking numbers.* Is your therapy practice benefiting from the recession with higher numbers than ever from stressed-out folks?
- *Annual stories—holidays, back-to-school, anniversaries.* These are great for press releases. How about writing seven massage tips for making Valentine's Day special? Or, five ways to de-stress for the holidays? And, if you are offering special rates for the holidays or back-to-school, those are also worth a release. By the way, lists of three, five, seven, and 10 seem to be the magic formulas for editors.
- *Business stars—executives who are amazing at what they do and have saved their companies millions of dollars.* Are you a therapist who used to be a CPA? Do you have someone on your team who came up with a way to make the business more eco-friendly? Those are notable characteristics that make editors take notice.
- *Success stories—progress and change.* Don't be afraid to share your successes. In fact, shout them from the rooftops!
- *Things that are the first, last, biggest, smallest, newest, or oldest* are noticed by the media. Are you the first therapist in your town to offer Ayurvedic services? Is your facility the largest or newest?
- *Fads and trends are notable as well.* Read newspapers and websites daily to see what people are talking about. If eco is the rage, talk up your green practices. If chocolate is hot, consider adding a service with cocoa, and then promote it as part of a trend.
- *Local events.* Any time you connect with your community, this is newsworthy. Be sure to let local media know about upcoming area events, specials, and seminars.

The Facts on Press Releases

We have talked about content. Here are some things to keep in mind about the style of releases and what editors like to see.

- First off, keep releases short. The majority of your releases should be no more than one page. You can use 10-point, single-spaced fonts. Arial and Calibri are preferable.
- Speak in layman's terms on your releases. Don't use industry jargon. Test this out by having a friend outside of the massage and spa industries read your release before you send. If your friend cannot understand it, you must adjust the language.
- Speaking of sending, there is no need to mail or fax releases nowadays. Simply create a digital template that includes your logo and write the release there. Send it as an e-mail attachment, or provide a link to the release in your online pressroom. You may also want to save the final version as a PDF so that the release cannot be altered. PDFs are also useful because they are simple to open, even if you include an image.
- Make your first paragraph a winner! That first paragraph should be able to stand alone— consider that most editors may read only that paragraph. Make sure it includes the who, what, when, where, and why of your story. Skip the spokesperson quotes in the first paragraph; save those for later because they are the icing on the cake.

9-2: Find It on the Web

To help you become an expert, you can find numerous articles and research findings at the following places.

The **Touch Research Institute** was the first center in the world devoted solely to the study of touch and its application in science and medicine: http://www6.miami.edu/touch-research/

The **Massage Therapy Foundation** advances the knowledge and practice of massage therapy by supporting scientific research, education and community service: http://www.massagetherapyfoundation.org/

Becoming an Expert

Subject matter experts are highly sought-after individuals who have valuable knowledge to share with the rest of the world. Establishing yourself as an expert in your field can pay off. To start, think about the aspects of massage therapy that most interest you and naturally draw your attention. These are areas in which you can become an expert. Although it will not happen overnight, your specific focus will begin you on the path to achieving expertise. Start by gathering all the information you can about your areas of interest, and spend time studying and researching. When it is time to take your continuing education classes, choose the ones that will expand your expertise. Having training and certifications in your chosen area helps cement your credibility when it comes time to set yourself up as an expert.

The Massage Therapy Foundation and the Touch Research Institute are useful resources as you seek to become an expert. They provide access to many articles and research papers about the benefits of massage therapy. Plan to visit their websites and access information relevant to the area in which you want to become a subject matter expert.

After you have built your skills and materials, letting others know you are an expert becomes extremely important. Networking is a great way to make your expertise known in your community. Plan on starting to show up at events and activities where your expertise is sought. There are numerous online communities you can join if you are initially nervous about showing up in person. Another way to let your expertise shine is to work with the press and allow yourself to be publicized. Before you begin contacting the press, it is good to know how to build a press release.

Building a Press Release

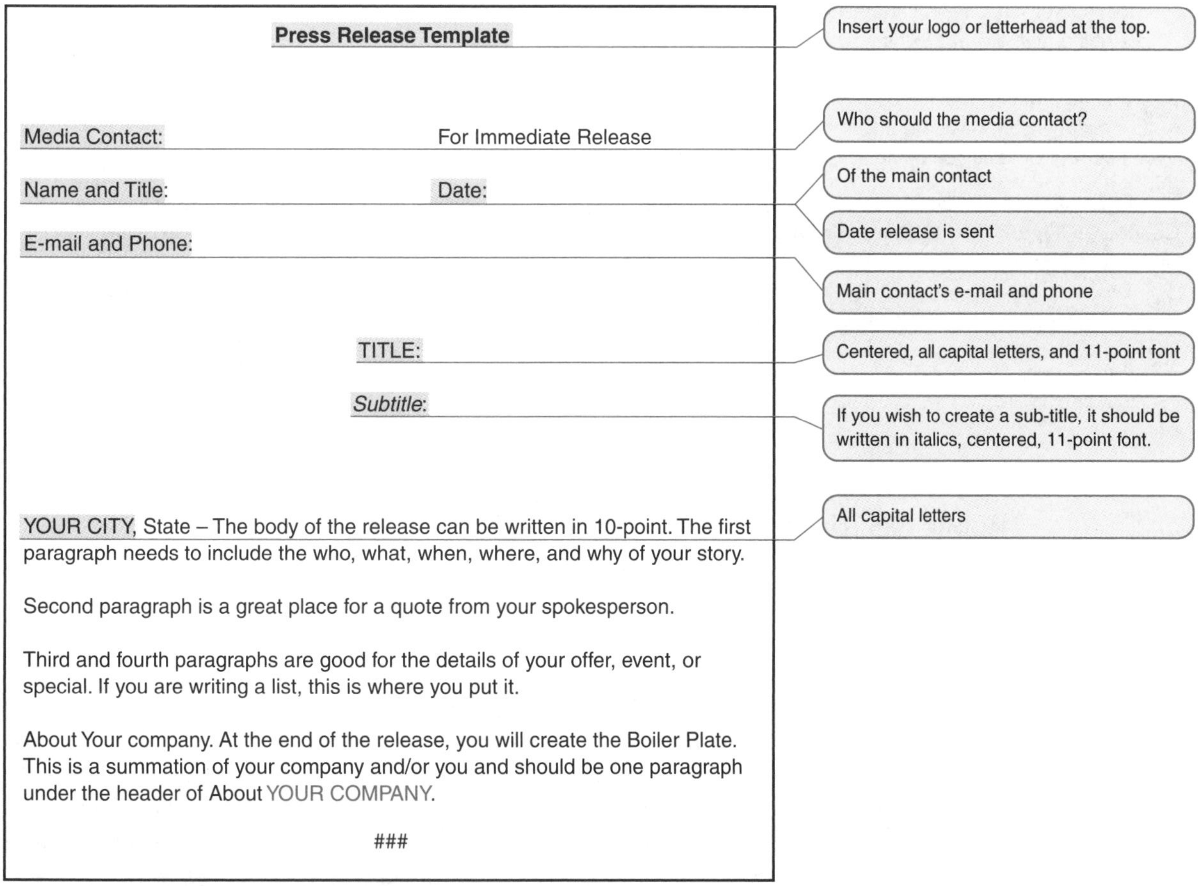

Press Release Template

Media Contact: For Immediate Release

Name and Title: Date:

E-mail and Phone:

TITLE:

Subtitle:

YOUR CITY, State – The body of the release can be written in 10-point. The first paragraph needs to include the who, what, when, where, and why of your story.

Second paragraph is a great place for a quote from your spokesperson.

Third and fourth paragraphs are good for the details of your offer, event, or special. If you are writing a list, this is where you put it.

About Your company. At the end of the release, you will create the Boiler Plate. This is a summation of your company and/or you and should be one paragraph under the header of About YOUR COMPANY.

###

Callouts:
- Insert your logo or letterhead at the top.
- Who should the media contact?
- Of the main contact
- Date release is sent
- Main contact's e-mail and phone
- Centered, all capital letters, and 11-point font
- If you wish to create a sub-title, it should be written in italics, centered, 11-point font.
- All capital letters

Figure 9–6 This template can be used to help you build your first press release.

Box 9.2 Sample Press Release

The Journey Into Wellbeing, National Health and Wellbeing TV Series, to Shoot Pilot Episode in Kentucky in October
Series Set to Air on PBS Stations Nationwide in 2013
Contact: Debra Locker

LEXINGTON, KY. — Kentuckians, prepare to inspire the nation's health transformation! The jokes about being a state made up of obese, sedentary people are ending soon. **The pilot episode of the national health and wellness series The Journey into Wellbeing will be shot entirely in Kentucky in mid-October.** To be carried on PBS stations nationwide, a panel of Bluegrass-based experts will be featured alongside health explorer Debra K. as she educates America that the **Bluegrass state is much more than horses, hillbilly hoedowns and hot browns... it's HEALTHY!**

As *The Journey into Wellbeing's* host and executive producer, Debra K. will travel to all 50 states and has selected the Bluegrass state to begin her Journey. "After spending 20 years in Kentucky and raising both my children here, I hold a special place in my heart for all things in the Bluegrass. As I've explored what the state has to offer over the past few months, I am so proud of all the creative wellness initiatives across the commonwealth. I believe every state has hidden gems of wellbeing and Kentucky felt like a great place to start."

A top-notch line-up of Kentucky's top wellness pros will share their tips for enriching lives of Kentuckians as well as all Americans. Segments to include:

- Bobby Benjamin, Executive Chef, La Coop, Louisville. Chef Benjamin will teach Debra K. how to redo traditional recipes in a healthier fashion.
- Lena D. Edwards, MD, FAARM, Balance Health & Wellness Center, Lexington. Dr. Edwards will provide Debra K. with her initial health assessment and offer tips to viewers on beginning their own healthy journey.
- Frontier Nursing University, Hyden. Debra K. treks off to Eastern Kentucky to explore the oldest and largest midwifery school in the nation.
- Molly Galbraith, Fitness Expert, J&M Strength & Conditioning, Lexington. Molly puts Debra K. through her paces and assigns a fitness grade, while offering simple tips for beginning a fitness journey.
- Janey Newton and Maggie Keith, founders and co-owners, Foxhollow Farm, Crestwood. Debra K. learns about bio-dynamic farming and the journey Foxhollow's leaders have taken to create a profitable organic farm.
- Eric Stephenson, owner of imassage, Inc. and national presenter, will offer Debra K. and viewers alike great self-care techniques on common ailments such as back, neck, and shoulder pain.

Debra K. adds, "From hiking at Natural Bridge, to redoing recipes in Louisville, and organic farming in Oldham County, we'll present Kentucky's wellness options in a positive, educational light that encourages viewers to begin their own health journey."

Described as one part Rachael Ray, one part Ellen DeGeneres, Debra K. is a former Fortune 250 marketing and sales leader, author of the soon-to-be-released text *Success from the Start,* executive director of the Destination Spa Group, and founder of the wellness education company imassage. "I'm an overworked, pudgy insomniac!" laughs Debra K. "I'm at that point in life where I recognize what I've been doing isn't good enough anymore. I'm sure many of you feel the same. I invite you to join me as we travel and uncover the secrets to living an energetic, vibrant life!"

Public Relations Success Stories

To give you some ideas on what has worked for other massage therapists, read the following stories that are found on the Web:

1. *Happy Muscles: Suggestions for Quick Relief* by Dimity McDowell, Published: December 1, 2009 in *The New York Times.*
   Topic: An Atlanta-based massage therapist offered her top three leg techniques for pain relief.
2. *Massage Goes to the Dogs in Two Rivers* by Cindy Hodgson, Published: September 13, 2010 in the *Herald Times.*
   Topic: This story focused on a massage therapist who took specialized training in canine massage. She went to work for a company called "Bark, Bath and Beyond" and set herself up as an expert in dog pain relief.

3. *Five Surprising Benefits of Massage: We know a massage feels good, but it can have a host of therapeutic advantages, too.* Posted by newsweek.com in September 2008.

   Topic: This article focused on the surprising benefits of massage, such as how regular massage can help underweight newborns gain weight, and the positive impact massage can have on high blood pressure.

See Worksheet 9-8

Writing Articles

Many of you might have a natural gift and interest in writing. If this is the case, writing articles for local publications can be a great public relations tool to market your business. It may be best to start by writing for local publications like the niche market papers and magazines. This form of promotion also helps with the process of establishing yourself as an expert. Your published articles can be used in resumes, included in your portfolio, framed and hung in your place of business, and referenced in press releases.

Before you contact the owner or publisher for your selected periodicals, plan on doing some homework first. Gather all the periodicals that your potential clients may be interested in, along with all the health and wellness publications. Take some time to review them, noting the topics and lengths of published articles. These will provide you some of the facts you need to write an **article query**. A query is an inquiry from a writer to an editor regarding the interest in publishing an article. It is usually presented in the form of a letter that outlines the proposed article. It is recommended that you keep your query to one page because many editors receive numerous queries and limited time to read them.

When the editors read your query, they will get a good idea about your level of professionalism, your writing ability, and whether you are familiar with their publication. A query is beneficial because it allows you to explore the idea and see if it will be accepted before writing the full article. If your article is not accepted, do not be discouraged—they may already have similar articles on file. One surprising benefit to submitting regular queries is unexpected work. You may be contacted to write an article on a chosen topic that the editor feels you can cover. This could be the beginning of a very rewarding relationship and also initiate your entry into other publications.

Writing a Successful Article Query

The opening to your query should be interesting, organized, and entertaining. Plan to open with a strong sentence that captures the reader's attention. This is often referred to as the "hook." Your query is the bait, and you are attempting to hook the editor's interest. Your opening statement can be a fact, a question you plan to answer, or a quote from someone you interviewed. Whatever it is, it must be bold and exciting. You would not want to start by introducing yourself or by disclosing that you are novice at writing. An example "hook" may be something like, "Roughly 8 million Americans have been diagnosed with fibromyalgia, a syndrome of chronic, widespread pain—did you know that a great, helpful solution is located just down the road? It is your local massage therapist."

Your opening statement is followed by your bid for publication, in which you explain exactly what you are proposing. Your bid can include your article title, its proposed length, and a summary of the article's content. Check for article submission guidelines to ensure you pitch the right word count for the article. A good example of a bid could be, "I'd like to offer you a 1,200-word article titled *'I never knew massage therapy could help with that.'* The article would discuss several common but problematic conditions people suffer and how massage therapy offers alleviation of symptoms."

Your second paragraph will expand on the topic you have selected. This is the section where you outline exactly what you plan to cover in your article. You want to be thorough, but not too wordy. Stick to an outline format to make your main points. Think through the flow of the article. Most likely, you will touch on the main points you wish to cover; these become your subtopics. Do not try to put in too many subtopics. In a proposed 1,200-word article, you most likely would have space for only three main points, allowing about 400 words per topic. An example of a subtopic explanation may look like this: "This article covers three main conditions: fibromyalgia, migraines, and cancer. It discusses and presents research validating the positive impact massage therapy has on these conditions. It will discuss the different modalities and techniques recommended for each condition and how readers can find a qualified therapist in their area." Within this section, you can talk about the readers who might find your article interesting and beneficial and list the reasons why. If you plan to use a quote, you can include it also in this portion of the query.

The end of your query is the opportunity to discuss your qualifications. In this portion, you summarize your training, certifications, skills, and level of expertise. This is also an opportunity to thank the editor for reviewing your submission and to state your availability and timeline for writing the article. Elaborate that if they are interested, you can deliver the article in a shorter period of time.

Within the query, be sure to include your full name, credentials, address, phone number, and e-mail address. Plan on including a self-addressed and stamped envelope for the editor's response. Just like a resume, the query should preferably be on letterhead, using good quality paper and envelopes. It is advisable to submit in a formal way using proper salutations and block-style writing. You can look these up on the Internet if you are unsure of how to do this.

See Worksheet 9-9

See Worksheet 9-10

Social Marketing for Success

The newest category of promotion to find its way into marketing plans is the effective use of social media to expand a business. At first, social media was viewed with skeptical eyes. Many companies were leery about committing time and money to an online effort, most likely because of their lack of knowledge about social marketing. However, with huge corporations jumping on board, the question for marketers is no longer "Should we do it?" but "How best can we make this work?"

A **social network** is an online community filled with friends, family, coworkers, and new acquaintances drawn to similar topics and themes. Through social networking, you can quickly share information and stay connected to your world of contacts in an informal way. Once viewed as a way for teens to expand their network of friends and connections, it has quickly expanded to include people of all ages (Fig. 9–7).

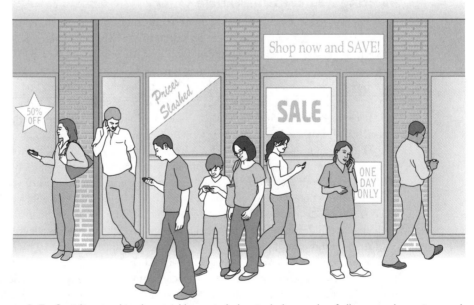

Figure 9–7 Social networking has quickly expanded to include people of all ages, and growing numbers are networking via their cell phones as well as their computers.

In March 2010, The *Web Trends Blog*[1] reported the following numbers of monthly unique visitors to these top social networking sites. One interesting fact is that MySpace, once the largest online social network site, continues to decline, losing about 13% of their visitors from the previous year. Also intriguing is that Twitter appears to be the fastest growing site, quadrupling their number of monthly visitors.

UNIQUE MONTHLY VISITS

- Facebook: 133,623,529
- MySpace: 50,615,444
- Twitter: 23,573,178
- LinkedIn: 15,475,890

Clarifying Your Social Media Objectives

Before you jump in and start setting up online profiles and writing posts, creating a strategy will prevent any missteps in representing who you are and what your business is all about. Once you go live on the Web, it is hard to remove or replace content. The most successful businesses recognize the importance of providing relevant and educational social media content that is useful for readers. Most people will not engage if a company is simply using this platform to talk about themselves and the specials they are running. They want to connect with like-minded individuals who are sharing information on interesting topics. These companies know that building a sense of belonging among followers is vital for amassing a huge following. When you plan to begin social marketing, know that your goal is to build a community—almost a family—of engaged members.

> When you plan to begin social marketing, know that your goal is to build a community—almost a family—of engaged members.

You will want to provide content that is honest and authentic, letting your personality shine. Write in a way that is conversational and encourages readers to respond. Resist posting content about sales, specials, and the offer of the week. This is boring and will discourage people from checking back in with you. The first part of your social networking strategy should be that quality always comes before quantity.

Formulating your plan includes assessing all the social sites you could potentially become involved with, observing activities similar to those you wish to engage in, and formulating your strategy by being very selective about the sites you choose to set up—all before you begin.

First, take a look at all the sites you can possibly become involved with. Conduct an online search with key words such as "top social networking sites." This will pull up reviews and lists of possible sites to join. Before setting up your own pages, become an observer. You can learn much from those who are already doing this well. Sign up for feeds with some popular social contributors and observe how they interact with their followers and how their followers interact with them. You can visit http://www.delicious.com and type "massage" in the search box. This will pull up some popular book-marked sites on massage. To search for popular massage blogs, visit http://www.technorati.com. In the search box, choose blog and type in the words "massage therapy." This will yield numerous blogs on massage that you can read and follow.

Prepare your social networking strategy by determining the stance you will take when presenting yourself to the world. Are you seeking to set yourself up as an expert, are you trying to attract like-minded people, do you plan to mostly engage current clients, or are you seeking to draw potential new clients to your sites? This is important because your intention becomes the filter through which you run all your topics and ideas. If you are setting yourself up as an expert in reflexology, you probably will not be sharing advice on canine massage. Most of your content, links, sharing, and data will relate to your main strategy.

There are many social sites to choose from. This chapter will highlight the most relevant and popular social networking vehicles—blogs, Facebook, Twitter and LinkedIn.

Blogs at a Glance

One way experts begin to share their expertise is through blogs. A **blog** is software that allows someone to post content on the Web. Often these are free or inexpensive to set up. You must commit to regularly filling it with relevant content, however, or it will be a waste of time.

The information in a blog generally resembles an article or typed letter. For those who are seeking to become known in the world, it becomes a great vehicle to achieve this. You do not have to be accepted or approved before publishing information. With blogs, you generally link your content to any other online vehicles you are using, such as social networking sites and websites. It is a fast way to get your information out there. Most blogging sites have great customization and editing tools. Blogs can become very vibrant with the use of design, color, video, and photographs. You can have fun creating your own unique look and feel.

If you choose to encourage engagement from your readers, you can allow them to post comments, share with others, and subscribe to your future posts. Regular blogging allows you to create quality content and make connections with people everywhere. The secret to blogging success is a continual inflow of relevant content posting. Too often, someone thinks creating a blog is a great idea but within a couple of months or weeks realizes how much work it is and abandons the site. Many times you may visit blogs and find that nothing has been posted for months or even years.

Successful blogging takes some strategy. Using keywords—words that are popular and favored by search engines—is one way to ensure that people find your content. Posting relevant, frequent information is another step to success. Becoming engaged in other people's efforts also links back to your blog and can help in building a following. As with everything else, before you begin, plan to observe blogging activity for a while and ensure that it is a fit for you. Keeping up with blogging and all the other social networking avenues can become time-consuming. To see if you are ready to become a dedicated blogger, begin writing articles, finding links, and locating relevant pictures, and put them into a text document. If you can regularly do this for a month without any problem, then you might be ready to tackle a blog. Then, once you create your blog, you will already have a month's worth of prepared content.

Facebook at a Glance

Originally started as an online connection among college students, Facebook has become a worldwide phenomenon, expanding to all parts of the world and capturing the interest of all kinds of people. Currently, it is the world's leader in online social connection, based on volume of use.

Setting up a profile allows you to post comments, pictures, blogs, and apps. You can use your mobile device to do this as well, capturing items of importance as they happen. Facebook can be used to expand relationships with people you currently know and to expand your network of new friends and followers. There are two ways to set yourself up on Facebook. You can create both a personal profile section and a business page. Some people started out with personal pages and then

---

9-3: Find It on the Web

Some common blogging sites to explore:

- **WordPress:** Their homepage says, "Web software you can use to create a beautiful website or blog. We like to say that WordPress is both free and priceless at the same time." http://www.wordpress.org
- **Blogger:** Their homepage says, "Create a blog. It's free." blogs.windows.com
- **Windows Live Space:** Their homepage says, "Make your own space on Windows Live. It's your place on the web to express yourself." http://blogs.windows.com

opened their business pages. They soon became concerned because there is a close association between the two, and often their personal page was a bit too personal for their business followers. Keep this in mind as you build your pages.

A business fan page has quite a bit of functionality and allows you to open your page up to a larger audience than just your personal friends. All updates that you post on your business page will also show up on the pages of your fans, expanding your reach.

> All updates that you post on your [Facebook] business page will also show up on the pages of your fans, expanding your reach.

Once you set up your profile, and before you post anything too serious, click your account link and explore the help center and privacy sections. These will immediately offer you guidance on how to set your pages up correctly and safely. Once you are comfortable and ready to create some excitement with your posting and events, you can begin to communicate directly with your fans and create a large following. To get started today, visit http://www.facebook.com.

LinkedIn at a Glance

LinkedIn has become known as the premier site for business professionals and connections. It is bit more formal than the other sites, and reaching out to others must be justified through common connections. Initially plan to spend some time familiarizing yourself with the culture and styles of communication before you jump in. In the search box, type in the word "massage" and take a look at the different types of profiles others have already set up. Notice how some of the massage therapists have asked clients to create recommendations for them. This is a great way to build credibility in your market. LinkedIn also allows you to promote events you plan to host or participate in. If you have built a community of like-minded individuals, it is also a great source of information. For example, you can post questions to other professionals about common complaints or specific techniques.

If you decide LinkedIn is where you want to be, pay special attention when setting up your profile. This becomes the personality and resume for you and your business. Upload a great picture, include links to all your other online content, and plan on updating it regularly. To get started on LinkedIn, visit http://www.linkedin.com

Twitter at a Glance

In a nutshell, Twitter is a social communications tool that allows you to post everything that is going on in 140 characters or less. Some call this micro-blogging. Like the other social networking sites, Twitter allows you to "friend," follow, post, and share. Twitter seems especially useful for networking with like-minded people and groups. Once you select groups to follow, you will have a continuous stream of current and relevant information about your selected topics. It is not really the best tool for targeting potential clients, but it can help keep you current with what is going on in your chosen fields of interest.

Twitter has created a whole new language describing the different activities people partake in. "Tweeting" is what posting is called; individual posts are called "tweets." "Re-tweeting" is when you tweet someone else's tweet. The terminology can be confusing at first. Certain symbols stand for certain things as well, so become familiar with using the @ and the #. There are some great online resources to help get you started.

The main objectives of Twitter are to get others to follow you and to follow others. You can quickly build a large group of people who are likely to see your information. One site, http://www.twellow.com, allows you to search for others by their industry. You can select the ones that look interesting and follow them. Usually, the more groups you follow, the more people will follow you.

If you decide to set up a Twitter account, you will quickly discover that you will need a Twitter management program, like the popular TweetDeck or Hootsuite. These are software programs that download to your computer and make managing your content much easier.

> See Worksheet 9-11

Social media may or may not be right for you. Before you jump in, you should know that daily commitment is required to keep it going. More than likely, you will not garner immediate clients through your social networking efforts. Instead, it can become a great tool to build your credibility in the industry, acquire large networks of like-minded people, and provide you with current and relevant information. Through this, you will find yourself becoming more involved in larger activities, which may ultimately lead you to acquiring new clients and a full practice. For social networking, beginning with this end in mind is helpful and will keep you from getting frustrated.

CHAPTER SUMMARY

Marketing is a powerful, essential ingredient for success as you start on your massage business journey. Finding the right medium to communicate your message is worth the time and effort of research. There are many ways to target your most likely customers, but not all advertising avenues are well suited to your business. Reaching out to your potential customers is rewarding when you employ your creativity to successfully forge a new connection. Public relations tactics, such as press releases, can further enhance your ability to reach your ideal audience and bring in loyal clients. Social media offers you more opportunities than ever to promote your expertise and your business, while expanding your network and exploring other interests. As you delve into the many possibilities of marketing, the challenge lies in finding the avenues that work best for you in your chosen market.

BIBLIOGRAPHY

1. Nations, D. (2010, March 15). The Top 10 Most Popular Social Networks. *Web Trends Blog*. Retrieved from http://webtrends.about.com/b/2010/03/15/the-top-10-most-popular-social-networks.htm.

REVIEW QUESTIONS

1. **Good marketing involves promotion, sales, product and service distribution, and:**
   a. Research
   b. Advertising
   c. Watching the competition
   d. Setting the highest price for your services

2. **Familiarizing yourself with the competition keeps you informed about where they are located, how much they charge, and:**
   a. How they position themselves in the community
   b. What ideas you can copy from them
   c. Prospective good employers
   d. Both a & c

3. **What is the best pricing strategy?**
   a. Charge what you think you are worth
   b. Charge the least you can without losing money
   c. Charge the most you can without deterring the clients you want
   d. List all of the things you want for your business in a budget, then back into how much to charge clients to cover all of these expenses

4. Which of the following is *not* something to consider when setting your price structure?
    a. Research how massage is priced in the area you plan to practice
    b. If fear is driving your decision
    c. The types of clients you hope to attract
    d. Cost-per-point (CPP)

5. Under what circumstances would you realistically consider charging more than the national average for a massage?
    a. If you specialize in a specific modality
    b. If you practice in a rural area
    c. If you are very hopeful you will fill your practice at any fee
    d. If you have a great faith in your gifts

6. Cheap prices attract cheap customers.
    a. True
    b. False

7. Price-sensitive customers are:
    a. Less likely to be loyal
    b. Harder to keep satisfied
    c. More likely to visit more often
    d. Both a & b

8. Why is specialization an important benefit in regard to marketing?
    a. You can more easily communicate what your business is
    b. You can attract clients more willing to pay for your specialization
    c. You can attract clients who will be more loyal and have higher satisfaction levels
    d. All of the above

9. When considering marketing options, keep in mind that marketing efforts will pull from the following two areas:
    a. Advertising and promotion
    b. Financial and energetic
    c. Emotional and intellectual
    d. Simple and complicated

10. Advertisements can be spoken, in video, or in print.
    a. True
    b. False

11. What is more important than finding the right delivery method for your message?
    a. Ensuring you target the right audience
    b. Ensuring you have the right message
    c. Ensuring you compliment traditional methods with nontraditional methods
    d. Keeping Facebook and Twitter accounts current

12. **What are the four points to consider when evaluating advertising proposals?**
    a. Finances, time, energy, and emotion
    b. Audience profile, reach, frequency, cost-per-point
    c. Advertising, promotion, public relations, and social networking
    d. National averages, competitors' advertisements, distribution, and discounts

13. **Which type of television advertising allows you to target more customized viewers and is often more affordable?**
    a. Cable channels
    b. Major networks (NBC, CBS, ABC, FOX)
    c. Sporting events, particularly men's basketball and football
    d. It's not possible to target customized viewers with television advertising

14. **Which traditional media outlet reaches the largest audience?**
    a. Local newspapers
    b. Local radio stations
    c. Television
    d. Websites

15. **Which type of traditional media advertisements can be created relatively quickly and start running almost immediately?**
    a. Event sponsorships
    b. Website banners
    c. Television commercials
    d. Radio spots

16. **Small, local businesses find newspapers an effective way to advertise, but newspapers have a short life span, so frequency is key.**
    a. True
    b. False

17. **Which of the following is often an effective nontraditional strategy for small businesses to reach both potential and existing clients?**
    a. Public relations
    b. Direct mail
    c. Direct e-mail
    d. Both b & c

18. **Word-of-mouth promotion will quickly fill your practice.**
    a. True
    b. False

19. **Which of the following is not a type of marketing promotion?**
    a. Connectors
    b. Discounts
    c. Sponsorship and event participation
    d. Group and club memberships

20. **Public relations are a paid form of self-promotion.**

    a. True

    b. False

21. **How many interesting or inspiring points should you include in a press release?**

    a. None, no one reads press releases anymore

    b. One point to keep the message simple and clear

    c. Three points that are woven into a compelling story

    d. Ten points to ensure the journalist reads at least one of them

22. **What form of promotion also helps with the process of establishing yourself as an expert?**

    a. Writing articles

    b. A well-rounded resume

    c. Writing a successful article query

    d. Meaningful and numerous Facebook posts and Tweets

23. **The most successful social networking businesses recognize the importance of:**

    a. Quantity over quality

    b. Sharing information about themselves

    c. Taking advantage of the free advertising social media offers

    d. Providing relevant and educational social media content

24. **What generally resembles an article or typed letter?**

    a. A Tweet

    b. A re-tweet

    c. A blog

    d. A LinkedIn recommendation

25. **A business fan page on Twitter allows you to open your page up to a larger audience than just your personal friends.**

    a. True

    b. False

26. **Which of the following social media tools is a great way to build credibility in your market?**

    a. Twitter hashtags (#)

    b. LinkedIn recommendations

    c. Facebook pictures

    d. Blog postings with key words

27. **Twitter is not the best social networking tool for targeting potential clients, but it can help you keep current with what is going on in your chosen fields of interest.**

    a. True

    b. False

Worksheet 9-1   Becoming Aware of the Competition

The following worksheet will help guide you in becoming aware of the competition. It is beneficial to initially understand the competition you might have so that you can make good decisions when setting up your practice. Your strategy is to differentiate yourself from others in a way that is meaningful and so that you stand out.

Your state board will most likely be able to provide you with an idea of how many therapists hold licenses in the market you choose. See if you can figure this out.

State: _____ Number of licenses in the state: _____

City: _____ Number of licenses in the city: _____

County: _____ Number of licenses in the county: _____

Start paying attention to what you see in the community. Build a short profile on each massage business you see.

Example:

Name of Business	Massage4You
Describe type of business	Large clinic that hires therapists as independent contractors
Location	Downtown location, close to many other businesses, friends who work there say they are always busy
Key marketing features	Most ads focus on the variety of massages offered. They never run discounts. They advertise gift certificates in all ads. Ads indicate all their MT's are Nationally Certified. They run ads in the local newspaper, have very bright signage, and are often at local events with massage chairs.
Personal comments	This might be a good place to start working. I would meet a lot of therapists and build my skills.

Name of business

Describe type of business

Location

Key marketing features

Personal comments

Name of business

Describe type of business

Location

Key marketing features

Personal comments

Name of business

Describe type of business

Location

Key marketing features

Personal comments

Worksheet 9-2   Pricing Research

The following worksheet provides you with some space to do pricing research. Take time to research your chosen marketplace and fill in some pricing details for different types of businesses. Find pricing on regular massage, longer sessions, and special modalities. Many businesses have a printed pricing menu you can take with you.

Day Spa	Massage Specialist: Rolfer/Prenatal/Cranial Sacral/etc.
Regular	Regular
Long	Long
Specialty	Specialty
Other:	Other:

Massage Franchise	Massages in offices: Chiro/Dr/etc.
Regular	Regular
Long	Long
Specialty	Specialty
Other:	Other:

Higher-End Spa	Other
Regular	Regular
Long	Long
Specialty	Specialty
Other:	Other:

Worksheet 9-3   Pricing Your Services

I would like to charge the following amounts for my massage services:

50 minutes:

80 minutes:

Specialty massage:

Are you confident enough now to set your prices at this level?   YES   NO
If yes, what makes you able to charge this amount?

If no, what do you feel you need to do to charge this amount?

Worksheet 9-4   Finding the Right Marketing Piece for Your Message

To fill in this worksheet, you will need to gather several local newspapers and magazines. Once you have several, glance through them. Pay attention to the types of articles running and see if you can figure out what type of reader the information might interest (the target market). Also pay attention to other advertisers. Use the below form to figure out whether this piece might be a fit for you.

EXAMPLE:

Name of publication:	Types of articles	Types of advertisers	Would this appeal to my client and why?
SENIOR Magazine	Medical screenings Recognizing stroke symptoms Health insurance laws Myofascial pain	Senior living Dentists Doctors, chiropractors Health supplements	Yes, I plan on working directly with those over the age of 50. All of the articles and advertisers are aimed at this audience. It might be a good idea for me to network with some of the local advertisers.
Name of publication:	**Types of articles**	**Types of advertisers**	**Would this appeal to my client and why?**
Name of publication:	**Types of articles**	**Types of advertisers**	**Would this appeal to my client and why?**
Name of publication:	**Types of articles**	**Types of advertisers**	**Would this appeal to my client and why?**

Worksheet 9-5   My Advertising Plan

Draft your early thoughts about how you can use advertising to market and expand your business.

Worksheet 9-6   Finding Your Future Clients

Similar to your work in the last chapter, spend a few moments writing down your ideas about where your potential clients might be going to shop, dine, hang out, and enjoy recreational activities. Once you have your list, plan on visiting these places to see what opportunities exist to promote your business.

Type of client I would like to work with:	These are places they are likely to shop, eat, and hang out. Note to self: I will go check these places out to see if there is opportunity to advertise and promote my business	Events I have found to explore further
Example: People who own dogs	Pet stores, veterinarians, grooming places, pet treat stores, parks, dog trails, pet play areas, shelters	"Pooch"tacular Bazaar and Dog Walk for Charity

Worksheet 9-7   My Promotions Plan

Draft your early thoughts about how you can use promotions to market and expand your business.

Worksheet 9-8   Press Release Ideas

To help begin the process of writing your first press release, enter on the left side of the worksheet some interesting topics. On the right side, enter the top three points you plan to focus on throughout the release

Example Topic: Are you ready for natural assistance for the stress that might be killing you?	1. Facts on the high level of stress in our society and how it is affecting our health negatively 2. The Touch Research Institute data on how massage reduces stress and quotes from you, the expert MT 3. Quote from a local doctor about how stress affects the body and what conditions he sees in local patients
Topic:	1. 2. 3.
Topic:	1. 2. 3.

Worksheet 9-9   Article Ideas

To help begin the process of writing your first article query, enter some possible "hook" topics.

Example Hook Topic:
Roughly 8 million Americans have been diagnosed with fibromyalgia, a syndrome of chronic widespread pain—a great preventive measure is down the road, your local massage therapist.

Hook Topic:

Hook Topic:

Worksheet 9-10   My Public Relations Plan

Draft your early thoughts on how you can use public relations to market and expand your business.

Worksheet 9-11 My Social Marketing Plan

Draft your early thoughts on how you can use social media to market and expand your business.

Chapter 10

Client Loyalty: Every Therapist's Pot of Gold

Repeat business or behavior can be bribed. Loyalty has to be earned.

–Janet Robinson

Outline

You will learn to ...

■ Create an overall experience that exceeds customer expectations
■ Assess client satisfaction
■ Calculate the lifetime value of a client
■ Help ease common anxieties in new and experienced clients
■ Perfect your intake process
■ Establish a safe, healing "therapeutic bubble"
■ Understand clients' verbal and nonverbal cues
■ Educate your clients at timely stages

Key Definitions

This chapter references several key terms, which are indicated in bold. For easy reference, these terms are briefly defined here:

Client experience: Encompasses every interaction customers have with a business and influences whether the customer will decide to return to the business again.

Client satisfaction: Degree of contentment a customer has with the product, service, or experience; often measured by repeat business and/or referrals.

Customer satisfaction assessment: Measurement to determine level of client satisfaction with the purchase and/or experience.

First contact: Any avenue potential clients use to make contact, usually because they have questions or are attempting to book an appointment.

Lifetime value: How much revenue a client would bring to you during the time as your customer.

Loyalty: A state of faithfulness to buy products, services, or experiences from one company or person.

Mindfulness: Fosters the attitude of living in the moment and enjoying each guest in an unhurried, relaxed state as the guest enjoys each service in a relaxed state.

Continued

Key Definitions—cont'd

Mirroring: Technique used to repeat back to clients their request, to ensure you understand their true desire.

Open-ended question: A question that is answered in the respondent's words, without pre-determined answers to select from.

Presence: A state of mind, free from distraction and practiced through mindfulness.

Rebooking rate: The percentage of clients who return and ask for you.

Service path: The journey a consumer takes while engaging with a business that offers something for sale. For massage, it encompasses the moment a potential client reaches out to gather more information about the therapist or business. It continues as the client arrives for the service, through the session and departure, and may even include some form of follow-up after the client has gone.

Therapeutic bubble: An analogy for the atmosphere created by a therapist to create a safe, healing environment with each client, which involves presence, unconditional positive regard, and treating each client as a unique person with specific needs.

Touch point: A critical interaction during the service experience.

Unconditional positive regard (UPR): Term coined by the humanist Carl Rogers, which is a blanket acceptance and support of a person regardless of what the person says or does. This acceptance of each person includes see that person in a positive light, as whole and complete person, despite personality challenges.

AN INTRODUCTION TO LOYALTY

Beyond marketing, there is another aspect of your new career to be explored fully. This is the experience you offer your clients. By now, you have more insight into what it takes to narrow your focus, choose marketing avenues wisely, and attract the clients you most want to work with. However, your work is not quite done. You must build an experience that satisfies your clients so completely they become raving fans of everything you have built— and become loyal to you. This intense **loyalty** results in many benefits that will sustain your business for as long as you continue to exceed their expectations.

Client Experience

What is a **client experience**? The term, having gained popularity over the past several years, encompasses every interaction customers have with a business. Every nuance of these interactions should be carefully viewed and assessed for importance because it can determine whether customers view their decision to hire you positively or regretfully (Fig. 10-1). This perception will also determine whether they are inclined to return and whether they will talk about their experience with friends and family, generating highly beneficial word-of-mouth advertising. As we explored previously, really smart businesses, both large and small, recognize the importance of truly understanding their customers. These businesses study, observe, and forecast the movements of their customers, and their efforts help them fully comprehend how and why customers access products or services. As a customer, you probably have some examples of when, during your interactions with businesses, they dropped the ball. For example, maybe you found the perfect washer. As you were preparing to order it online, the process became very cumbersome; you gave up in frustration. If this company does not become aware of the issues you experienced during this phase of the buying process, it will most likely lose many sales. It might be the greatest washer in the world, but the buying experience is getting in the way of allowing people to experience it. You also probably have some great memories of companies that got it right. They surprised you with their level of attention, and you left feeling like you would definitely go back

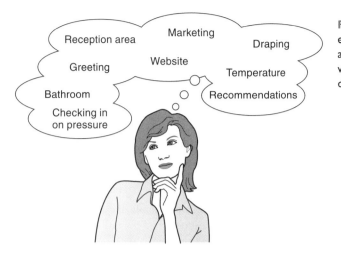

Figure 10–1   A customer experience is defined as all the events and activities your customer interacts with in their efforts to achieve a desired result from your business.

and may even tell others about your experience. If it was a service misstep, maybe the company recovered so well that you were even more satisfied with your overall experience.

Experiential Strategy

Once you decide on your target customer groups, you begin to strategically build an experience that will exceed customer expectations. In other words, what carefully chosen tactics will you put in place to create a unique massage experience? Answering this question will affect every aspect of your business, including the type of employees you hire and your printed collateral materials, communication processes, pricing, and services offered.

To help ensure a consistently exceptional experience for your clients, it is wise to map out the experiential path and define actions you plan to take for each step of the journey. This may sound challenging, but this chapter will help you along this path of discovery. After you become clear on your decisions, it will become easier to build the actions and processes, ensuring something flawless for your clients. Also, going through this process makes it easier if you are in the position to hire or train others. Because you have thought through every step, you can create training materials that are clear and understandable. An example of this is the way you decide to answer your business phone. Once defined, it becomes very easy to do and to train others how to do it. It also makes it easier to hold yourself and others accountable for times when things start to move away from what you have decided is a key element of the massage experience you offer.

To begin this process, think through the natural massage path. A short version of a massage experience path could look something like this: Somewhere, a potential client has decided she needs a massage, so she goes to the Internet and finds a therapist near her. After calling and booking her appointment, she reads more on the website to educate herself. She arrives, receives her massage, and departs. What would it feel like if you broke each step of this process down and identified what is most important to deliver at each phase? It would feel like success.

There are ways you can strategize and customize your experience for your clients. The first is through observation. Pay close attention to all the details of your client interactions and the processes you have built for them to go through. You can learn a great deal just by paying attention. A great retail example is shown by businesses that have started placing bathroom trash cans closer to the door. As society has become more germ-phobic, these businesses noticed that their customers want to have paper towels in their hands when opening the bathroom door. To accommodate this and to save their cleaning staff from having to pick up piles of paper towels, they simply moved the trash cans closer to the doors. This keen observation, although going unnoticed by most customers, alleviates discomfort for the customer who has opened the door and has no option but to toss the paper towel across the bathroom and hope they make a basket. This type of behavior can be noted only through observation. If asked about what could be done to improve a business, most customers would not mention moving a trash can.

Another example is of a grocery store that was not paying attention to the experience it was offering customers. This particular store just built a new section featuring a grab-and-go restaurant area. They spent millions expanding their current infrastructure to meet a new growing demand for fast, convenient food to go. However, they missed several key details. One issue they didn't foresee was in the sitting area. They had nice tables, encouraging on-site eating, and an area for trash, encouraging customers to clear the trash from their tables. Unfortunately, the plates provided on the food bar were larger than the hole in the trash cans. This was such a simple thing but remained completely unaddressed for quite some time. Imagine your frustration if you go to throw away your plate and it doesn't fit. More than likely, you would leave your items on the table. If the store workers are not paying attention, they might wonder why they have to constantly waste valuable time and resource dollars by having employees clean up after people. However, by simply sitting in the eating area for a short period of time, they would have observed the problem and corrected it quickly, saving their customers some frustration and their employees from unnecessary work.

Some companies go so far as to hire families to be observed by members of their organization. The family goes about their daily activities while the observers pay close attention to their patterns, behaviors, and frustrations. This has resulted in the creation of new products that meet the changing needs of the modern family. Now, you might not want to ask your clients if you can hang out in their houses so that you can observe any challenges they face that may result in the need for massage, but you can observe many things about them during your interactions with them. When you pay attention at this level, purposely seeking to understand client behavior, you will have some keen insights that can help you deliver something exceptional.

Hone Listening and Observation Skills

Pay attention to what clients are saying and doing. They often leave you clues about what makes them happy and what dissatisfies them. You can discover some gems of information by honing your listening and observation skills. As they talk, listen for common themes in what they are saying. Are there things you hear often from many clients? If so, there may be an opportunity to create an experiential item that makes your service unique. Keenly observing their actions will provide you with information about what they may be seeking. Many clients are not even aware of what they would like from their experience, but their actions will tell you. As you become better at being an experiential detective, you will discover things that will really make a difference.

Real Life Scenario: Listening to Your Clients

Patricia recently moved her practice to a new location. The new location was in a strip mall surrounded by many other businesses. She felt this new location would bring her more business because of the higher amount of people in the area. After being in her location for a while, she was a bit disappointed that her practice was not growing as quickly as she hoped. She began to pay close attention to what new clients were saying when they came in. She observed that, more than usual, new clients were apologizing for being a bit late for their first appointments. Now that she was paying attention, she heard the answer begin to emerge. Instead of just assuming they couldn't find her place because they were new, she paid more attention and discovered that because her center was located between two larger businesses, her sign was not as visible as it could be. To make matters worse, she noticed that every day one of the stores put out a big tent sign, which partially blocked her entrance. She addressed these issues to help make it easier for new clients to find her and also began telling them on the phone which two stores she was between. This simple observation resulted in more people noticing her business and fewer people being late and frustrated. This simple experiential improvement had a positive effect on her business.

Real-Life Scenario: Observe Your Clients

Mario is a therapist who caters to corporate employees. He has his office set up in an area that is surrounded by business offices. He has done a great job networking with the offices and has a full practice of business people. He began to notice that he often knocked on the door of the treatment room before people were ready for him to come in and that they seemed to take a long time coming out. Having worked in massage for many years, he couldn't figure out why this group seemed to take longer. He began paying attention to the way his room was set up and noticed that his clients were trying to place all their items on the chair he provided them. This had worked great in the past, but because these people were in business attire and often were returning to work, they were taking extra precautions not to wrinkle their clothing. He also noticed that while they came in with all their jewelry, he couldn't see where they had placed it. He surmised that they were taking the time to carefully place it in their purses. Quickly seeing what might be causing delay and a bit of worry, he added several features to his treatment room, including shirt and pants hangers, small covered dishes for jewelry, and a cubby space for shoes, laptop carriers, and other miscellaneous items. This thoughtful action improved the time problem, and several clients remarked that they hadn't seen another therapist take such care with their business clothing—a differentiator that makes a difference.

THE IMPORTANCE OF CLIENT SATISFACTION

Many companies have made great strides in measuring the success of their experience. They do this through **customer satisfaction assessment**. These results become the report card for the experience they deliver. More than likely, a business has asked you to complete a satisfaction survey, written, online, or on the phone. Be thankful when you are asked for this feedback because this means the company is truly interested in how they are doing and what they can do to improve. There are valid reasons for companies to take the time to inquire about their performance.

> "The difference between a highly satisfied customer and a satisfied customer can drown a business" —*The Service Profit Chain*

There are significant differences between being satisfied and being highly satisfied with an experience. In fact, as reported by the Service Management Group (SMG), a firm specializing in measuring and analyzing customer satisfaction, if your customers indicate they are satisfied with their experience, they are just as likely to visit a competitor as they are to return to you.

> Highly satisfied customers . . . are twice as likely to return as those who are merely satisfied, and highly satisfied customers are three times more likely to recommend the business to friends and family.

The Difference Between Satisfied and Highly Satisfied

When analyzing the results of their satisfaction scores, many businesses make an error—assuming that a satisfied customer is good enough to return and good enough to tell their friends and family (Fig. 10-2). This assumption is wrong.

Research shows that less than half of satisfied customers say they are highly likely to return to a business, meaning most of them probably will not come back. Less than one third would recommend that business to someone else—meaning no word-of-mouth benefits. Highly satisfied customers, however, are twice as likely to return as those who are merely satisfied, and highly satisfied customers are three times more likely to recommend the business to friends and family. From this, you can gather that merely "satisfying" customers is not enough.

If you leave a client anything less than highly satisfied, potentially half of them will never come back to you. Businesses that unknowingly group their customers together (satisfied and highly satisfied) are probably losing more customers as a result of this assumption than they are aware (Fig. 10-3).

Placing the Bar on the Right Rung

Another key to your long-term success as a massage therapist is ensuring you are striving for the highest levels of satisfaction. When you are aware that mere satisfaction is not enough, then nothing but the best will do. You will create everything hoping to achieve this

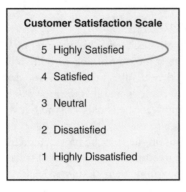

Customer Satisfaction Scale

5 Highly Satisfied

4 Satisfied

3 Neutral

2 Dissatisfied

1 Highly Dissatisfied

Figure 10–2   This illustration demonstrates a typical rating scale for a customer experience. Customers are asked to rate their satisfaction with an element of the experience, such as friendliness of staff. Many companies combine their satisfied and highly satisfied scores and assume they are doing much better than they really are. Research shows that there is significant difference between customers within each group. The focus for your business should be on achieving the highest number of scores in the highly satisfied ranking.

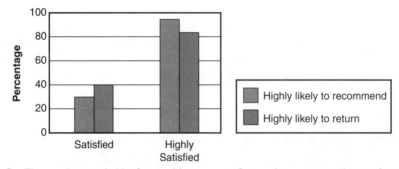

Figure 10–3   This graph, provided by Service Management Group, demonstrates the significant difference between a satisfied and a highly satisfied customer. A customer's likelihood to recommend and return is a key indicator of customer loyalty, vital to your long-term success. (From Service Management Group, Inc. (2007). *Five Things We Learned From Talking to 100 Million People.*)

level, and you will reap the rewards from doing so. Setting your satisfaction bar on the right rung is a necessary step in the process of improving client satisfaction, earning repeat business, and receiving referrals from clients. But that rung is high: it is a flawless, present-centered experience (Fig. 10-4).

Assessing Satisfaction

Once your experience is defined and launched, it is important to constantly assess results and adapt your experience accordingly. Assessing **client satisfaction** is one way to do this. Even if you are a one-person operation, collecting feedback from your clients is valuable. As you have discovered, most massage clients do not voice complaints—they just do not return. They may be very hesitant to approach you and say that you did something that was not right for them, especially for a service as intimate and sometimes sensitive as massage therapy. To prevent this from happening, become proactive in addressing concerns and soliciting feedback. It is much easier for them to talk to you through an alternative method, such as feedback forms.

It is recommended that you gather all responses anonymously. Although it may be tempting to match comments to clients, overcome the urge to do this. This discreet process allows your clients to truly express what makes them happy or unhappy and how likely they are to return to you. Often, your most satisfied clients will be happy to associate themselves with their responses and write in their names. It is more important to gather authentic answers than to fix an individual problem. Gathering this information is key to solving problems and ensuring that clients keep coming back.

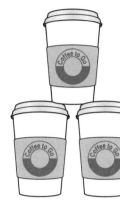

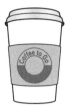

Figure 10–4   For Starbucks, moving customers from satisfied to highly satisfied is worth millions of dollars to their bottom line. (Data from http://www.customerservicemanager.com/the-power-of-highly-satisfied-customers.htm.)

Satisfied Customer

Visits 4.3 per month
Spends $4.06 per visit
Stays a customer for <u>4.4 years</u>
Lifetime value = $921.78

Highly Satisfied Customer

Visits 7.2 per month
Spends $4.42 per visit
Stays a customer for <u>8.3 years</u>
Lifetime value = $3,169.67

Ensuring Anonymity

To ensure privacy, you must be sensitive about collecting feedback. There are several methods to consider. The following ways allow you to integrate a client feedback program into your practice:

1. Give out a pre-created feedback form with postage that can be mailed at the clients' convenience. To save costs, you can rotate giving them to new and returning clients. Or, you can do this in bursts, whereby every client receives a form for a month, and then you don't do it again for a few months.
2. Have a professional receptacle in the waiting room for feedback and check it only once a week. Try to resist checking it after each client to ensure that client responses truly are anonymous. If you can't resist the temptation to read each card after each client leaves, do not respond to any problems indicated because this will break your promise of anonymity.
3. Create an online survey in which responses can be gathered and analyzed at your leisure. There are several inexpensive sites that allow you build and edit surveys.

Questions to Include in Your Survey

There are several important questions that should be included in every satisfaction measurement form. The first is, **"Please rate your satisfaction with your overall experience."** The total

---

10-1: *Find It on the Web*

- Zoomerang offers a free introductory service and has an expanded service for an affordable amount: http://zoomerang.com/signup/
- Survey Monkey, an affordable online option, offers surveys that are easy to build and analyze: http://www.surveymonkey.com
- Constant Contact is an e-mail marketing, event management, and survey site: http://www.constantcontact.com

percentage of responses that indicate high satisfaction to this simple question is your final grade and a measurement of your success. This question allows your clients to assess the entire experience and assign a score they feel matches their time with you. Your goal is to achieve a high percentage of clients marking highly satisfied with overall experience. When adding up your scores, you will take the number of clients who have given you the highest satisfaction level, which is your score, and compare this to the amounts in every other response.

Understanding Satisfaction

One hundred surveys were collected. The responses to the question, "How satisfied are you with your overall experience?" were as follows:

- 68 gave a 5 = highly satisfied

Great job! These clients are most likely to return for more massage and tell their friends and family about you.

- 22 gave a 4 = satisfied
- 6 gave a 3 = neutral

Although it is tempting to be happy with these scores, there is a good chance you will never see these clients again.

- 3 gave a 2 = dissatisfied
- 1 gave a 1 = highly dissatisfied

Fortunately, this number is small. Unless they have no other choice, they will not be back. Your overall satisfaction score is 68—your opportunity rests primarily with the 22 who were satisfied with their experience. There were many things about their visits that they liked, so it is easier to focus on improvements that will move your 4s to 5s. Remember, of the 32 who were less than highly satisfied, most will not return to see you whether or not changes are made to improve the experience.

Other questions that are important to include in your survey are, **"How likely are you to return?"** and **"How likely are you to refer (your business) to friends and family?"** These two questions are indicators of loyalty. Because massage is so personal, you will not receive as high scores on the "likely to recommend" question. Some people are just not comfortable talking to others about massage. The importance of these two questions is to compare these scores from the clients who are highly satisfied with those less than highly satisfied. You should see a significant drop in the percentages.

Other questions you can include on your survey pertain to all aspects of the massage. You can include questions on the booking process, knowledge of therapist, pressure level, comfort with the environment, and how the client felt about being asked to return. The most important parts to ask about are the areas that have the most likelihood to decrease satisfaction if not handled correctly. Keep it short and simple and feel free to change questions as time goes on.

Another important feature of satisfaction assessment is **open-ended questions**. Many businesses surveying their customers will only leave a space for general comments. You can go deeper than that, however, and explore the nuances behind their answers by encouraging more specific feedback. Two great open-ended questions are, **"If you marked "highly satisfied" for question 1, please describe what caused you to be so highly satisfied"** and **"If you marked "satisfied" or below for question 1, please tell us what we can do to improve our service."** These pointed questions get to the heart of what is working and what is not (Fig. 10-5). Do not take each individual

Your Massage Company

Anonymous Massage Evaluation Form

Rate you Satisfaction with an (x)	Highly Satisfied	Satisfied	Neutral	Dissatisfied	Highly Dissatisfied
1) Overall satisfaction with the massage experience					
2) Setting the appointment					
3) Therapist was a good listener					
4) Therapist delivered the massage I asked for					
5) Comfort with draping for modesty					
6) Level of pressure used during the massage					
7) Massage started and ended on time					
8) Noise level during the massage					
9) Room the massage was held in					
10) Overall professionalism of the therapist					

If you WERE highly satisfied with this massage experience (#1), please indicate what in particular caused your high level of satisfaction.

If you WERE NOT highly satisfied with your overall experience (#1), please indicate what can be done to improve the massage experience.

POINTERS:

☐ You can build your own evaluation form using this as a template. I recommend using some or all of the questions from above. The first question is the most important.

☐ You are striving for only the highest levels of satisfaction from your clients. Anything less than a five for the first question (Overall Satisfaction) means they might not return to you for another session.

☐ Look for common themes in comments, rather than personalizing individual responses. If you notice that many clients mark you lower on a couple of the questions, then this is where you should focus your energy on improvement.

☐ The open-ended question allows the client to fully express those things that caused high or low levels of satisfaction. Look for themes in this area as well. Be thankful when a client writes for you, because most massage clients will never voice complaint, they simply will not come back.

☐ It is important that this form remain anonymous for the client so they give you authentic answers. Create a way for them to return the form without identifying who is returning it. You can create mailers, online surveys, or simply have a drop box in your waiting room that you review on a weekly basis.

Figure 10–5   This is an example of a satisfaction form that can be used for massage clients. It is an in-depth exploration of the elements of the massage experience.

response and try to make changes; instead, look for trends in responses and make changes accordingly. Also, remember that you will never please everyone, and there are some clients you probably prefer not to work with again.

What Is a Good Score?

Currently, there is not much benchmarking for the massage industry. Usually, the most thorough assessments are done by spas, where massage is often grouped with other services or the massage service has just one assessment question. To give you an idea of other industries, some companies have successfully moved their overall satisfaction scores into the 90% range. This is a great accomplishment for them, especially for companies that serve millions of customers. Reaching a score in the mid or upper 90s is rare, especially for large companies. Higher scores are more attainable for small businesses because they can quickly adapt and make immediate changes.

For your business, focus primarily on improving your experience to raise your scores. You are where you are—whether that is in the 60% or 90% range. The first step is to get an idea about where you are and to seek to improve that top score by moving your satisfied guests to being highly satisfied. If you are above 80% for guests in the highly satisfied area, then you are doing very well. If you have a very high overall satisfaction score and your practice is not full, it is not because you aren't doing a great job, but because the word is not out enough—you need marketing and promotion!

BUILDING LOYALTY BUILDS SUCCESS

There are numerous benefits to be gained by placing a strong focus on earning repeat business not only from a personal standpoint, in the form of self-confidence and the satisfaction of knowing you are helping improve the long-term wellness of your clients, but also economically. Garnering high satisfaction from your clients is the first step toward earning loyalty. When you consistently deliver a superb experience, clients are much more likely to return. Set your bar on the right rung—high satisfaction—and you will be on your way to earning repeat visits.

> Garnering high satisfaction from your clients is the first step toward earning loyalty.

Benefits of Loyalty

There are specific ways you can determine whether your clients are loyal to you. The first measurement is your **rebooking rate**—the percentage of clients who return and ask for you. If you work in a business that tracks this, what they are really tracking is loyalty. They assess this score because they know the importance of return behavior. The really great companies figure out the "secrets" of their high rebooking therapists, and teach other therapists how to do this as well. Some companies offer incentives for return behavior. This encourages employees to figure out what it takes to exceed customers' expectations so that they return. This is a smart move for a company, if handled correctly.

Another strong indicator of loyalty is when you notice clients begin recommending your service to others. This is extremely valuable because a personal referral for a service, especially one as sensitive as massage, establishes instant credibility. The referring clients are putting their stamp of approval on you. Also, these referrals will come in with higher expectations, so it is important to deliver superior service to keep their business and also reflect well on the referring client.

Loyal clients also have a tendency to spend more and upgrade more often. When you have clients who love what you do, they are often the ones most likely to upgrade their service time and try other services you offer. Your most loyal clients are more receptive to purchasing other items from you as well, such as products and gift certificates.

Lifetime Value of a Client

For independent contractors and entrepreneurs, one way to ensure that your focus is always on loyalty is to assess the **lifetime value** of your clients. Lifetime value is how much revenue a client would bring to you during her time as your customer. By placing the focus on what this client means to you long-term, you are encouraged to address problems or spend a little additional money to earn that client's repeat business. For example, although a cashier at McDonald's may see a dissatisfied customer who will not return as only a $4.23 immediate loss, in reality, if that customer never returns, much more is lost—the thousands of dollars he would have spent if he had stayed a customer through his lifetime. For massage business owners, this concept is important because rebooking is vital to business success. So, let us do the math.

Lifetime Value Defined

My loyal client, Susan, visits me on average every other week. She has been coming to me for 2 years and has no intention of stopping anytime soon. During our time together, she has bought gift certificates from me, referred coworkers, and upgraded to longer sessions on occasion. She always tips me at least $10. What is her lifetime value to my business?

$65 x 26 = $1,690	She spends this annually for her massage
$65 x 10 = $650	She buys at least ten gift certificates for special occasions yearly
$15 x 5 = $75	She upgrades to an $80 massage at least five times annually
$65 x 16 = $1,040	She refers at least four people per year, who become loyal and visit at least 4x/year
$10 x 26 = $260	She tips at least $10 per session

Annual Value of Susan = $3,715

Susan remains a client for 6 years, making her lifetime value $22,290.

This is only a basic estimate. It does not capture other referrals who also become loyal and the numerous other people she talks to and who eventually come in even after she is gone. If you were to include these amounts, your most valuable clients would be worth well over $30,000 to your business during their time with you. This is an amount worth keeping in mind as you decide how to interact with your most loyal clients. Imagine Susan has a concern that could be rectified with a gift certificate—isn't that worth saving the potential loss of her as a $30,000 client? If you viewed each client loss as a potential $30,000 walking away, would you do things differently for them?

Now, how many loyal clients would it take for you to feel comfortable with your income? Eight loyal clients like Susan would bring you an annual amount of about $29,720. This would be your base income, and when you add in less loyal clients, you could be making two to three times as much. Acquiring eight loyal clients is very achievable and should be your minimum goal.

> It is much easier, not to mention more economical, to keep clients than to constantly try to attract new ones.

When you start to view each client in this way, it makes it easier to take the extra step to ensure they have a great experience. You can do the math to determine which clients are your most loyal and thus most valuable. It is much easier, not to mention more economical, to keep clients than to constantly try to attract new ones. When faced with big decision about investing in clients, think of this number and make your decision accordingly.

Cost Differences Between New and Return Clients

There is significant difference between the cost of acquiring a new client and the process of encouraging that client to return. Think back to all the ways you can market your practice. Many of these things cost a significant amount of money. Now think about creating an experience designed to encourage loyalty. There might be some initial investment in things designed to completely satisfy your chosen clients, but this is primarily an upfront cost. If you have an unclear strategy and experience, then you will constantly be spending money and energy on trying to get new clients because you are not building a loyal base.

Imagine the bucket in Figure 10-6 is your business. The role of your marketing is to fill the bucket with customers. Once the customers are in the bucket, your business, they will decide whether they will stay in (loyalty) or fall out (nonloyalty). The role of the experience is to deliver on your marketing promises and to plug the bucket, keeping as many customers loyal as possible. It costs as much as seven times more to be constantly marketing and filling the bucket. If the experience is mediocre, holes develop, and the customers leak out. When the experience delivers, the customer stays, and marketing costs are much less. It is up to the people delivering the experience to keep highly satisfied customers coming back. For spas, massage clinics, and therapists responsible for getting their own clients, that means you are responsible for keeping these clients exceptionally satisfied and returning.

THE MASSAGE SERVICE PATH

A **service path** is the journey a consumer takes while engaging with a business that offers something for sale. For massage, it encompasses the moment your potential clients reach out to gather more information about who you are and what you offer. It continues as they arrive for their service and through the session and their departure and may even include some form of follow-up after they are gone. This experiential journey will determine how your clients view your business. Every step of their journey should be viewed with an analytical eye. You must use the proverbial "see what they see" to understand their journey. One fact remains true for all massage clients: even if every step of their journey is blissful, if you have not perfected the art of giving an exceptional massage, you will always be seeking new clients. Also, perfection does not usually depend on how great your technique is. Instead, it lies within the softer subtleties of your greeting, your presence, your communications skills, and your attention to the clients' current state of mind. You can have the best-looking marketing materials and clinic, but if you are not present with your clients, they probably will not be back. As we prepare to travel with a massage client through their journey, be thinking of ways you would take this information and make it useful for the practice you will be building.

> One fact remains true for all massage—even if every step of their journey is blissful, if you have not perfected the art of giving an exceptional massage, you will always be seeking new clients.

Joining Clients on the Spa Massage Service Path

Now, we will travel with clients through their massage journey, exploring crucial **touch points** along the way. Because many of you will at some point be an employee, we will travel with a guest through

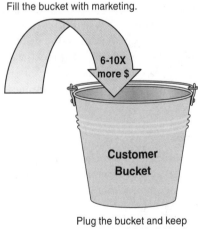

Fill the bucket with marketing.

6-10X more $

Customer Bucket

Plug the bucket and keep your practice full by delivering a flawless experience.

Figure 10–6 Imagine this bucket is your business. You pay money to fill your bucket with clients through your marketing and promotional efforts. When the customers arrive in the bucket (your business), you want to have an experience that keeps them from leaking out of the bottom. When you have built this type experience, your bucket will fill with happy customers. Average experiences result in leaks, and your bucket will never be full.

the spa massage experience. If you are in business for yourself, think of these ideas and how you would apply them to your own massage experience.

A touch point is a critical interaction during the service experience. Within each touch point, you will find ideas for personalizing your service. These particular touch points were selected because they are likely to cause the highest levels of satisfaction when handled expertly. The great news is that most of these ideas will not cost a lot of money because they are primarily behavioral in nature. They are simple techniques that can be learned and taught to others. We will begin our journey with the client contacting a spa to either book an appointment or to solicit more information.

Touch Point 1: First Contact

For massage clinics and spas, **first contact** is any avenue a potential client uses to make contact, usually because they have questions or they are attempting to book an appointment. A good philosophy at this phase is to maintain informative, easy-to-navigate communication between the potential client and the person answering the phone. If you are the person answering the phone, you will quickly acclimate to the most common questions and adapt your answers to fit. If you have employees who are not massage therapists, you should consider spending time listening to their responses and offering guidance on how to answer questions. Many spas have a training book that helps front-desk staff answer questions.

Another method of first contact is through the Internet. Many spas and massage clinics are moving toward online booking. Frequently asked questions (FAQs) should be accessible on the website to assist clients in making the decision to book. After the booking is complete, consider e-mailing the client a professional confirmation response that highlights important details.

Treat New Guests Differently When They Contact You

When an inquiry comes in from a newer client, consider using language that specifically alleviates some of the "newbie fears." The top fears of spa guests are in the areas of nudity, tipping, communicating complaints, and transitions. Making an effort to alleviate these concerns in subtle ways will pay off by increasing satisfaction scores. You would never greet a guest by saying you are happy to take their tips. Instead, recognize there is confusion around this and make it easy for them to figure it out for themselves. Some ideas to consider are having written materials, e-mails, graphics, or mailers that help communicate this for you. Have content focused on important information, process explanation, and fear alleviation. If your booking system allows, enter any relevant notes when the guest checks in so that you can reference the conversation later.

Knowledgeable Responses

Another important way to ensure a great first contact is by having a knowledgeable person answer the phone and smoothly navigate any questions. This initial conversation often determines whether the guest books or not. Consider having these employees attend service and product training, and even experience the treatments themselves, so that they acquire a high level of knowledge for all aspects of the business. Keep a service binder with detailed descriptions of the treatments near the phone. If the person answering the phone is not familiar with the types of modalities offered and the therapists that excel in certain areas, then the guests are being set up for disappointment even before they arrive. Many companies find creative ways to continually educate their frontline staff about their products and services. If you are the only person answering the phone for clients, take note of any questions you were not able to answer and find answers to these questions for future use. During slow times, encourage your practitioners to spend time with the front-desk people, answering their questions and educating them about services.

Provide Smooth Access

Another opportunity area lies in how your guests make purchases. You must make it easy to buy your services. This sounds like such a simple concept, but many companies make purchasing very difficult for potential customers. Think of a time when you were trying to book something and were put on extended hold because the front desk was busy, or you were purchasing something online and the site malfunctioned halfway through the process. These are experiential issues you want to avoid. If your front-desk person cannot navigate check-ins, check-outs, phone calls, and technician transitions, consider increasing staff or using a call service to assist during busy times. Some spas have all their calls managed by a call center, freeing their front-desk staff to perfect the art of personal interaction. This first or last contact can have immense repercussions on satisfaction if things are not running smoothly. If you are the only person answering the phone for your massage business, then simply pay attention to any areas for concern on the potential client's behalf. For example, if you are not always available to take calls because you are giving sessions, you may be losing valuable revenue.

Your "First Contact" Mantra

See Worksheet 10-1

Your mantra for the first contact phase should be something like, "I am professional, I make it easy for my clients to book an appointment, and I have educated answers for their questions." When you can deliver this, then your guests are ready to transition to the next phase of the service path.

Touch Point 2: Ready or Not, Here They Come

The decision to visit your business has gone smoothly. Your guest booked easily; all questions were answered efficiently; and she received an e-mail containing information on draping, tipping, and what to expect during the visit, alleviating some concerns she had about her first, upcoming massage experience. Your guest prepares for her visit and arrives with high expectations. What is waiting for her? What will her first impression be? It will be a lasting impression, so pay attention to everything she will see and do.

It is up to you whether the experience creates a loyal guest or something less. If it is less, you may never see this guest again, and she will probably not tell you why. Spa-goers say they are looking for confident employees and a smooth, informative intake. The first face-to-face interaction sets the tone for the rest of the visit.

Recognize Returning Guests

Returning clients are gold mines for businesses. Find ways to recognize and express your appreciation for return behavior. For spas, train your staff to thank clients for returning, demonstrating that they recognize their value. You receive bonus points if the receptionist discusses their previous visits and treatments. Everyone likes to be remembered and valued. Massage therapists in private practice have an even greater opportunity to remember clients and their treatments, letting them know that they recognize their value and appreciate their business. Find creative, inexpensive ways to reward loyal clients.

Use Kid Gloves for New Guests

If a new guest is checking in, take special care to ensure he is comfortable with all aspects of his visit. Also consider putting a new guest process in place. This can include escorted transitions, a thorough explanation of processes, and an active way to identify areas of unease. To alleviate confusion about tipping, you can have subtle ways to communicate whether or not you accept tips. Your draping policy can be clearly outlined in a welcome kit. Use pictures to show what professional draping looks like. This will go a long way in reducing any anxiety he might experience about undressing.

Your "Ready or Not Here They Come" Mantra

See Worksheet 10-2

Your mantra for the second contact phase should be something like, "I will welcome you when you arrive. Everything you see and experience will match what you expected. If you are new, I will make an extra effort to ensure you feel safe and comfortable. If you are returning, you will know I appreciate you." When you can deliver this, your clients are ready to transition to the next phase of the service path.

Touch Point 3: Managing Wait Time and Transitions

Spa-goers and massage clients can have a high level of discomfort with waiting and transitioning between services. These are the moments when guests are left to their own devices waiting for their service, transferring between services, or trying to figure out where to go for what. These apprehensions can be managed by trained employees who recognize that the discomfort is usually a result of insecurity about what comes next. There are some specific tactics you can implement to increase comfort during waits and transitions.

Guide Transfers

Never just point guests in the direction they should go. Find ways to ensure they are clear on where to go, what their options are while they are there, and what comes next. Be specific so that they do not feel unsure or abandoned as time passes. Use caution with loyal guests because they can become irritated if you overexplain to them. Build systems to help your employees determine what level of explanation is needed for each client. It is recommended that you walk with guests for part of their journey so that they are not nervous about going to the wrong place or not being where they are supposed to be.

Sell Products Carefully

Eighty-five percent of guests report being uncomfortable with sales tactics. Selling a $50 product is not worth changing a highly satisfied customer to being just satisfied because an employee tried to hard-sell the product of the week. The International SPA Association (ISPA) 2006 Consumer Report[1] discusses this dynamic in detail. Two product categories identified in the report that spa-goers preferred were (1): products that continue the "most distinctly well done service experiences" and (2) products that "re-create spa ambiance at home."

If you do sell, guests prefer to hear about unique, customized recommendations from the therapist working with them. Remember that they are seeking relief from something—making them feel pressured to buy can ruin an experience. For massage therapists, this means staying focused on the products you truly believe are beneficial to your clients. Pain relief creams, soaks, skin emollients, and aromatherapy are examples of products you might be comfortable in recommending. If you can relate the product to the therapy you are providing to the client, then it comes across less as a sale and more as a wellness aid.

Your "Wait Time and Transition" Mantra

See Worksheet 10-3

Your mantra for the third contact phase should be something like, "I will take care of you even when you are in the waiting room. I will ensure you know exactly what is coming next on your journey with me. I will pay attention to your actions and respond when I think you need help." When you can deliver this, then your clients are ready to transition to the next phase of the service path.

Touch Point 4: Warm Welcome

Guests have now passed through the first phase of their experience. They have actively selected your business, decided which services they would like, and navigated the earliest phases of arrival and waiting. This guest has decided to have a massage, so we will transition her into the care of the caregiver. As the guest moves from process to relaxation, an optimal environment would ensure consistent experiences while allowing service providers the creativity to adapt to the client's changing needs.

A warm, professional greeting from their therapist will set the tone for the middle phase of their journey.

The majority of spa-goers begin to feel "settled in" during the earliest stages of their treatments. A warm, professional greeting from their therapist will set the tone for the middle phase of their journey. The few seconds it takes to make a first impression will affect the rest of their journey, especially for new guests. Guests want to feel like a name, not like a number on your docket today.

Use an Authentic Greeting

So, how do we ensure that the rest of their journey brings them what they were hoping for? It begins the moment you open the door to the waiting room and introduce yourself. The greeting should be authentic and include an introduction using the guest's name, a handshake, eye contact, and a smile. Body language communicates even more strongly than words (Fig. 10-7). Imagine you are an apprehensive guest sitting in the waiting room. Your therapist walks in, gives a limp handshake, does not make eye contact with you, and simply says, "Follow me, please." Although there is nothing glaringly wrong with this, it can be so much better and authentic if each client is purposely viewed as an individual by a therapist who is present with each person. Consciously use these few seconds to set the tone of how you will care for the guest once she is in the treatment room.

Employ Unconditional Positive Regard

Unconditional positive regard (UPR), a term coined by the humanist Carl Rogers, is blanket acceptance and support of a person regardless of what the person says or does. For the therapists walking into the waiting room, the suspense of who is waiting for them can be just as uncertain as it is for the guest. It is important for practitioners to suspend any judgments based on who they see sitting there. UCP means accepting each person as whole and complete and seeing that person in a positive light, despite personality challenges.

Modeling this positive regard will create a climate of acceptance and belonging throughout the spa. Growth is nurtured through acceptance. This concept can be hard to keep in place. Imagine you are walking in to greet your client, and something about the person pushes your buttons. Old perception filters emerge, and if you are not careful, you may begin to treat this person differently based on whom they seem to be. If the client is in any way threatening beyond just your personal perception, then take precautions as necessary.

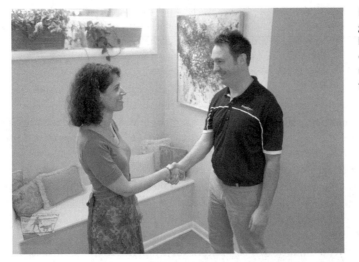

Figure 10–7   An authentic greeting will help your clients begin to have a great experience. Make eye contact, smile, use their name, and make them feel welcome.

Your "Warm Welcome" Mantra

See Worksheet 10-4

Your mantra for the fourth contact phase should be something like, "I will make sure that within your first few moments of meeting me, you will feel welcome and seen. My demeanor will help you begin to relax, and you can begin to anticipate the work we will do together." When you can deliver this, then the clients are ready to transition to the next phase of the service path.

Touch Point 5: Professional Intakes

Conducting a professional intake has several benefits. It allows you to go through any concerns you need to address with the client while establishing yourself as an expert. As you learn to improve your intake process, know that you will face challenges. If you work for a busy massage clinic, you might face time constraints. Also, know that the guests are highly attuned to the amount of time you spend with them, and they pay attention to the time before they get on the table as well. You can create a smooth process to effectively gather the information you need to deliver an exceptional massage. You most likely will use the few minutes available to discuss expectations, identify health concerns, alleviate nervousness, and get agreement on the treatment. Establishing these boundaries early will provide the structure the guests seek so that they can relax, knowing exactly what to expect. In general, spa-goers appreciate therapists who verbally disclose the structure of the treatment. Guests will be much more inhibited if they feel unsure about nudity, draping, and pressure levels. Knowing that 80% of communication is nonverbal, a perceptive therapist customizes services based on unspoken cues as well.

Recognize That Nudity Is a Top Concern

After you have discussed any pertinent medical information, you can use the time allotted for the intake to clearly explain the procedure of getting undressed and on the table. Let them know they can undress to their comfort level. Clearly communicate that their modesty will be maintained with proper draping. You can communicate this by saying that in your experience about half of clients choose to completely undress and about half choose to leave their underwear on. Let them know that either way is fine and that they will be honored at all times. This allows them to comfortably fit with a sizeable percentage regardless of what they choose.

There are varying beliefs on level of draping. If unsure, err on the side of caution and make the effort to improve your draping skills. A drape is a boundary that should not be crossed and often is a legal requirement. Think twice before allowing your hands to go underneath a drape, even if is an area you feel is safe. It is not your perception that matters—it is the guest's.

Mirroring to Clarify Expectations

Another way to increase guests' satisfaction is to deliver the massage they were expecting. That sounds easy, but you may be surprised how many complain of not receiving what they came for. During the intake, you have a great opportunity to communicate understanding of what they are seeking. There is a simple technique you can use that allows clients to recognize that they have been heard and that you plan to deliver what they are seeking. This technique is called **mirroring**.

Step 1: Listen

During the intake, ask the guest what type massage she would like to receive. Specifically ask if there are any areas of the body the guest would like addressed or avoided. Listen to what they are asking. *Example:* I would like a full body massage. My neck has been hurting lately, and if it is fine with you, I would like some extra time spent on my feet.

Step 2: Mirror Back

After the client identifies what she is seeking, mirror this back to her so that she knows her concerns were heard. *Example:* So, you would like to have a full body massage, some work that will specifically alleviate the tension you feel in your neck, and extra attention and time for your feet. Is that correct? The client will either agree or clarify further.

Step 3: Get Agreement

Once you have mirrored correctly, you will get agreement from your client. *Example:* Yes, that is exactly what I am looking for. If you did not get it right, this is your opportunity to further explore the client's needs and make another attempt to get agreement before you begin the work.

Step 4: Deliver

Now you must deliver what the client has asked for. It is vitally important to deliver what the guests are requesting—not what you think they need. Although therapists may make suggestions, ultimately guests will be dissatisfied if they do not receive what they perceived they would.

Solicit Input

While the guests are still dressed, let them know you will be tracking their responses to pressure, room temperature, and comfort during the treatment. This will allow them to process this when they are less vulnerable. Invite them to give feedback on anything that would make their experience better. When inquiring about therapeutic pressure levels during a Swedish massage, use the terms "light," "medium," or "firm." Avoid using the term "deep" when referring to pressure unless the treatment is named deep-tissue massage.

Your "Professional Intake" Mantra

See Worksheet 10-5

Your mantra for the fifth contact phase should be something like, "I will educate you on the undressing policy and make you comfortable with your decision. I will listen for why you are here and what is going on with your body. I will paraphrase this back to you so that you know I listened and understood what you said." When you can deliver this, then your guests are ready to transition to the next phase of the service path.

Touch Point 6: The Therapeutic Bubble

The **therapeutic bubble** is an analogy for the atmosphere created by therapists to encompass themselves in a safe, healing environment with each client. A healing relationship is special. As we have touched on in previous chapters, it involves presence, unconditional positive regard, and treating each client as a unique person with specific needs. The therapeutic bubble is the place where these qualities come to life; it is the protective circle surrounding the moments of interaction between the therapist and the person on the table receiving the work. Just two people are contained within: the therapist, who is helping the recipient receive what she has come in for, and recipient, who is able to go to the place she was seeking. It is during these moments of interaction that the success of the entire industry rests. It is in these moments that miracles can happen—miracles the therapist might never see. They can manifest at the guests' home as they demonstrate more patience with their children, or perhaps the guests can move in a way they haven't been able to for some time. It is also in these moments that disaster can strike, and missteps can lead to someone never seeking the therapeutic benefits of massage ever again.

Much is at stake during this part of the journey. There is an obvious power differential during this phase. What other business asks customers to take their clothes off, lay face down, and allow a total stranger to touch their body? The experience a therapist should create is: "I am your guide on this journey, you are safe, and I will seek to deliver what you are looking for." Establishing rapport guides the guest's nervous system toward a resting place and away from the fight-or-flight state. The sense of "being transported" is one of the most alluring features of the massage experience. If a guest does not feel safe and comfortable, the sympathetic nervous system (fight or flight) will inhibit the relaxation response, resulting in lower satisfaction and less wellness benefit.

Do No Harm

The ISPA conducted extensive research to understand what motivates people to visit spas and discovered that for all spa types, fully half of guests are seeking to reduce stress. With stress reduction as a key motivator, it is imperative that the spa and massage experience avoid inducing additional stress. Harm can be imposed in many ways, the most obvious being to cause pain during the massage. Even the most experienced massage client may have difficulty finding her voice and asking you to lighten up. Sometimes just asking, "How's that pressure?" is not enough. An easy way to get your guests to provide guidance is to check in on pressure the first time using this method— "Would you like me to stay here, apply more pressure, or go lighter?" This simple question prompts them to give you exact guidance instead of mumbling that everything is fine.

There are more subtle ways therapists can impose pain on their guests. One common way is to talk unnecessarily during the massage. There have been many dissatisfied clients who reported they couldn't relax because the therapist kept talking. Also, not following the agreement made in the intake can impose pain on others, and the guests may leave feeling like they have been misled. Not focusing your attention on a client is another subtle way of imposing pain on others.

The Power of Presence

Presence is a state of mind, free from distraction and practiced through mindfulness. **Mindfulness** fosters the attitude of living in the moment and enjoying each guest in an unhurried, relaxed state as the guest enjoys each service in a relaxed state. Spa-goers crave a structured service flow managed by authentic personnel who make them feel like individuals worthy of time and attention. This is especially true for first-time guests, who may feel out of place in the spa habitat. Distracted therapists can make guests feels as if staff is simply going through the motions. Presence speaks loudly: "My focus is here with you right now."

The modern spa requires "spa stamina," which is achieved when energy remains steady throughout the day. To maintain your energy, consider establishing a quiet area to regroup and become present as needed during the day. To start each session, take a moment to become grounded and consider beginning a stretching regimen. These few moments can center and prepare you for the sessions ahead. Infusing your environment with the practice of mindfulness (present-centered attention) is a powerful way to have a lasting, positive impact on guests and coworkers.

When a group of massage recipients are asked, "How many of you have had a massage when the therapist wasn't really there with you?" most will raise their hand. It is difficult to stay fully engaged with each client. Your mind will tend to wander. You might start thinking about what to do for dinner, where your kids are, or any number of distracting things. This is normal, but when you find yourself doing this, know that the person beneath your hands is sensitive and may be picking up on your lack of focus. Gently bring yourself back to the therapeutic bubble you have created, to ensure that you maintain presence with each client.

Communicate

Finding the right amount and type of communication during the massage session is sometimes difficult. Some guests talk during the whole session, whereas others seem not to want to talk at all. By paying attention to verbal and nonverbal clues, you can pick up on what they seem to need in the moment. If you do find yourself communicating, aim your words at improving their experience. For example, educate them about the work, tell them what you are seeing in their body, or check in on their comfort. Avoid discussing your personal life. Because many guests are uncomfortable with voicing their concerns, therapists must sharpen their intuitive and communication skills to ensure guest satisfaction.

Your "Therapeutic Bubble" Mantra

See Worksheet 10-6

Your mantra for the sixth contact phase should be something like, "I understand you are seeking some form of relief. I will conduct myself in a way that helps guide you toward the relief you are seeking in this moment. I will remember that working with you is safer than working on you. I will ensure that I am not causing you any pain or discomfort." When you can deliver this, then your guests are ready to transition to the next phase of the service path.

Touch Point 7: Educate at Timely Stages of the Interaction

Information is empowering! Part of being in a therapeutic environment with clients is discerning how to communicate information in a way they understand. It is important to find ways to offer insights that your guests are open to. Most people seeking relief are interested in what the contributing factors are, what they can do to make improvements, and what you recommend for them going forward. For example, imagine that you were experiencing nausea and headaches on a regular basis and you sought out a doctor to help you. She will more than likely ask you questions about your habits and symptoms, discuss what may be causing your issues, and prescribe some sort of further work or medication. Often, she will ask that you come back to see her within a certain period of time. You would be highly disappointed if she communicated nothing and only gave you a prescription. The most successful therapists understand the importance of educating their clients at timely stages. Education is vital and becomes a precursor to recommending that they come back for more work.

Peer Profile 10-1

Tara Thompson, LMT
Omaha, Nebraska

Value of Teaching

I've been in practice as an LMT for 5 years. I feel my decision to become a massage educator has been the most instrumental in helping me achieve success as a therapist. Early on, I was lucky enough to be asked by someone while I was in massage school to assist in continuing education. I'm also an instructor at a massage school, and both experiences have helped me with confidence as a therapist and in perfecting my techniques. Educating others has helped me stay mindful and aware of the ever-changing and evolving field. Also, getting involved in teaching so early in my own career pushed me to a level that I may not have experienced otherwise. I consider myself extremely blessed and grateful to have had the opportunities I have.

My experience as an instructor has helped me tremendously in being professional and educating my clients. Taking the time to explain to my clients why I'm doing the techniques I'm doing and what I think is the best "plan of action" has kept my practice full. Educating clients on the benefits and importance of massage has helped tremendously with my rebooking rate and keeping clients on a maintenance plan. I've found that my passion for education in general helps with client loyalty because it gives clients more value out of a session. My advice to other therapists is to not be afraid to pull out resources and show your clients how you came to the specifics of their session. When dealing with a client and addressing conditions, whether chronic or acute, you need to show results to build loyalty. Once you can do that, your client will shout it from the mountain tops. They will stay with you and want to tell everyone they know about it! Build short-term loyalty by showing results, and this will turn into a long-term loyalty.

It's easier to entice past clientele to come back than to find all new clients. Checking in with your clients by phone, e-mail, mail, or text is very important to sustaining a strong practice. Clients love that you are thinking of them and care about their well-being. I know that honesty, education, suggestion, and loyalty (my loyalty to my clients) are required for my success in my practice.

Collecting and using client recommendations can be useful too. Here's an example of what one client had to say about my practice. I use these type quotes (with their signed permission) on my website and in my marketing materials. "I highly recommend Tara for massage work. From the first visit it was obvious Tara has a lot of knowledge and skill; she is also very professional before, during, and after every single visit, doing justice to her profession! I am currently going to her for intensive work on a running-related injury (IT band) and trust her recommendations completely. Thanks, Tara!" —Heather

Word-of-mouth is my best advertising. If you treat your clients with respect and as a name and not a number, you will gain respect and positive feedback. Karma is another great way to trust in your practice. I wish you the best of luck as you seek to build a loyal base of happy clients.

Educate During the Intake

Depending on the setting in which you work and the level of connection you have established with a client, the intake provides you with the opportunity to begin the education process. This sort of education is in addition to the necessary questions such as those regarding contraindications, medications, and injuries. It could include information about applied pressure levels, the importance of secure draping to feel comfortable on a massage table, the approach of your particular modality, or the human autonomic nervous system (fight or flight versus rest and digest). Attempt to keep the information in small, digestible pieces. Take into account how much experience a client may have in receiving massage. Using time wisely is important so that the client does not feel as though time is being taken away from the hands-on portion of the session. Having said that, some of the most powerful learning a client can experience in a therapeutic massage session can actually take place off the table.

For example, a new client coming to you for a relaxation massage may comment about how stress is having dramatic effects on his life. A skilled therapist may take an opportunity to explain the parasympathetic nervous system (rest and digest) and how regular massage can reduce stress levels and the amount of sympathetic (fight or flight) stimulation he is receiving. With this understanding, the client may choose to not only receive regular massage but also look for other ways to bring parasympathetic stimulation into his life through methods like yoga, meditation, and active relaxation techniques.

Educate During the Session

The hands-on portion of a massage provides countless opportunities for education. Depending on the intention for the session and the client's availability to engage in conversation, it is best to keep the dialogue focused. This sort of education could include explanation of musculature, connective tissue, trigger points, and agonist/antagonist muscle relationships. Clients will be curious about what is going on in their body and will look to you for professional insight.

For example, a client may state during the intake that she has no specific physical aches or pains. However, after you contact her mid-back/rhomboid muscles on the table, she begins to complain of sensitivity and referral pain to her ribcage. You may ask her permission to spend a few minutes explaining the relation of trigger points to referred pain. Palpating the area during the education will give the client a "felt sense" understanding that she may not have had if you were merely explaining the concept in conversation.

Educate at Departure

As clients depart a massage, there is an opportunity to obtain and share more information. This may require you to invite them to give you a minute to check in with them, as opposed to them rushing back out into their lives. The departure is all too often a missed opportunity for therapists. It can be used as so much more than, "Please remember to drink a lot of water and here is one of my cards. It was a pleasure to work with you and please call me if I can help you again."

Contrast that with: "Let's take a moment to have you stand up and test the range of motion in your arm again. What do you notice as you move your arm around? Has anything changed from before the session began? Please remember that as I described in the session, your connective tissue begins to gel when you sit for long periods behind your desk. Here is one simple stretch I would like you to try. I would invite you return again in a week for a follow-up session to build on the work we did today. Would you be open to me following up with you in a few days to see how you are feeling?"

Which therapist would seem more knowledgeable to you? With which one might you develop a deeper sense of trust? As with any other health-care provider, clients are looking to you to provide them with a professional recommendation about when to return and what potential benefits may come from an investment of their time and money.

Remember that it is always appropriate, at any stage of a session, to ask permission from the client to take some time to explain beneficial information. It may seem to be a simple question: "Would you be interested in taking 5 minutes at the start of the session so that I can explain what connective tissue is and how the myofascial massage approach I use will address your specific needs?" When you ask permission, the clients have the power to make their own choice.

Your "Educate at Timely Stages" Mantra

See Worksheet 10-7

Your mantra for the seventh contact phase should be something like, "I will seek to find the right moments to offer you education on your specific needs. I will keep this information highly inform-ative and present it in a way you understand." When you can deliver this, then your clients are ready to transition to the next phase of the service path.

Touch Point 8: Do Sweat the Smaller Things

It is so easy to ruin an experience if you do not pay attention to annoying little details. Think about some recent experience when small details got under your skin—the restaurant table that wobbled, the clear plastic case that was impossible to open, or the soda machine that would not take your dollar bill. These all are small things, but all have the potential to distract from the experience sought. For massage therapists, these annoying details are often seen as not that important. However, paying attention to every detail of the environment, from the lighting to the music, from the temperature to the smells, will ensure a better chance of allowing your clients the experience they are seeking. Also, the higher price that you charge for a massage, the higher will be the guests' expectations for a pristine experience. Any aspect that proves incongruent runs a risk of degrading the overall view of the experience.

See What They See

Therapists should occasionally run a "shoes and cobwebs" check. Take a few moments and lay on the massage table. Lie face down and notice what you see. This is what your clients see when they are on the table. A dirty floor or carpet will not be pleasant to stare at for 30 minutes. Look closely at the shoes you wear during the massage. What are they communicating to your guests? If they are dirty and unkempt, this communicates something less than positive. Many spas have shoe requirements for this reason. Also, take the time to lie facing the ceiling. Is it clean and free of cobwebs, or is it cracked and dirty? This communicates with the guest about the cleanliness and health of the business they are visiting. We get very accustomed to our environment, which is why it is good to occasionally scan your treatment room with a critical eye. Verify that your product bottles, decorations, and fur-niture are clean and look professional. Your intent is to promote and encourage healing. It is worth the extra time and expense to create an atmosphere that allows healing to happen.

Hear What They Hear

It may be impossible to create a noise-free zone, but it is ideal. You do not have control over construction, neighbors, or traffic. But you can exercise caution with the things within your control. Music should be an enhancement to the experience—something that resides in the background, helping soothe guests while they are on their journey. If the guests seek relaxation, stimulating music would be incongruent. The process of letting the mind go can be hindered by certain sounds. It is recommended that you have music free of lyrics because the human mind tends to try to follow words. Choose music that matches the type of work you are doing. If it is highly engaging, therapeutic work, you can choose stronger music that will not detract from the work you are doing. Make efforts to minimize hallway noises by placing signs that encourage silence. A quiet environment helps guests relax into their experience.

Guarantee Functionality

When things break, it is sometimes inconvenient and costly to replace them. For a customer seeking relaxation and relief, these small malfunctions can result in their inability to achieve what they came for. For massage therapists, these problems usually happen with equipment such as table warmers, face cradles, electric tables, product pumps, and lighting. It is recommended that you regularly perform checks to ensure they are all in proper working order. A damaged or misaligned face cradle is rarely something guests will complain about, yet it can ruin their ability to rest their head properly during the treatment (Fig. 10-8).

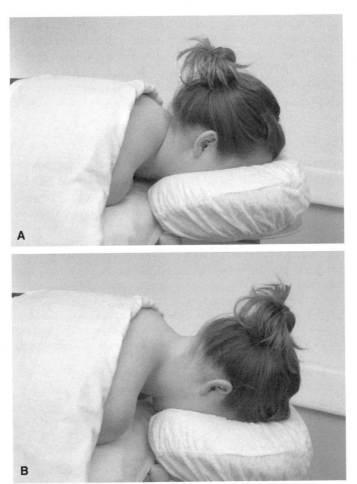

Figure 10–8   (A) Improper neck angle can ruin an entire session for a client. **(B)** Ensure the neck cradle allows the next to slightly relax at a downward angle.

Your "Sweating the Smaller Things" Mantra

See Worksheet 10-8

Your mantra for the eighth contact phase should be something like, "I will minimize things within your environment that might discourage you from relaxing. I promise all things will be in good working order and that you will have a pleasant view, no matter which way you are facing." When you can deliver this, then your guests are ready to transition to the next phase of the service path.

Touch Point 9: Professional Recommendations

At this stage, things can break down for many therapists. When it comes to confidently recommending a client to return, many defer their power to the clients and let them decide when it is time to come back. When asked about this, many therapists admit that they feel like they are selling something. Often, too, they feel a simple lack of confidence in their training or skill. Imagine what would happen if the mindset of all massage therapists could shift to a paradigm of, "This service is so beneficial for you, I would be causing harm by not recommending that you come back." Not only would we see a lot healthier society receiving regular massage, but there would also be far more successful massage therapists. So, how do you become comfortable with encouraging repeat visits?

Using Research to Build Your Confidence

During the past decade, the expansion of available research has brought a higher level of credibility to massage therapy. Staying current with recent findings helps you to communicate effectively and ethically with clients. There is much information on the benefits of massage for stress, headaches, muscular issues, and even some diseases. Staying familiar with these findings helps you confidently make recommendations to clients who are exhibiting the concerns you have read about. With this knowledge, you can communicate directly to your clients about the issues they are experiencing and be able to recommend their revisits using facts as validation. It is also recommended that you have some common findings typed up into a professional document, with the sources cited. You can use these as handouts for clients who are experiencing similar problems. This takes the pressure off of you to make recommendation based on what you "think."

Box 10-1. Study: Massage Helps Treat Low Back Pain

Massage may be serious medicine, at least when it comes to treating persistent low back pain, a new study shows. Low back pain is one of the top reasons people seek medical attention in the United States, and it is notoriously tough to treat.

The new study randomly assigned 400 adults with moderate-to-severe low back pain lasting for at least 3 months to weekly whole-body massages for relaxation, weekly massages that focused on specific muscle problems around the lower back and hips, or usual care.

People assigned to the usual care group were tracked by researchers, but they dealt with their back problems on their own. The approach could include, for instance, taking pain medications or muscle relaxants, seeing doctors or chiropractors, having physical therapy, or simply not doing anything.

After 10 weeks, participants in both massage groups reported greater average improvements in pain and functioning compared with those in the usual care group. And the type of massage they received didn't seem to matter.

Daily functioning, for example, improved, on average, between 2 and 4 points on a 23-point scale. Average pain improved about 2 points on a 10-point scale.

But for a substantial minority, however, the improvements were much greater.

At the end of the 10-week intervention, 36% and 39% of patients in the massage groups said their pain was nearly or completely gone, compared with 4% in the usual care group.

The study was funded by the National Center for Complementary and Alternative Medicine. It's published in the *Annals of Internal Medicine*.

Modified excerpt from article published on *WebMD Health News*.

10-2: Find It on the Web

These sources are available for you to research and stay current with the benefits of massage.

- **American Massage Therapy Association:** *Research Citations on the Efficacy of Massage.* This is a sample of research on the efficacy of massage, which was developed in 2001. http://www. amtamassage.org/infocenter/research02.html
- **Associated Bodywork and Massage Professionals:** *Massage Therapy Fact Sheet.* This brief listing of research on the benefits of massage was published in 2009. http://www.massagetherapy. com/_content/images/Media/Factsheet1.pdf
- ***International Journal of Therapeutic Massage and Bodywork: Research, Education, and Practice*** (IJTMB). This online journal is an open-access, peer-reviewed publication intended to accommodate the diverse needs of the rapidly expanding therapeutic massage and bodywork community. http://www.ijtmb.org
- **Massage Therapy Foundation:** Massage Therapy Research Database. This database contains more than 4,800 records, including both indexed and nonindexed journal citations. http://www. massagetherapyfoundation.org/researchdb.html
- **Mayo Clinic:** The mission is to empower people to manage their health. It is accomplished by providing useful and up-to-date information and tools that reflect the expertise and standard of excellence of Mayo Clinic. http://www.mayoclinic.com/health/massage/ SA00082
- **Touch Research Institute at the University of Miami School of Medicine:** The Touch Research Institute has conducted more than 100 studies on the positive effects of massage therapy on many functions and medical conditions in many different age groups. http://www6. miami.edu/touch-research/Research.html

---

Filling Your Practice With Treatment Planning

A three-session massage treatment (see Fig. 8-5) plan has many advantages over a one-session "wait and see how you feel before you book another" approach. In a three-session series:

- Clients can see cumulative results because of a realistic time-line and strategy.
- Client and therapist have a proper window of time to establish safety and trust (rapport), which is vital in any healing relationship.
- Reinforcing good behaviors within a 3-week period leads to a higher likelihood of creating habits. Establishing a new habit takes about 21 days.
- Clients stay focused on the expectation of feeling better, increasing a potential placebo effect.
- Studies have shown that written goals have a tremendous rate of success.

In addition, individual therapists and spas increase revenue in a way that does not cost money!

Your "Professional Recommendations" Mantra

See Worksheet 10-9

Your mantra for the ninth contact phase should be something like, "I recognize that massage is extremely beneficial for you. I will customize a recommendation based on your unique needs and confidently explain when and why you should return to see me." When you can deliver this, your clients are ready to transition to the next phase of the service path.

Touch Point 10: Gone, but Not Forgotten

The experience for guests does not end after they pay their bill and head back to their hectic lives. There are many ways to continue the positive feelings while encouraging loyalty.

(Continued on page 371)

Peer Profile 10-2

Eric Stephenson, LMT, NCTMB
Director of Education for imassage, Inc.*

Fill Your Practice With Treatment Planning

We are at a perplexing intersection in the evolution of massage therapy in America. More people than ever are experiencing massage, research is validating its benefits, and it is slowly being integrated into our healthcare system. Simultaneously, with the economy limping along, people are finding it increasingly difficult to pay out of pocket for preventative healthcare.

This conundrum has many therapists searching for ways to attract and retain clients in an effort to stay in practice. Treatment planning could be an answer.

Treatment planning is a win/win for client and therapist. In practical terms, the goal is to keep clients healthy and our practices thriving. By engaging and empowering clients within a structured format, therapists have the potential to increase therapeutic results while simultaneously building a sustainable practice.

The concept of a multi-session treatment plan approach is nothing new in the medical field. However, from my observations, it is not widely practiced in our profession. Almost without exception, mainstream and complementary healthcare providers give clients specific instructions about rebooking and treatment options. Clients want to know when and why they should return. We will explore an approach for massage therapists that provides simple guidelines for our profession.

My intention is to provide a simple template for:

■ working with a new or existing client for three sessions within a three-week period, and
■ establishing a monthly maintenance schedule thereafter.

This is not an exploration of the various techniques that are part of assessment (active and passive range of motion testing, muscle testing, standing assessment, etc.). Also note that a treatment plan is not a substitute for, but rather is used in conjunction with a full client health history form with SOAP noting.

Return on Investment

The two biggest reasons clients give for not receiving regular massage are time and money. The three-session series educates a client about the positive cumulative health effects of scheduling massages closely together and then following an ensuing maintenance plan. The theory is that if properly educated, many clients are willing to invest the time and cost for three sessions, especially if the investment results in a noticeable improvement in their presenting condition.

This approach may be applied with any modality. In my practice, it works especially well with a sub-acute or chronic problem using various Deep Tissue methods. Applying heat and pressure to connective tissue activates the thixotropic and piezoelectric qualities of fascia. More frequent sessions increase the range, ease, and quality of motion, hydration of muscle tissue/fascia, and overall parasympathetic tone. By agitating tissue continually within a short period, habitual distortion patterns have less chance of setting in between sessions.

Printed originally in the September 2009 issue of *Massage Magazine*.
*A continuing education and consulting company dedicated to helping massage therapists extend their careers. See http://www.imassageinc.com

A three-session treatment plan has many advantages over a one-session "wait and see how you feel before you book another" approach. In a three-session series:

- Clients can see cumulative results due to a realistic time-line and strategy.
- Client and therapist have a proper window of time to establish safety and trust (rapport) that is paramount in any healing relationship.
- When client sessions and simple homework are reinforced within a three-week period, it is much more likely to become a habit. Establishing a new habit requires approximately 21 days.
- Clients stay focused on the expectation of feeling better, increasing a potential placebo effect.
- Studies have shown that written goals have a tremendous rate of success.

This all sounds good in theory, but how do we confidently integrate this approach into our practice?

Selling vs. Sharing

Many therapists are uncomfortable with the idea of proactively selling their services. In conversations with therapists across the country, a common question is how to recommend regular visits without feeling like a salesperson. I believe a large part of the answer is a paradigm shift away from the idea of selling toward one of sharing our gifts with a world in need.

When working with a team of therapists to refine this skill, I invite them to recognize their gifts, offer them in good faith, and detach emotionally from the client's choice. As humans, relatively few of us do well with rejection. However, when therapists view a treatment plan as a preventative measure that will benefit clients rather than a service that is being "sold," the therapist feels empowered. We offer our gifts to the world, and the world decides if it needs what we have to offer. In the words of author, Andrea Adler: "When we come from a place of love, of service, people will never have the impression that we are selling them a bill of goods that they don't want."

Engage and Empower

Belief inspires hope. Hope begins with the therapist's attitude and beliefs about the efficacy of massage therapy. Does your verbal/non-verbal communication express hope? Clients are looking for inspiration and the chance they may find relief through massage therapy.

Tracey Moon, Massage Program Director at Duke Integrative Medicine on belief and hope: "If we can skillfully do this, I believe we can change the world. Really! Clients come in all the time with limiting beliefs due to their 'DNA,' an old injury that they will 'have to live with,' a knee that the 'doctor said would not be able to run again.' How can we honor their beliefs and offer hope, inspiration to a new way of thinking with ease and kindness?"

After communicating a hopeful message to clients, we then seek to educate them. Information is empowering and involves the client in their healing process. Asking permission to take 10 minutes of the first session to speak about the approach of your particular modality and the structure of the three-session format establishes your expertise. Remember to keep it simple, though. Find simple terminology to explain complicated anatomical and physiological concepts, and reinforce the concepts with visual aids such as reference books and wall charts.

Strengths and Resources

In a therapeutic model, it is all too easy to continually focus on what is wrong. While most people are looking for some kind of relief from a presenting condition, don't let that be your immediate focus. Instead, step back and ask your client, "What is working well with your overall health, and where do you feel strong in your body?" At first, most clients may find this surprising and possibly irrelevant. But by always looking for the next positive answer, you reframe the focus and offer a unique perspective, one that the client has possibly never experienced in a health-care setting.

A resource might be an at home yoga practice, a daily meditation practice, or walking on the treadmill for a few minutes each night after putting the kids to bed. Simply, it is a proactive step toward health.

Presenting Complaints

Where is the primary complaint? How might you distill the information into one or two common themes within a three-session format? Refrain from taking on too much. By keeping the focus simple, you make the best use of time.

Short- and Long-Term Goals

Ultimately, all goals are subjective and individual. Treatment plans offer a way to achieve client-centered goals. Encourage clients to think about realistic goals that want to come out of the first three sessions, usually as it relates to their immediate complaint. Goals must be quantifiable and tracked throughout ensuing sessions. Reducing the level and duration of pain might be an example of a measurable short-term goal. Playing 18 holes of golf comfortably could be the ultimate aim.

Beyond the initial complaint, what improvement is the client seeking to make in his or her overall sense of well-being? How would the client imagine massage therapy as part of his or her long-term preventative health care? Why might this approach be worth the investment?

Therapeutic Objectives

As a therapist, it is important to remember that treatment plans need to work toward addressing the client's goals. Therapists understand the body's distortions and how they might be worked with. By education and invitation, we may seek permission to proceed with a certain approach; however, the client's informed consent is of utmost importance. Any sort of imposed force in a therapeutic setting will be met with resistance, usually to the detriment of the healing relationship and possibly harming both therapist and client. Because each person has a unique set of presenting conditions and outcome goals, a routine approach to every situation is often limited.

The Three-Session Series

1. **Preparing the Way:**

   Here, we look for the path of least resistance into the client's system, usually with direct contact to an area of complaint in order to alleviate pain. In the words of Ron Kurtz: "If a therapist can show that he or she understands the immediate situation, something in the client will relax and allow the process to unfold further." Preparing the way means listening to a client's request and then delivering touch within the client's comfort level.

2. **Exposing the Complaint:**

   By scheduling the second session within a week of the first, the cumulative effects of massage on the body's systems increase exponentially. As connective tissue is mobilized through the addition of heat and pressure, working with it again within a short time period keeps it from returning to its chronic condition. Clients will usually complain of problems in their locked-long, inhibited muscles. This session looks beyond localized pain to the cause.

   As a society, we live in a flexion-addicted existence. The unforgiving effects of gravity coupled with computer use, driving, and watching television set the body up with shortness in the anterior torso and hips. Interestingly enough, these are the two areas most therapists report being the most uncomfortable with and the least trained to address. Muscles such as pectoralis minor, subscapularis, sternocleidomastoid, scalenes, psoas, and the abdominals all may be involved but usually are not the site of the initial complaint.

3. **Integration**

   This is a fusion between the first two sessions. Humans do well with slow, organic change. When our nervous system receives too much input, it has a tendency to recoil. Integration is not an end but a springboard into regular maintenance sessions.

Ultimately, the final goal is to educate clients about pain and stress patterns in their own lives. Through self-tracking, clients are able to determine how often they need massage to avoid the effects of stress and pain in their daily lives. This empowered decision comes from the inside-out opinion of the client, rather than from the outside-in opinion of the therapist. Furthermore, this self-guided decision goes a long way toward helping clients make preventative massage part of their routine. All conditions remaining constant, a client will be able to find a window of time that he or she remains relatively pain free. Encourage clients to book regular appointments within this window.

Approach the idea of treatment planning with playful curiosity, staying flexible to the changing needs of the client. Begin with the simple format outlined here, and over time, customize the approach to fit your practice.

Finally, remember that the gifts you bring to this profession are unique and needed by a part of your community. There are clients waiting for you.

Follow-Up

According to an ISPA consumer report,[2] many spas don't phone guests after a visit to ask about their experience. However, when guests were asked, they enthusiastically indicated they would appreciate a follow-up phone call. This is a huge missed opportunity in defining the client experience. If you are unable to follow up with all guests, at least attempt to ensure new guests are contacted. One note: guests do prefer if the call is from someone who has the power to change things.

You might follow up with a nice mailer, thanking your guests and inviting them to return. If you have captured their birthdays, you might even create a system so that all previous clients receive a birthday card with an incentive to return.

Your "Gone, But Not Forgotten" Mantra

See Worksheet 10-10

Your mantra for the tenth contact phase should be something like, "Even though you are gone, I remember you and will let you know I valued our time together." When you can deliver this, then congratulations—you have just completed a superior experience!

WHAT TO DO WHEN THINGS GO WRONG

This particular touch point will not occur with every guest but must be included. As hard as you try, there will be times when the service experience falls short in some way. When clients bring this to your attention, be thankful. Most guests will not voice complaints—they will just never return. On average, 65% of customers who report problems are less than highly satisfied with the resolution. Interestingly, for those customers who are highly satisfied with resolution, a full 84% report a high likelihood to return, showing signs of greater loyalty than a highly satisfied customer who did not experience a problem.[3] It is worth the effort to recover when things go wrong.

Empower Responses

For spas and massage businesses, consider building a service recovery structure that gives employees latitude to make decisions that immediately appease guests. Some of the biggest companies have figured out the value in letting the frontline people fix problems. There is nothing more annoying than waiting in a line of people for the cashier to get a manager to fix a problem. It is bad for the employee, the person with the problem, and everyone else who is affected by the wait. Also, make it easy for your employees to say yes. The last thing a smart business wants to do is win the argument and lose the customer.

Customize Resolutions

Recognize that every person is different and has a unique definition of the solution to the problem. A free gift certificate will not please everyone. Consider asking the question, "What can we do that would make this situation better for you?" You might be surprised to find that just because you ask, the person does not require anything more. Your willingness to compromise may be enough. Have options available to ensure each guest is highly satisfied with the resolution offered.

Fire Problem Clients

See Worksheet 10-11

In the end, some guests may simply drain more financial and energetic resources from you than you can possibly recoup. When you identify them as such, do not hesitate to professionally fire them. Those of you with employees will improve morale by taking a stand against problem guests. For yourself, you will free up the resources you are applying in constantly managing problem clients. It is amazing how much easier you will find your practice to fill once you let them go.

CHAPTER SUMMARY

Every massage therapist can benefit enormously from client loyalty. Obtaining that loyalty is worth your time, effort, and creative energy. Always let your clients, especially your repeat clients, know how much you appreciate their choosing you. Taking the time to assess your clients' satisfaction creates an outstanding opportunity for you to learn what works and what doesn't. Customize your touch points to complement your style and address the specific needs of your client base. A smooth, informative intake process sets the stage for an exceptional massage experience and allows your guests to relax in the certainty that you have truly heard them and are taking their needs into consideration. When you attentively listen to what you clients tell you, verbally and nonverbally, you have a greater chance of successfully creating the all-important "therapeutic bubble" upon which the entire massage industry is based. Knowing when to back away when things do not go as planned is also important. The power to create a soothing, safe, and beneficial interaction between you and your clients is literally in your hands!

BIBLIOGRAPHY

1. International SPA Association. (2006). *ISPA 2006 Consumer Report: Spa-Goer and Non-Spa-Goer Perspectives.* Lexington, KY: International SPA Association.
2. International SPA Association. (2006). *ISPA 2006 Consumer Report: Spa-Goer and Non-Spa-Goer Perspectives* Lexington, KY: International SPA Association.
3. Service Management Group, Inc. (2007). *Five Things We Learned from Talking to 100 Million People.* (http://www.smg.com)

REVIEW QUESTIONS

1. **Which of the following most determines whether customers view their decision to hire you positively or regretfully?**
   a. Price
   b. Overall satisfaction with the client experience
   c. Technique and skill
   d. Recognizing return guests

2. Strategically building a customer experience that exceeds their expectations affects:
   a. Hiring decisions and communications
   b. Insurance coverage
   c. Record-keeping and data collection
   d. Personal relationships

3. Which of the following is the best place to start strategizing and customizing the client experience?
   a. Observation
   b. The intake process
   c. Mirroring technique
   d. Unconditional positive regard

4. When listening to clients, what are you listening for in regard to increasing client loyalty?
   a. An opportunity to sell them a unique retail product
   b. An opportunity to create an experiential item that makes your service unique
   c. Common themes in what clients are saying
   d. Both b & c

5. Where do many businesses make an error when it comes to customer satisfaction surveys?
   a. Not asking enough questions
   b. Assuming a satisfied customer is a loyal customer
   c. Not keeping results anonymous
   d. Both a & c

6. Research shows that _____ of satisfied customers are highly likely to return to a business.
   a. 10%
   b. Less than half
   c. 75%
   d. 100%

7. Once you define and launch your optimal client experience, it is important to continue the plan as you have outlined it with unwavering resolve.
   a. True
   b. False

8. Which of the following shows sensitivity and guarantees anonymity when collecting feedback from customers?
   a. Asking open-ended questions
   b. Personally interviewing the client after the massage
   c. Personally interviewing the client before and after the massage
   d. Distributing pre-created feedback forms with postage for the client to return by mail

9. Which of the following should be asked on every satisfaction measurement form?
   a. Please rate your experience in the relaxation area
   b. Please rate your experience during the intake
   c. Please rate your satisfaction with the overall experience
   d. None of the above

10. **Which of the following questions is a good indicator of loyalty?**
    a. How likely are you to visit a competitor of ours?
    b. How likely are you to return?
    c. Please rate your satisfaction with the technique of the therapist
    d. Please describe what caused you to be so highly satisfied/dissatisfied

11. **What is the first step toward earning customer loyalty?**
    a. Garnering high satisfaction from your clients
    b. Conducting a satisfaction survey
    c. Determining the lifetime value of a client
    d. Both b & c

12. **What is a good measurement of customer loyalty?**
    a. Rebooking rate
    b. Clients recommending your service to others
    c. High percentage of satisfied customers
    d. Both a & b

13. **It costs as much as _____ times more to be constantly marketing to get new clients than to retain new ones.**
    a. Two
    b. Seven
    c. Fifteen
    d. It doesn't cost any more to get new clients than to retain new ones

14. **Which of the following is not a part of the service path?**
    a. Arrival for the massage
    b. The treatment
    c. The departure
    d. What clients tell their friends after their treatment

15. **Top fears of spa guests include:**
    a. Communicating complaints and transitioning between services
    b. How much they will pay for their service
    c. Slipping or falling in the facility
    d. Not being heard or understood

16. **Which of the following would be a good idea to do for new guests?**
    a. Give them a notecard with a price range for their service, tips, and retail products
    b. Wear protective gloves during the treatment
    c. Give them a welcome kit that includes a copy of the draping policy
    d. Show them video footage of a bad draping procedure

17. **What communicates more strongly than words?**
    a. Marketing visuals and graphics
    b. Price
    c. Body language
    d. Unconditional positive regard

18. When a client identifies what she is seeking and you repeat it back in your own words, what is that an example of?

    a. Therapeutic bubble

    b. Mirroring technique

    c. Unconditional positive regard

    d. A welcome mantra

19. What is the protective circle that surrounds the interactions between the therapist and the client receiving the massage?

    a. Therapeutic bubble

    b. Healthy bubble

    c. "Do no harm" mantra

    d. Protective bubble

20. When it comes to increasing customer loyalty, don't sweat the smaller things, such as cradle angle and foot attire.

    a. True

    b. False

21. Advantages of treatment planning include clients seeing cumulative results because of a realistic timeline and strategy as well as:

    a. Client and therapist have a proper window of time to establish safety and trust

    b. Increases revenue

    c. Reinforces good behavior

    d. All of the above

Worksheet 10-1   Customizing Touch Point 1: First Contact

What will you do to customize this touch point? Think of things that will be easy to implement, are cost efficient, and will have the most positive impact on the client.

Idea	Why This Is a Good Idea

Worksheet 10-2   Customizing Touch Point 2: Ready or Not, Here They Come

What will you do to customize this touch point? Think of things that will be easy to implement, are cost efficient, and will have the most positive impact on the client.

Idea	Why This Is a Good Idea

Worksheet 10-3 | **Customizing Touch Point 3: Managing Wait Time and Transitions**

What will you do to customize this touch point? Think of things that will be easy to implement, are cost efficient, and will have the most positive impact on the client.

Idea	Why This Is a Good Idea

Worksheet 10-4   Customizing Touch Point 4: Warm Welcome

What will you do to customize this touch point? Think of things that will be easy to implement, are cost efficient, and will have the most positive impact on the client.

Idea	Why This Is a Good Idea

Worksheet 10-5   Customizing Touch Point 5: Professional
Intakes

What will you do to customize this touch point? Think of things that will be easy to implement, are cost efficient, and will have the most positive impact on the client.

Idea	Why This Is a Good Idea

Worksheet 10-6   Customizing Touch Point 6: The
                    Therapeutic Bubble

What will you do to customize this touch point? Think of things that will be easy to implement, are cost efficient, and will have the most positive impact on the client.

Idea	Why This Is a Good Idea

Worksheet 10-7   Customizing Touch Point 7: Educate at Timely Stages of the Interaction

What will you do to customize this touch point? Think of things that will be easy to implement, are cost efficient, and will have the most positive impact on the client.

Idea	Why This Is a Good Idea

Worksheet 10-8 | Customizing Touch Point 8: Do Sweat
the Smaller Things

What will you do to customize this touch point? Think of things that will be easy to implement, are cost efficient, and will have the most positive impact on the client.

Idea	Why This Is a Good Idea

Worksheet 10-9 Customizing Touch Point 9: Professional Recommendations

What will you do to customize this touch point? Think of things that will be easy to implement, are cost efficient, and will have the most positive impact on the client.

Idea	Why This Is a Good Idea

Worksheet 10-10   Customizing Touch Point 10: Gone, But
Not Forgotten

What will you do to customize this touch point? Think of things that will be easy to implement, are cost efficient, and will have the most positive impact on the client.

Idea	Why This Is a Good Idea

Worksheet 10-11 Responding to Service Failures

How will you respond to service failures? Think about the most common complaints massage clients might have and think through how you would rectify these problems for them.

Common Problem	What I Would Do to Correct It

Appendix

Answers to Review Questions

CHAPTER I

1. **d.** All of the above
2. **a.** Mental discipline; meditative practice
3. **b.** Keeps you more in the present moment and better able to make decisions based on reality
4. **c.** Intention; action
5. **d.** Both a & c
6. **c.** Unhappiness and discomfort
7. **d.** Intention
8. **a.** Well-defined purpose
9. **a.** True
10. **b.** Natural tendencies
11. **d.** Both b & c
12. **b.** False
13. **a.** True
14. **a.** It allows understanding of how you prefer to receive stimulation
15. **b.** Reflect, take action, then reflect again
16. **c.** 75%
17. **d.** Those in the management position come from a thinking preference, and the therapists come from a feeling preference
18. **d.** Both a & c

CHAPTER 2

1. **c.** At a very early age (childhood)
2. **a.** Understand your current financial status
3. **d.** All of the above
4. **c.** Easier it is to borrow money
5. **b.** Tax returns filed with the Internal Revenue Service
6. **b.** False
7. **d.** Make arrangements to get caught up with companies you owe money and are behind in payments
8. **a.** True
9. **a.** Avoid putting charges on your credit card that you cannot pay off with short notice
10. **c.** 7 years
11. **d.** Both a & b
12. **d.** All of the above
13. **d.** Both b & c

14. **b.** Part-time
15. **b.** 15 to 20 percent
16. **d.** Credit score
17. **c.** Nonpay incentives
18. **b.** Massage franchise
19. **b.** False
20. **c.** Insurance
21. **d.** All of the above

CHAPTER 3

1. **c.** Vary depending on where a therapist plans to practice
2. **a.** True
3. **d.** All of the above
4. **a.** A limited amount of time
5. **b.** Are recognized by a majority of states
6. **b.** False
7. **c.** 500
8. **d.** Professional or trade association membership
9. **d.** All of the above
10. **d.** Both a & c
11. **d.** All of the above
12. **b.** National and state associations
13. **a.** Liability insurance
14. **c.** Client safety and privacy
15. **a.** Body; intuition
16. **d.** All of the above
17. **a.** Ensure data are documented, saved, and accessible for as long as they have value
18. **b.** Recycle private records

CHAPTER 4

1. **c.** Inner guidance and external circumstances
2. **b.** The closer you move toward a misalignment with your moral compass
3. **a.** Make decisions
4. **b.** Uncertain
5. **d.** Integrity and values
6. **a.** Enforce your personal boundaries
7. **d.** Diffused, semi-permeable, and rigid
8. **c.** Rigid boundary
9. **a.** True
10. **a.** Clearer
11. **d.** Both b & c
12. **b.** False
13. **b.** Unconscious representation
14. **a.** Foundational ethics
15. **c.** Thought, documentation, and constant management
16. **a.** True
17. **d.** Both a & b
18. **c.** Guiding external perceptions
19. **b.** False

20. **d.** Marketing materials and advertisements
21. **a.** Constant assessment and refinement of the ethical beliefs you hold

CHAPTER 5

1. **b.** Building physical stamina and professional skills
2. **d.** Both a & c
3. **d.** Consistent job duties and opportunities
4. **a.** To reinforce the image of the company and ensure consistency
5. **b.** Variable pay
6. **c.** Workers compensation and/or disability insurance
7. **c.** If massage appointments are not booked as expected, therapists are released from duty early or assigned other duties for their shift
8. **b.** False
9. **b.** Training is limited to technical skills
10. **a.** Clean the changing or relaxation areas
11. **a.** To review and plan for professional goals with your manager
12. **d.** Security
13. **a.** Your personal vision and mission statement
14. **c.** Company principles, age, size, and who you'd be reporting to
15. **d.** Both a & b
16. **c.** Management skills
17. **d.** Traits
18. **b.** Have a friend read and edit your resume
19. **a.** True
20. **d.** Stay aware of your nonverbal communication to ensure positive messaging
21. **b.** Draft and be ready to ask effective, informative questions of the interviewer
22. **a.** True
23. **d.** Both b & c
24. **c.** Health care facility
25. **b.** 20
26. **a.** Spas
27. **d.** Both b & c

CHAPTER 6

1. **b.** Independent contractor
2. **d.** If the employer controls or directs only work results, the worker is generally considered an independent contractor.
3. **a.** Behavioral, Financial and Relationship of the Parties
4. **a.** To be in compliance with IRS regulations regarding taxes and withholding
5. **d.** Both a & c
6. **c.** Agreement/contract
7. **b.** Other businesses who temporarily contract your services
8. **d.** All of the above
9. **a.** Business license(s) and insurance
10. **c.** Office administration and tax preparation
11. **a.** Value of service and market rates
12. **b.** False
13. **b.** Alone; self-motivated
14. **c.** Pay bills and save receipts, invoice and bill clients, complete tax returns

15. **d.** All of the above
16. **d.** Identity or employee theft
17. **b.** False
18. **a.** Quality of their work
19. **c.** Initiative
20. **b.** Treating and honoring all people with respect
21. **b.** False

CHAPTER 7

1. **a.** Small business owners
2. **c.** Jobs in other professions
3. **b.** 28 percent business-related tasks/72 percent performing massage
4. **c.** Widespread growth of new, unproven techniques
5. **a.** True
6. **d.** A well-crafted exit strategy
7. **d.** They remember it is all about them and take what they do lightly
8. **d.** Both b & c
9. **b.** Purpose
10. **a.** Sole proprietorships
11. **a.** Kiva
12. **b.** False
13. **a.** Clearly define expectations and put them in writing
14. **c.** Micro loan
15. **a.** Bank loan proposal and application
16. **b.** Client concerns about privacy, safety, and comfort
17. **c.** Chiropractors, fitness centers, and salons
18. **d.** All of the above
19. **a.** True
20. **a.** You don't control the environment and can be put in less than ideal situations
21. **d.** Food and beverage
22. **c.** Answer larger business questions, such as whether to sell retail products or accept insurance
23. **d.** Communication, management, and planning
24. **a.** True
25. **d.** Include a description of the business, including marketing, financial, and management information

CHAPTER 8

1. **a.** Marketing preparation and selecting marketing avenues
2. **d.** Both a & b
3. **c.** Narrow your target and be very specific about the kind of clients you want
4. **b.** To become experts at fewer things
5. **a.** True
6. **a.** Skillfully choosing your clients
7. **d.** All of the above
8. **d.** To keep their products/services relevant and understand their guest perceptions
9. **b.** Nearly half
10. **c.** Ages 55+
11. **d.** Both b & c
12. **b.** Treat pain

13. **d.** Both a & c
14. **a.** Inexpensive way to gather information about your clients
15. **b.** Singing a customized chant to every client
16. **d.** Translating your accomplishments into specific benefits for your client
17. **d.** Both b & c
18. **c.** If you plan to work with other businesses or employ another person
19. **d.** All of the above
20. **a.** Business card

CHAPTER 9

1. **a.** Research
2. **d.** Both a & c
3. **c.** Charge the most you can without deterring the clients you want
4. **d.** Cost-per-point (CPP)
5. **a.** If you specialize in a specific modality
6. **a.** True
7. **d.** Both a & b
8. **d.** All of the above
9. **b.** Financial and energetic
10. **a.** True
11. **b.** Ensuring you have the right message
12. **b.** Audience profile, reach, frequency, cost-per-point
13. **a.** Cable channels
14. **c.** Television
15. **b.** Web site banners
16. **a.** True
17. **d.** Both b & c
18. **b.** False
19. **b.** Discounts
20. **b.** False
21. **c.** Three points that are woven into a compelling story
22. **a.** Writing articles
23. **d.** Providing relevant and educational social media content
24. **c.** A blog
25. **b.** False
26. **b.** LinkedIn recommendations
27. **a.** True

CHAPTER 10

1. **b.** Overall satisfaction with the client experience
2. **a.** Hiring decisions and communications
3. **a.** Observation
4. **d.** Both b & c
5. **b.** Assuming a satisfied customer is a loyal customer
6. **b.** Less than half
7. **b.** False
8. **d.** Distributing precreated feedback forms with postage for the client to return by mail
9. **c.** Please rate your satisfaction with the overall experience
10. **b.** How likely are you to return?

11. **a.** Garnering high satisfaction from your clients
12. **d.** Both a & b
13. **b.** Seven
14. **d.** What clients tell their friends after their treatment
15. **a.** Communicating complaints and transitioning between services
16. **c.** Give them a welcome kit that includes a copy of the draping policy
17. **c.** Body language
18. **b.** Mirroring technique
19. **a.** Therapeutic bubble
20. **b.** False
21. **d.** All of the above

Index

Page numbers followed by b indicate box. Page number followed by f indicate figure

A

AAIM. *see* American Association of Integrative Medicine (AAIM)
AANP. *see* American Association of Naturopathic Physicians (AANP)
Ability(ies), 140, 149, 152, 201
ABMP. *see* Associated Bodywork and Massage Professionals (ABMP)
About.com, for resume templates, 154
ACA. *see* American Chiropractic Association (ACA)
Academic Consortium for Complementary and Alternative Health Care (ACCAH), 167
ACCAH. *see* Academic Consortium for Complementary and Alternative Health Care (ACCAH)
ACSM. *see* American College of Sports Medicine (ACSM)
Action
    definition of, 3
    taking, 13–14
Adaptive skills, 140, 152
Additional insured endorsements (AIEs), 76
Advertising. *see also* Nontraditional advertising; Traditional media advertising
    acquiring proposals, 306–307
    creating focus in, 306b
    definition of, 303, 306
    discounts and, 306, 307f
    services, 114
Advice, small business entrepreneurs and, 223b
Aetna, 194
Agreement, of Massage Therapy Independent Contractor, 188–191b
AHA. *see* American Hospital Association (AHA)
Ahh That's the Spot Massage, 54
AHMA. *see* American Holistic Medical Association (AHMA)
AIEs. *see* Additional insured endorsements (AIEs)
AINM. *see* American Institute of Naturopathic Medicine (AINM)
Airports, income working at, 55

Alabama, liability insurance requirements in, 86
Alignment, meaning of, 149
Alignment process, 8
All Hospital Jobs, 161
AllLaw.com, 192
Alternative Therapy Association (ATA), 167
American Airlines, 111
American Association of Integrative Medicine (AAIM), 167
American Association of Naturopathic Physicians (AANP), 169
American Chiropractic Association (ACA), 169
American College of Sports Medicine (ACSM), 167
American Holistic Medical Association (AHMA), 169
American Hospital Association (AHA), 166, 169
American Institute of Naturopathic Medicine (AINM), 169
American Massage Therapy Association (AMTA)
    on average earning of massage therapists, 161
    on challenges facing professionals, 220–221
    code of ethics, 89–90, 107b
    consumer research, 277
    on current massage market data, 241
    on future clients, 277–278
    health care and, 167
    health insurance benefits, 193
    on income of massage therapists, 47, 47b
    learning events, 282–283
    listing service for members, 311
    "Massage is a healing art as well as a science," 151–152
    on massage therapists in health-care settings, 166
    as national association, 83, 84
    on number of massage therapists, 160
    on percentage of independent contractors, 219
    personal security tips from, 91
    professional liability insurance, 239

research on benefits of massage, 367
    security tips, 91
    on state boards and requirements, 78
    state chapters, 196–197
    2010 Massage Industry Research Report, 4
    web site, 194
American Naturopathic Medical Association (ANMA), 169
American Orthopaedic Society for Sports Medicine (AOSSM), 169
American Society of Association Executives (ASAE), 85
AMTA. *see* American Massage Therapy Association (AMTA)
AMTA Massage Therapy Industry Fact Sheet, 47
Animal massage
    associations on the web, 56
    income working for, 56
ANMA. *see* American Naturopathic Medical Association (ANMA)
Anthem BlueCross and BlueShield, 194
Anxiety, clients and, 279
AOSSM. *see* American Orthopaedic Society for Sports Medicine (AOSSM)
Appearance
    interview and, 157, 157b
    personal, 117, 119
    in policies and procedures, 143b
Appendix, in business plan, 242
Article ideas (worksheet), 339
Article query, definition of, 303
ASAE. *see* American Society of Association Executives (ASAE)
Assessment
    of associations, 85
    of client satisfaction, 348–352
    of personal financial behavior, 41, 41f
Associated Bodywork and Massage Professionals (ABMP), 3, 47
    code of ethics, 89, 107b
    consumer research, 277–278
    description and website, 82
    on focus of Wellness Centers, 166
    licensure of therapists, 76–77
    listing of massage modalities, 282
    listing service for members, 311
    on massage clinic, 163